Genetics and Hearing Impairment

Edited by
Alessandro Martini MD, Andrew Read PhD and
Dafydd Stephens FRCP

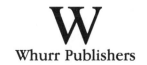
Whurr Publishers

© 1996 Whurr Publishers Ltd
First published 1996
by Whurr Publishers Ltd
19B Compton Terrace,
London N1 2UN,
England

Reprinted 1999

British Library Cataloguing in Publication Data
A catalogue record for this book is available from the British
Library.

ISBN 1-897635 29 X

Printed and bound in the UK by Athenaeum Press Ltd,
Gateshead, Tyne & Wear

Contents

Foreword

About 4 years ago, when we were planning to update our text, Hereditary Hearing Loss and Its Syndromes, several confrères commented that it was a parlous time to write a text book. At that juncture, molecular genetics was beginning to discover hearing loss or those involved in hearing loss were becoming aware that molecular genetics was a powerful tool with which to investigate hereditary deafness. Clinical investigations had done about as much as they could in defining genetic heterogeneity. Molecular genetics could simply do it much better. The point that these sceptics made was that one should wait until some sort of quietus was reached - until the dust settled after this information explosion. In part, their point was a valid one. As authors, we agonised that no matter how careful and all-encompassing was our monitoring of the current literature, major discoveries would be announced within days after publication. And so it was - and so it ever will be! In the October 1995 Hereditary Deafness Newsletter, there are listed 16 mapped genes for non-syndromic hearing loss. I am sure that the authors will be updating the galley proofs until the deadline imposed by the publisher has been breached.

Hereditary hearing loss is important - about 1 per 1,000 births. If a child is born deaf, in about one third of the cases it is genetic, and syndromal hearing loss constitutes a large fraction of these examples. In spite of the frequent occurrence of genetic hearing loss, the 1976 text of Konigsmark and Gorlin was the first to comprehensively address the subject. During the next two decades, until our 1995 second edition, no additional texts were published.

This book represents a very welcome addition. It represents a distillation of the very latest by the very best. Each author is an authority on the subject of her/his chapter(s). Further, the text can be read at many levels and both the neophyte and the seasoned investigator will treasure this volume. It was not the purpose of the editors to be all encompassing, but each of the entities the book addresses is covered in depth. In order to write this foreword, I read a large portion of each section so that I could get a taste of the entire spectrum of this work. This book is a sumptuous feast. Pull up to the table and enjoy!

Robert J Gorlin

Preface

The aim of this book is to provide a broad and up to date overview of genetic hearing loss for audiologists, otolaryngologists and clinical geneticists. It does not set out to be a comprehensive description of syndromes in the way of Gorlin's fine text (1995), but to provide an easily read sourcebook for those students and clinicians with an interest in this field. We are, furthermore, most grateful to Professor Gorlin for his kind and generous foreword.

The book comes in five sections. The first gives a background for the reader, providing an introduction to auditory function, basic genetics and genetic techniques relevant to this field. This is followed by a section providing an introduction to the audiological aspects of genetic hearing loss. The third section covers most of the commonest syndromes associated with hearing loss, and the fourth is concerned with non-syndromal hearing losses with different modes of inheritance. The final section deals with approaches to the management of individuals with genetic hearing loss, and encompasses genetic counselling, rehabilitation and surgery.

As a reflection of our desire to look at this field as a whole, we have amalgamated all the references at the end, as many key references are featured throughout the book. We also include a glossary of audiological and genetic terms used throughout the book, which may not be familiar to some readers.

The contributors, all experts in their fields, have been asked to produce a short, succinct and completely up to date review of their particular topic, although the speed of change in this field is such that there will have inevitably been some developments between the chapters being written and the publication of this book.

We are grateful to our contributors for their enthusiasm and efficiency in providing what we hope will be a useful overview of this field that should provide a sound basis for future work. We are also indebted to the Amplifon foundation, which organized an international meeting on genetic hearing loss, which provided the inspiration for the production of this book.

Alessandro Martini,
Andrew Read and
Dafydd Stephens

Contributors

Edoardo Arslan
Department of Audiology and Phoniatrics, University of Padua, I-35128 Padua, Italy

Peter Beighton
Department of Human Genetics, Medical School, University of Cape Town, South Africa

Kirk Beisel
Center for Study of Human Communication Disorders, Boys Town National Research Hospital, Omaha, Nebraska, USA

Susan Bellman
Department of Audiological Medicine, Great Ormond Street Hospital, London WC1N 3JH, England

Stephen DM Brown
MRC Mouse Genome Centre, Harwell, Didcot, Oxon OX11 0RD, England

Han G Brunner
Department of Human Genetics, University Hospital of Nijmegen, 6500 HB Nijmegen, Netherlands

Elisa Calzolari
Institute of Medical Genetics, University of Ferrara, I-44100 Ferrara, Italy

Luigi Clauser
Department of Craniomaxillofacial Surgery, Regional Hospital, Vicenza, Italy

Paul Coucke
Department of Medical Genetics, University of Antwerp (UIA), 2610 Antwerp, Belgium

Cor WRJ Cremers
Department of Otolaryngology, Nijmegen University Hospital, 6500 HB Nijmegen, Netherlands

Camillo Curioni
Maxillofacial Surgery Clinic, University of Ferrara, Ferrara, Italy

Bruno Dallapiccola
Department of Medical Genetics, University of Rome 'Tor Vergata', I-135-00133 Rome, Italy

Frank Declau
Department of Otolaryngology, University of Antwerp, 2610 Wilrijk, Belgium

Michael J Dixon
School of Biological Sciences, University of Manchester, Manchester M13 9PT, England

D Gareth R Evans
Department of Medical Genetics, St Mary's Hospital, Manchester M13 0JH, England

Nathan Fischel-Ghodsian
Department of Pediatrics, Cedars-Sinai Medical Center, Los Angeles, California 90048, USA

Mary Francis
Welsh Hearing Institute, University Hospital of Wales, Cardiff CF4 4XW, Wales

William J Kimberling
Center for Study of Human Communication Disorders, Boys Town National Research Hospital, Omaha, Nebraska, USA

Alessandro Martini
Audiology-ENT Department, University of Ferrara, Ferrara, Italy

Rita Mingarelli
Department of Medical Genetics, University of Rome 'Tor Vergata', I-135-00133 Rome, Italy

Claes Möller
Department of Otolaryngology, University Hospital, S-58185 Linköping, Sweden

Robert F Mueller
Yorkshire Regional Genetics Service, St James' Hospital, Leeds LS9 7TF, England

Valerie E Newton
Centre for Audiology, University of Manchester, Manchester M13 9PL, England

Eva Orzan
Department of Audiology and Phoniatrics, University of Padua, I-35128 Padua, Italy

Alan Palmer
MRC Institute of Hearing Research, University Park, Nottingham NG7 2RD, England

Agnete Parving
Department of Audiology, Bispebjerg Hospital, DK 2400 Copenhagen, Denmark

Christine Petit
Department of Human Molecular Genetics, Institut Pasteur, 75724 Paris cedex 15, France

Silvano Prosser
Audiology-ENT Department, University of Ferrara, Ferrara, Italy

Andrew P Read
Department of Medical Genetics, St Mary's Hospital, Manchester M13 0JH, England

William Reardon
Mothercare Unit of Paediatric Genetics and Foetal Medicine, Institute of Child Health, London WC1N 1EH, England

Alberto Sensi
Institute of Medical Genetics, University of Ferrara, I-44100 Ferrara, Italy

Richard JH Smith
Department of Otolaryngology, University of Iowa, Iowa City, Iowa, USA

Karen P Steel
MRC Institute of Hearing Research, University Park, Nottingham, NG7 2RD, England

Dafydd Stephens
Welsh Hearing Institute, University Hospital of Wales, Cardiff, CF4 4XW, Wales

Richard C Trembath
Department of Medicine, Therapeutics and Genetics, University of Leicester, Leicester LE2 7RT, England

Guy van Camp
Department of Medical Genetics, University of Antwerp (UIA), 2610 Antwerp, Belgium

Paul van de Heyning
Department of Otolaryngology, University of Antwerp, 2610 Wilrijk, Belgium

Patrick J Willems
Department of Medical Genetics, University of Antwerp (UIA), 2610 Antwerp, Belgium

Acknowledgements

Chapter 9

This work was partially supported by MURST 1994 - 95.

Chapter 13

This chapter is an amended and updated version of a paper published in *Seminars in Hearing,* with permission of the Editor.

Chapter 15

We would like to thank our collaborators Professor K Britton and Dr P Phelps for providing us with perchlorate discharge and Mondini figures respectively; Professor Sir D Williams for guidance concerning the association between Pendred syndrome and malignant change in the thyroid gland; Miss Rebecca Coffey for careful and painstaking proof reading. Our work on Pendred syndrome is supported by the Medical Research Council.

Chapter 20

This work is dedicated to the memory of John J Wasmuth; friend, collaborator, mentor.

I should like to thank all the Treacher Collins families for their co-operation. I should also like to thank collaborators in the laboratories of Drs John Wasmuth (especially Dr Stacie K Loftus), Katherine Klinger, Greg Landes and Rakesh Anand; members of my own laboratory (Jill Dixon, Sara Edwards, Amanda Gladwin and Rahat Perveen) and clinicians who provided patient samples. The financial support of the Wellcome Trust (grants number 036797 and 044684), the Medical Research Council (G9010336CB and G9204430), the Hearing Research Trust and the Independent Order of Odd Fellows is gratefully acknowledged.

Chapter 21

I acknowledge Jacqueline Levilliers for her constant and friendly help. I thank Jean-Pierre Hardelin and Viki Kalatzis for critical reading of the manuscript, and members of the GMRDSH ('Groupe méditerranéen de recherche sur les dèficits sensoriels héréditaires') for their contribution.

Chapter 25

The author wishes to thank Dr Han Brunner (Department of Human Genetics, University of Nijmegen) for his constructive comments.

Chapter 26

This work was supported by NIH/NIDCD grants DC01402 and DC02273.

Part I
Background

Chapter 1
Basic mechanisms of hearing and hearing impairment

KAREN P STEEL and ALAN PALMER

The auditory pathway

The auditory system extends from the pinna of the external ear to the auditory cortex of the brain, with neural interconnections to several brain centres that enable correlation of auditory information with other sensory inputs and/or mediate reflex actions. Genetic defects may affect any part of the system, but most genetic hearing impairment in the population affects the inner ear, and so this introductory chapter will focus mainly on inner ear function.

Figure 1.1 illustrates the peripheral part of the auditory system. The pinna and the outer ear canal act as a channel for sound to reach the middle ear, and these structures have resonances which serve to increase the sound pressure levels at particular frequencies that reach the eardrum (tympanic membrane). The outer ear also plays a part in sound localisation, by enhancing sound from particular directions and providing spectral cues for sound source position.

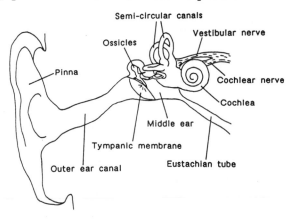

Figure 1.1 The human outer, middle and inner ear. (reprinted from Steel and Brown, 1994, with permission)

3

The middle ear contains a chain of three small bones (the middle ear ossicles): the malleus, connected to the tympanic membrane; the incus; and the stapes, which inserts into the oval window of the inner ear. These ossicles, together with the tympanic membrane, serve to transmit the sound energy to the inner ear. This is not a trivial process. The impedance of the inner ear fluids at the oval window is much greater than the impedance of the air. Without some means of matching these acoustic impedances the transmission of sound energy into the inner ear would be very inefficient and most of the energy would be reflected back out again. The middle ear acts as a pressure amplifier and produces a good impedance match, and hence efficient transfer of sound energy into the inner ear. This is achieved in three ways. The major contribution arises because the tympanic membrane has a much greater area than the oval window of the inner ear, which allows force to be collected over a wide area and delivered to a small area, thus increasing the applied pressure by about 35 times. Further pressure amplification is provided by the lever action which results from different lengths of the ossicles (1.15x) and by deformation or buckling of the tympanic membrane (2x). Other factors also influence the transmission of sound through the middle ear, and the efficiency of transmission at different frequencies is a major factor shaping the audiogram.

Contraction of muscles which connect the malleus and stapes to the middle ear wall stiffens the ossicular chain, reducing the energy transmission. These muscles are activated by reflexes and may protect the ear against very loud sounds or reduce the interfering effects of internally generated sounds. The middle ear cavity is air filled and is maintained at atmospheric pressure by periodic opening of the Eustachian tube which connects the middle ear cavity to the nasopharynx.

The inner ear can be divided into two parts: the cochlea which contains the auditory receptors, and the vestibular part containing the balance and gravity receptors. The receptor cells, or hair cells, in both auditory and vestibular parts of the inner ear are basically very similar, and all respond to deflections of the stereocilia that extend from their upper surfaces. The stereocilia of hair cells in the sacculus and utriculus are deflected when the gelatinous otolithic membrane, to which they are attached, moves due to gravity when the head position is altered. Hair cells in the cristae of the semicircular canals respond to the motion of the fluids in the canals caused by angular motion of the head.

The cochlea consists of a bony tube spiralling around a central core (the modiolus) divided by a central partition along its length (see Figures 1.1 and 1.2). The partition (the basilar membrane) vibrates when sound energy is introduced into the cochlea. The spiral arrangement has presumably evolved to allow the development of a long basilar membrane in a small space inside the head. The auditory hair cells are arranged in four rows along the length of the basilar membrane and

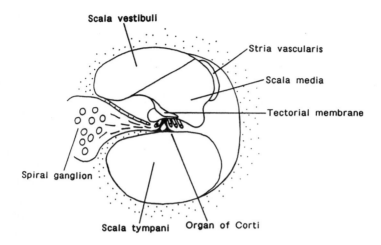

Scala vestibuli

Stria vascularis

Scala media

Tectorial membrane

Spiral ganglion

Scala tympani   Organ of Corti

Figure 1.2 A cross-section of one turn of the cochlear duct, showing the sensory hair cells within the organ of Corti, the pillar cells (black), the stria vascularis on the lateral wall of the cochlear duct, and the spiral ganglion, containing the cell bodies of the afferent neurones of the auditory nerve. The duct is divided into three channels: scala vestibuli and scala tympani contain perilymph and scala media contains endolymph. Reprinted from Steel and Brown, 1994, with permission.

their stereocilia are topped by the gelatinous tectorial membrane. The hair cells and their supporting cells on the basilar membrane together are called the organ of Corti (Figure 1.3). Sound induced vibration of the basilar membrane causes a shearing motion between the tops of the hair cells and the tectorial membrane which in turn deflects the stereocilia.

We shall focus upon the stimulation and responses of the cochlear hair cells in the rest of this chapter, but much of our knowledge of their function has come from studies of vestibular hair cells. As the hair cells of the cochlea and vestibular system are so similar, it is perhaps not surprising that genetic defects affecting cochlear hair cells often also affect vestibular hair cells. What is surprising is that vestibular dysfunction is often undetected in people with hereditary hearing impairment until clinical tests are performed.

Cochlear hair cells connect via a synapse at the hair cell base with the dendrites of bipolar neurones situated in the modiolus at the centre of the cochlea. The axons of these neurones form the cochlear nerve which projects to the central nervous system and terminates in the cochlear nucleus in the brainstem. The cochlear nucleus processes the sound evoked responses and passes the information to higher brain centres via several parallel output pathways, which appear to subserve different hearing functions (Palmer, 1995).

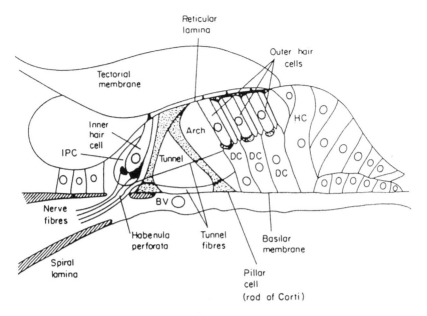

Figure 1.3 Cross section through the organ of Corti illustrating the three rows of outer hair cells and single row of inner hair cells. Some of the supporting cells are labelled: DC, Deiters' cells; HC, Hensen's cells; IPC, inner phalangeal cell. The upper surface of the organ of Corti appears to be strengthened by various intracellular cytoskeletal elements, forming the reticular lamina. In some immature specimens, a blood vessel (BV) is still present below the basilar membrane, but in most cases this atrophies as the cochlea matures. Reprinted from Pickles, 1982, by kind permission.

Organisation of the cochlea

One half of the cochlea is further divided along its length by another membrane forming three chambers. The three chambers extend the length of the cochlear duct, and are called the scala vestibuli, the scala media, and the scala tympani. Figure 1.2 shows a cross-section through one turn of the cochlear duct, illustrating the arrangement of the three scalae. Scala vestibuli and scala tympani are filled with perilymph, a fluid that is high in sodium and low in potassium like most other extracellular fluids. Scala media, in contrast, is filled with a very unusual fluid, the endolymph, which is high in potassium and low in sodium (like the intracellular fluids of neurones). Endolymph is the fluid that bathes the upper surface of the organ of Corti, which gives a clue to why it has such a high potassium level. The current through the sensory hair cells which is modulated during transduction (the process of changing the mechanical energy of sound vibration to an electrical signal) is predominantly a potassium current, with positive potassium ions moving from the endolymph into the sensory hair cells.

Another feature of the endolymph in scala media is that it is maintained at a high positive resting potential, around +100mV in a mouse, for example. This resting potential, called the endocochlear potential, creates a large potential difference across the tops of the hair cells, between the positive endolymph and the negative potential maintained inside the hair cells (as in neurones), and this large potential gradient is essential for normal hair cell function. Both the endocochlear potential and the high potassium, low sodium composition of the endolymph are generated by ion pumps in the stria vascularis on the lateral wall of the cochlear duct (see Figure 1.2). The endolymph is thus the ionic battery for the organ of Corti, and is maintained by the stria. The stria has a generous capillary supply, and consists of marginal cells on the lumenal surface (facing the endolymph), and basal cells separating the stria from the underlying connective tissue. Scattered in between these two layers are the intermediate cells, which are modified and specialised melanocytes (pigment cells). Although it was once believed that the marginal cells were primarily responsible for generating the endocochlear potential, recent evidence suggests that the situation is not that simple, and intermediate cells are known to play an essential role in generating the potential.

The organ of Corti is illustrated in Figure 1.3. The hair cells are characterised by the bundles of stereocilia on their upper surface (Figure 1.4). There are two distinct types of hair cell. A single row of inner hair cells and three rows of outer hair cells extend along the length of the cochlear duct. The inner hair cells are flask shaped cells surrounded by supporting cells, and are the primary receptor cells; they receive 90 - 95% of the afferent innervation of the cochlea (Spoendlin, 1972) and so account for most of the activity of the cochlear nerve. The outer hair cells differ from the inner hair cells in being long and cylindrical in shape, with their lateral walls contacting fluid filled Nuel spaces. Most of the innervation of outer hair cells is efferent. The lateral walls of the outer hair cells are characterised by the presence of a network of subsurface cisternae, and the lateral membranes contain an unusually high density of non-lipid inclusions (Gulley and Reese, 1977; Forge, 1991). These outer hair cells are primarily motor cells. When isolated in vitro and stimulated by applying an alternating current across the cell, they will contract and elongate at a rate at least as fast as lower frequencies of sound (e.g. up to 13 kHz, Gale and Ashmore, 1995). The motor that drives this length change is known to be located in the lateral cell membrane, and is thought to be the non-lipid molecules embedded in the lipid cell membrane, but the identity of the motor molecule is not known. The motion of the outer hair cells enhances the vibration of the basilar membrane (see below).

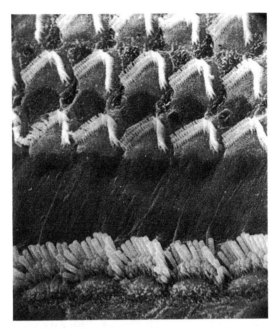

Figure 1.4 A scanning electron micrograph illustrating the surface of the organ of Corti, with each hair cell having a neatly arranged bundle of stereocilia on its upper surface. The tectorial membrane has been removed.

The hair cells are supported by a variety of distinct types of supporting cells in the organ of Corti (Figure 1.2). Two rows of pillar cells, packed with microtubules which presumably give them considerable rigidity, separate the inner from the outer hair cells, and Deiters cells which sit below the outer hair cells extend microtubule filled processes to the upper surface of the organ of Corti and support the upper ends of the outer hair cells. The upper surface of the organ of Corti, formed by the tops of hair cells and supporting cells joined together by tight junctions, is strengthened by the presence of dense arrangements of cytoskeletal elements, such as actin filaments, within the top part of each cell. The stereocilia are embedded in these strengthened plates, called cuticular plates, at the tops of the hair cells. The whole structure of the organ of Corti looks as if it has been designed to faithfully transmit tiny vibrational movements of the basilar membrane to the tops of the hair cells with the minimum loss of energy through absorption by flexible components.

The normal stimulus for a hair cell is a deflection of its stereocilia. Stereocilia are joined to each other by several different types of lateral link and also by a linkage across their tips (the tip link: Figure 1.5), a fine flexible thread which extends from the tip of one stereocilium to the side of the next tallest stereocilium (Pickles et al., 1984). The upper end of the tip link is embedded in the membrane at a characteristic thicken-

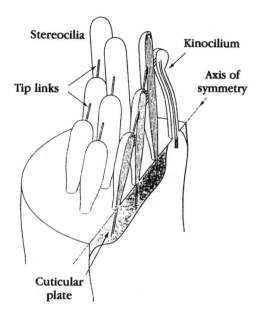

Stereocilia

Tip links

Kinocilium

Axis of symmetry

Cuticular plate

Figure 1.5 A diagrammatic representation of the stereocilia bundle of a hair cell, illustrating the strengthened cuticular plate into which the stereocilia insert. The stereocilia have an actin core, with the orientation of the actin fibres shown by the parallel lines. Each of the shorter stereocilia extends a fine tip link to the side of the adjacent stereocilium. The kinocilium has a structure typical of other cilia found elsewhere in the body, and is present in vestibular hair cells throughout life but in cochlear hair cells only at immature stages of development. Reprinted from Pickles and Corey, 1992, by kind permission.

ing called the insertional plaque. The recognition of these tip links was a milestone in our understanding of hair cell function, because it led to the development of a model of how the hair cell might transduce the mechanical energy of sound into an electrical change. The model assumes that there is a transducer channel that is sensitive to mechanical distortion at one or other end of the tip link, and that when stereocilia are deflected, the tension on the tip link exerts force directly upon the transducer channel, increasing the probability that the tranducer channel will be in the open state. When the stereocilia are deflected in the opposite direction, the probability that the channel will be in the closed state is increased. Over the 100 or so transducer channels on a single hair cell, this causes modulation of the potassium current passing through the top of the hair cell, which is reflected in a change in the hair cell intracellular potential. Depolarization of the hair cell increases the intracellular calcium resulting in a release of neurotransmitter from the synapse at the hair cell base, triggering a neural action potential in the afferent neurone.

This model of auditory transduction is different from the transduction processes in other sensory systems such as the olfactory and visual systems, which employ a second messenger cascade to amplify and transmit the signal. Auditory transduction needs to employ direct gating of the transducer channel because auditory hair cells can respond to frequencies up to 100 kHz or more, which is far too fast for a second messenger to act. The model accounts for the asymmetrical response to deflection of the stereocilia in opposite directions (larger depolarizations than hyperpolarizations) by assuming that only 15% of the channels are open in the resting position. Thus, there are more channels available to be opened when the stereocilia are deflected from rest in an excitatory direction than are available to be closed when the stereocilia bundle is deflected in the opposite direction. We know practically nothing about the molecular basis of hair cell transduction, although there is evidence that a myosin motor is involved in long term adjustment of the tension of the tip link (Hudspeth and Gillespie, 1994; Solc et al., 1995). The 'tip link' model is widely accepted as the most likely mechanism for auditory transduction, although it has not yet been proven (Hudspeth and Gillespie, 1994).

Mechanics and responses of the cochlea

The basilar membrane varies in width systematically along the length of the cochlear duct: it is widest at the apex and narrowest at the base. This, together with other systematic differences along the length of the duct, leads to a variation in stiffness of the basilar membrane. Pressure variations in the air (sound waves) after amplification by the middle ear, lead to pressure variations in the cochlear fluids. Increases in pressure at the oval window cause the round window to move out, and decreases cause it to move in. These alternating pressures across the basilar membrane cause it to move up and down producing a wave like motion (a travelling wave) which appears to move from the base toward the apex of the cochlea. The passive mechanical properties of the basilar membrane, including its stiffness gradient, lead to a peak in the amplitude of its vibration occurring near the base of the cochlea for high frequency sounds, and moving progressively toward the apex for lower frequency sounds.

This variation in the position of the peak basilar membrane deflection performs a passive filtering action, such that the base of the cochlea responds preferentially to high frequencies and the apex to low frequencies, and this passive filtering can still be measured post-mortem. However, the basilar membrane in a living mammal is actually far better tuned (i.e. the range of frequencies causing a particular part of the basilar membrane to vibrate is much narrower and the amplitude of the vibration is higher) than can be accounted for by the passive mechanical properties. The limited spatial extent of the basilar membrane movement in vivo increases the ability of the sensory hair cells to respond preferentially to specific frequencies depending on their place along the cochlear duct. A number of different observations (including otoacoustic emissions described later) have led to the suggestion that the minute motions of the basilar membrane are locally amplified by some form of feedback process, which, since it is not present post-mortem must involve active processes. What is this active amplification process and how does it work?

The answer is likely to be that the outer hair cells, which when isolated in vitro can be shown to change their length in response to electrical stimulation (as described earlier) and can also respond to changes within the cochlea caused by sound stimuli by contracting and expanding *in vivo*. These length changes are thought to augment the movement of the basilar membrane. The enhanced movement of the basilar membrane occurs only over very restricted spatial regions, and being an active process is highly susceptible to disruption. The appropriate trigger for outer hair cell contraction *in vivo* is not known, and could be mechanical, electrical or chemical changes that occur initially in response to the passive movement of the basilar membrane.

The responses of the cochlear receptors can be recorded either by single cell recording techniques (which are technically very demanding), or by measuring their summed activity at some distance, using gross electrodes. Intracellular recording has shown that inner hair cells respond to a single tone with a small oscillating (ac) change in the resting potential at the tone frequency (for low frequencies), combined with a steady (dc) shift in the cell's resting potential which is maintained for the duration of the stimulus (Russell and Sellick, 1978). This dc change in resting potential is a direct reflection of the nonlinearity (asymmetry) of the response to deflection of the stereocilia and at higher frequencies is the only component measured, due to the low-pass filtering action of the hair cell membranes. These voltages, which are as sharply tuned in frequency as the basilar membrane vibration, are responsible for increasing the probability of release of transmitter from the base of the cell into the synaptic cleft, eventually initiating an action potential in the afferent neurone. Inner hair cell responses vary between the base and apex of the cochlea, with the ac component of the response predominating in apical hair cells, while the dc component is the major component in basal inner hair cells (Russell and Sellick, 1978; Cheatham and Dallos, 1993). The gross correlate of the hair cell receptor potential change during stimulation is the summating potential, a dc shift in potential maintained for the duration of a stimulus, which can be measured with an extracellular or extracochlear electrode (Dallos et al., 1972; Dallos, 1986; Harvey and Steel, 1992).

The ac and dc voltage responses in outer hair cells are smaller than in inner hair cells. However, in response to a tone, a gross electrode measures a large potential (the cochlear microphonic) which reproduces exactly the sound waveform. The cochlear microphonic is thought to represent the summed ac responses of the outer hair cells and as such can be used as an indicator of their function. The cochlear microphonics recorded using a gross recording electrode reflect local outer hair cell activity, so an electrode placed on or near the round window of the cochlea will reflect basal turn outer hair cell activity (Patuzzi et al., 1989; Dallos and Cheatham, 1976).

A by-product of the active amplification of the basilar membrane motion is the generation of sound (otoacoustic emissions) by the organ of Corti, which can be measured using a microphone in the ear canal. Measurement of otoacoustic emissions has recently been introduced to assess cochlear function, since they appear to reflect outer hair cell activity in a place-specific manner: an emission at a particular frequency represents outer hair cell activity at that frequency place on the basilar membrane (Kemp, 1978).

The neurones which synapse with the base of the hair cells project to the brain via the cochlear (or 8th) nerve, and responses of individual fibres of this nerve have been extensively studied (see for example Kiang et al., 1965). Cochlear nerve fibre responses are sharply tuned (i.e. show narrow frequency filtering), with the most sensitive thresholds at a particular frequency (known as the characteristic or best frequency) for an individual neurone reflecting the position of its connection to a hair cell along the length of the basilar membrane (Liberman, 1982). An example is shown in Figure 1.6. The neural response has a shape very similar to that of the basilar membrane motion, with both showing a sharply tuned tip and broadly tuned tails. The sharply tuned region of the nerve fibre response is critically dependent on the active processes that permit sharp basilar membrane tuning, and these are highly susceptible to trauma (see Figure 1.6). The broadly tuned region of the neural response is similar in shape to the passive mechanical movement of the basilar membrane. The cochlear nerve can be thought of as a bank of narrow filters, spanning the whole hearing range of the animal, with best frequencies corresponding to the point of innervation along the basilar membrane. The gross correlate of activity in these cochlear nerve fibres is the compound action potential, which can be measured in response to transient sounds with an extracochlear electrode. This gross response represents the synchronous firing of an action potential in many cochlear nerve fibres, originating from a restricted part of the basilar membrane that depends upon the stimulus frequency used. The threshold of the compound action potential response follows those of single cochlear nerve fibres (Johnstone et al., 1979).

Finally, the functional integrity of central auditory nuclei can also be

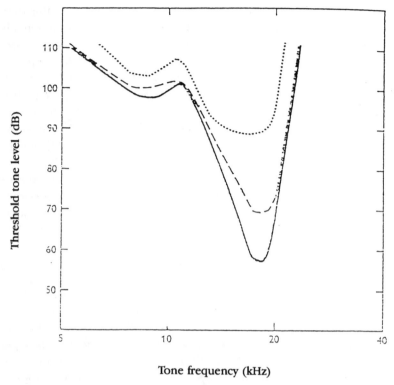

Figure 1.6 The response area of a typical auditory neurone, with threshold plotted as a function of stimulus frequency, showing the sharply tuned tip and broadly tuned tail of the normal response (solid line). The best frequency of this particular neurone was about 18 kHz. The dotted response area was obtained during hypoxia, illustrating the loss of the sharply tuned tip in an impaired neurone. The dashed response area was obtained during recovery from the hypoxia. Modified from Evans (1975), with permission.

assessed using gross electrodes. The evoked potentials recorded by such electrodes in response to transient sounds are extremely useful clinically as they are non-invasive. The waveform of the evoked response to stimulation with clicks consists of distinct components which reflect activity occurring at progressively higher levels of the auditory pathway, but not in any simplistic fashion.

Pathology of the auditory system

Traditionally, hearing impairment has been divided into two main types: conductive, in which the conduction of sound to the inner ear is affected by abnormalities of the outer or middle ear, and sensorineural, which includes any interference with cochlear function or neural responses. Mixed hearing impairment involves both a conductive and a sensorineural component. It is fairly straightforward clinically to distinguish conductive from sensorineural impairments by comparing thresholds to air conducted sound with thresholds to bone conducted sound, delivered by direct vibration of the skull. Bone conduction largely bypasses the middle ear and therefore gives an indication of cochlear function irrespective of the performance of the middle ear, while air conduction thresholds represent the combined action of the middle and inner ears. A purely conductive impairment is unlikely to raise thresholds by more than about 60 decibels at the most, so any impairment greater than this must involve a sensorineural component. A number of syndromes feature malformation of the outer ear or pinnae set low on the head, and these anomalies may be severe enough to affect conduction of sound to the middle ear. The most common genetic middle ear defect is otosclerosis, a dominantly inherited condition with low penetrance, that produces a slowly progressive conductive hearing loss as a result of excess ossification eventually leading to fusion of the stapes to the oval window.

A further distinction that can sometimes be made in clinical practice is between cochlear and retrocochlear lesions. If the cochlea appears to respond normally to sound stimuli (assessed by gross electrode measurements of cochlear function), but there is an abnormality apparent in a more central part of the auditory system (judging from behavioural responses or the auditory brainstem response), then a retrocochlear impairment is likely. Neurofibromatosis type II is one genetic condition that can lead to vestibular schwannomas, which in turn compress the auditory nerve and cause retrocochlear hearing impairment. Although there must be many genes involved in the development and functioning of the central auditory system (from the auditory nerve upwards), hearing impairment associated with central auditory system dysfunction seems to be relatively rare in the human population. This may be because the development of the central auditory system probably involves many of the same genes as does the development of the rest of the central nervous system, and mutations in such genes might be more likely to be lethal at a very early stage and are therefore not seen.

Inner ear defects, which account for the vast majority of cases of human genetic hearing impairment, can be divided conveniently into three broad categories that reflect fundamentally different mechanisms of interference in the development and function of the ear: morphogenetic, cochleosaccular and neuroepithelial abnormalities (Steel and Bock, 1983; Steel and Brown, 1994).

In morphogenetic defects, there is an early interference in the development of the inner ear, at a time when the inner ear is still in the process of changing from a simple ovoid cyst into the complex multichambered form of the mature inner ear. This interference leads to a malformed shape of the inner ear. The malformation can range from a slight constriction of one of the semicircular canals (the lateral canal is the most frequently affected) or a slight widening of the internal acoustic meatus through which the auditory nerve leaves the inner ear (as in X-linked mixed hearing loss, *DFN3*, Phelps et al., 1991), to the formation of a grossly distorted cyst bearing little resemblance to the normal inner ear. There is often asymmetry between the two ears. The neural tube in the developing mammal is known to have an influence on the morphogenesis of the inner ear (Deol, 1966), and some genes that have been identified as underlying morphogenetic defects are expressed only in the neural tube, and not in the inner ear. Morphogenetic defects in humans are detectable by imaging techniques such as CT scanning, and probably lead to a wide range of hearing impairments in different individuals depending on the extent of the malformation.

In the other two groups of genetic inner ear defects, the gross shape of the labyrinth develops normally, but there are abnormalities in the development and differentiation of different cell types within the inner ear (Figure 1.7). In cochleosaccular defects, there is a primary abnormality of the stria vascularis. As described earlier, the stria generates the endocochlear potential and the high potassium level in endolymph, both of which are vital for normal hair cell function. In cochleosaccular defects, the stria does not function normally. This dysfunction can be demonstrated in two ways. Firstly, by light microscopy, Reissner's membrane, the thin membrane that separates scala media from scala vestibuli (Figure 1.3), with increasing age can be seen to collapse on to the organ of Corti, suggesting a problem with fluid homeostasis, which in turn implicates strial function (e.g. Mair, 1973). Secondly, the measured endocochlear potential is often reduced or absent (i.e. near zero) in mammals with cochleosaccular abnormalities, again suggesting a strial dysfunction (Suga and Hattler, 1970; Steel et al., 1983). The lack of an endocochlear potential leads to a moderate to severe hearing impairment. For example, mice with no endocochlear potential have thresholds of over 100 dB SPL. The primary strial dysfunction usually leads to secondary hair cell degeneration.

A clue to the mechanism involved in strial dysfunction comes from the observation that many mammals with this form of hearing impairment have syndromal hearing impairment associated with a pigmentation abnormality, as in deaf white cats, Dalmatian dogs, various mouse mutants with white spotting of the coat, and also in humans with pigmentation anomalies. The white spotted areas of the skin or coat are devoid of the melanocytes that produce pigment, and when the stria vascularis is examined, this too is lacking in melanocytes in animals with no measurable endocochlear potential (Cable et al., 1994). In partly spotted mice, with some melanocytes in their strias, a positive endocochlear potential is recorded but it may not be as large as normal

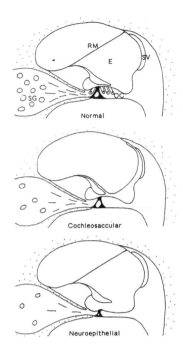

Normal cochlea

RM, Reissner's Membrane

SV, Stria Vascularis

E, Endolymph

SG, Spiral Ganglion

OC, Organ of Corti, with sensory hair cells

Stippled areas, bone

Cochleosaccular defects

• Primary SV defect

• Endocochlear potential reduced or absent

• RM may sometimes collapse

• Hair cells degenerate

• SG cells degenerate

Neuroepithelial defects

• Primary OC defect

• SG cells degenerate

• SV normal

• Endocochlear potential normal

• RM in normal place

Figure 1.7 Illustration of the key features of cochleosaccular and neuroepithelial inner ear defects. Top: the normal cochlear duct. Middle: cochleosaccular defects, showing thin and abnormal stria vascularis, occasional collapse of Reissner's membrane, secondary damage to the hair cells, and long term retrograde degeneration of cochlear neurones in the spiral ganglion. Bottom: neuroepithelial defects, showing a primary organ of Corti abnormality leading to hair cell degeneration and ultimately supporting cell degeneration, retrograde degeneration of auditory neurones, but normal stria vascularis structure and function.

(Cable et al., 1992). These observations suggest that melanocytes are essential for normal strial function (see Steel (1995) for further discussion). Cochleosaccular defects may presumably also be caused by defects in other cell types in the stria, but these have not yet been so clearly defined as in the case of pigmentation defects associated with hearing impairment.

The last major category of inner ear abnormality is the neuroepithelial group. In these, the primary defect lies in the neuroepithelia of the inner ear, including the organ of Corti in the cochlea and the various sensory cell patches in the vestibular part of the ear. The stria functions normally. Hair cells ultimately degenerate, but in those mutants that have been most carefully studied, there are usually some developmental defects that can be detected long before the onset of degeneration, suggesting that the degeneration is not a cause of hearing impairment, but is a secondary consequence of the mutation. Recently, the gene involved in the *shaker-1* mouse mutant has been identified by positional cloning as a myosin VII gene (Gibson et al., 1995). This is the first gene to be identified in which mutations are known to cause neuroepithelial defects of the inner ear. The observation that the *shaker-1* locus encodes an unconventional myosin gene suggests that genes encoding other cytoskeletal proteins may be candidates for other mutations causing neuroepithelial hearing impairment. The myosin VII gene was also found to be mutated in cases of Usher syndrome type IB (Weil et al., 1995), which is associated with profound hearing loss. The hearing impairment in neuroepithelial abnormalities is often severe or profound.

Conclusions

The inner ear, and particularly the cochlea is an extremely complicated organ which has evolved a range of specialised mechanisms to achieve its astonishing sensitivity to the frequency and amplitude of sounds. It is perhaps not surprising therefore that hearing impairments (to varying degrees of severity) are common. While some of these pathologies are undoubtedly a result of environmental factors, such as noise exposure and ototoxic substances, a large proportion involve some kind of genetic defect; even the severity of hearing loss due to environmental factors may involve hereditary susceptibility factors. Identification of the genes involved in hereditary hearing loss not only holds out the promise of prophylactic action, but will also reveal much about the complicated developmental processes which produce the normally functioning ear.

Chapter 2
Basic genetic mechanisms

ANDREW P READ

This chapter is intended for non-geneticists. The idea is to give a quick overview of the main concepts and terminology used by geneticists, which hopefully will make the genetic content of later chapters accessible to non-specialist readers. Molecular genetics is not intrinsically difficult, and anybody with a basic grasp of what molecules and cells are can arrive at a working understanding. The main obstacle is simply the number of different molecules and interactions involved in genetic programming of cells and organisms. This is an inevitable reflection of the huge complexity of living organisms as molecular machines. However, a few basic ideas go a long way in molecular genetics, and I have tried to outline these. The outline is of course very incomplete and omits many fascinating subtleties, but hopefully it is not misleadingly simplified. Further details may be found in numerous textbooks. I recommend particularly two fairly short general textbooks of medical genetics (Connor and Ferguson Smith, 1994; Mueller and Young, 1995), and two texts specifically on molecular genetics (Malcolm and Emery, 1995 (a small book) and Strachan and Read, 1996 (a large comprehensive book)).

Genes in pedigrees

Classically genes are inferred by studying the pattern of inheritance of a character (a *phenotype*). Starting with Mendel, most of the properties and behaviour of genes were worked out from results of breeding experimental organisms, without any clear idea of what genes might be physically. For each *locus* (type of gene), an organism has two *alleles* (alternative versions of a gene), one inherited from each parent. The two alleles may be the same (*homozygous*) or different (*heterozygous*). Characters that are seen in the heterozygote are *dominant,* and those seen only in the homozygote are *recessive* (note that dominance and recessiveness are properties of characters, not genes, despite the common bad habit of talking about dominant genes etc.).

Across a population, a given gene may have only one allele, two different alleles, or a very large number of different alleles, but any one person has only two alleles. Genes behaving in this way are described as *autosomal*. *Sex-linked* genes are inherited according to slightly different rules. The rules of Mendelian inheritance became self evident once the behaviour of chromosomes during formation of sperm and eggs was understood (see below).

As non-experimental organisms with small families and long generation times, humans are not well suited to this type of analysis. Single pedigrees are seldom extensive enough to prove a given mode of inheritance beyond doubt. However, certain patterns can be recognised, as follows.

Autosomal dominant inheritance

Affected people normally have one affected parent; in a mating of affected x unaffected, each child has a 50% chance of being affected (Figure 2.1a). For most human dominant diseases, affected people are heterozygotes. Sometimes a character shows imperfectly dominant inheritance, such that occasionally a person who carries the gene does not manifest the expected character. This is called *non-penetrance*, and reflects the influence of other genes or of the environment on the character. Penetrance may be age related, as in adult onset hearing loss.

Autosomal recessive inheritance

Affected people are homozygous for the abnormal gene. Their parents are usually phenotypically normal carriers (Figure 2.1b). Recessive conditions can become very frequent in multiply inbred genetic isolates, where many people carry a particular abnormal allele. Such kindreds have been crucially important for mapping recessive profound hearing loss (see Chapter 21).

X-linked inheritance

Men (44, XY) have only one X chromosome, which they pass on to all their daughters but none of their sons. This gives the characteristic pattern of X-linked inheritance. X-linked characters cannot be dominant or recessive in men, because there are no heterozygotes. For reasons connected with the phenomenon of X-inactivation (see Connor and Ferguson Smith, 1994; Strachan and Read, 1996), even in women the distinction between dominant and recessive is less clear cut than for autosomal characters; nevertheless, one can in principle distinguish

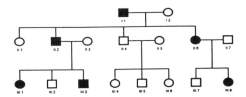

a.

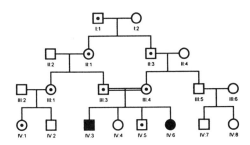

b.

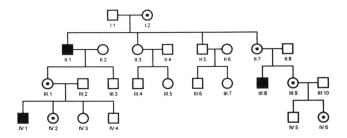

c.

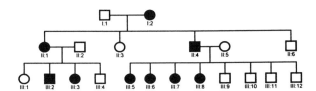

d.

Figure 2.1 Mendelian pedigree patterns. a. autosomal dominant; b. autosomal recessive; c. X-linked recessive; d. X-linked dominant. Pedigrees are often ambiguous, or do not conform to any of these patterns. See Chapter 26, Figure 26.1 for the pedigree pattern expected for a mitochondrially determined character. Squares represent males, circles females; filled-in characters mark affected people.

X-linked recessive and dominant pedigree patterns (Figure 2.1c, d).

Y-linked inheritance is not seen, because the Y chromosome carries very few genes, other than those determining maleness.

Although over 5,000 Mendelian human characters are known, the great majority of genetic or part-genetic human characters do not follow these simple Mendelian pedigree patterns. Usually more than one genetic locus is involved, and often environmental factors as well. Such characters are variously called *polygenic, oligogenic* or *multifactorial*, and are a major focus of human genetic research at present.

Genes on chromosomes

Like Mendel's genes, chromosomes come in pairs and one of each pair, picked at random, is passed on by a parent to a child. The mechanics of meiosis explain Mendelian segregation. During mitosis (the normal cell divisions that convert a fertilised egg into a fully grown adult) the 46 human chromosomes are exactly copied, so that every nucleated cell of a person contains a complete copy of all the genes and chromosomes. Chromosomes are normally observed in dividing cells at the metaphase of mitosis. At this time each chromosome consists of two sister chromatids, united at the centromere. The sister chromatids will separate in the next stage of mitosis (anaphase), and each chromosome then remains as a single chromatid until the DNA is replicated before the next cell division. Cytogeneticists are able to stain chromosomes in a reproducible pattern of dark and light bands. This greatly aids identification of each chromosome, and also forms the basis of the nomenclature of chromosome regions. Band 2q35 means chromosome 2, long arm (q; short arm = p), band 3, sub-band 5 (see Connor and Ferguson Smith (1994) or Strachan and Read (1996) for ideograms of the human karyotype with all bands numbered.)

A chromosome consists of a single immensely long double helix of DNA (typically 50 – 150 million base pairs), packed around a scaffold of proteins. Long before the molecular details of chromosomes were understood, genetic analysis had shown that genes form an unbranched linear array along a chromosome. Humans have perhaps 80,000 pairs of genes, so the average chromosome carries maybe 3,000 – 4,000 genes.

In addition to the chromosomes in the nucleus, the mitochondria in cells contain DNA. The mitochondrial genome is only 16,569 base pairs long and comprises 37 genes. Mitochondrial genes are important in the context of this book because *mutations* (changes in code sequence at the molecular level) in some of them can cause hearing loss (see Chapter 26). Sperm contribute no mitochondria to the fertilised egg, and so mitochondrial genes are inherited only from the mother. This produces an unusual matrilineal pedigree pattern for mitochondrial inheritance (see Figure 26.1).

Genes as DNA sequences

Genes are DNA sequences that specify characters, normally by specifying the sequence of aminoacids in a protein. Genes are expressed by *transcription* (synthesis of an RNA molecule containing the genetic message) followed by *translation* (construction of a polypeptide following instructions in the genetic code of the messenger RNA or mRNA). A few genes specify the structure of molecules of RNA that are functional in themselves, and are not translated. Three nucleotides of DNA or mRNA specify one aminoacid according to the genetic code (Table 2.1). The mechanism by which this is done involves complex interactions of the mRNA with ribosomes, transfer RNA and many other factors. The details need not concern us here.

Table 2.1 The genetic code.

UUU F (Phe)	CUU L (Leu)	AUU I (Ile)	GUU V (Val)
UUC F (Phe)	CUC L (Leu)	AUC I (Ile)	GUC V (Val)
UUA L (Leu)	CUA L (Leu)	AUA I (Ile)	GUA V (Val)
UUG L (Leu)	CUG L (Leu)	AUG M (Met)	GUG V (Val)
UCU S (Ser)	CCU P (Pro)	ACU T (Thr)	GCU A (Ala)
UCC S (Ser)	CCC P (Pro)	ACC T (Thr)	GCC A (Ala)
UCA S (Ser)	CCA P (Pro)	ACA T (Thr)	GCA A (Ala)
UCG S (Ser)	CCG P (Pro)	ACG T (Thr)	GCG A (Ala)
UAU Y (Tyr)	CAU H (His)	AAU N (Asn)	GAU D (Asp)
UAC Y (Tyr)	CAC H (His)	AAC N (Asn)	GAC D (Asp)
UAA STOP	CAA Q (Gln)	AAA K (Lys)	GAA E (Glu)
UAG STOP	CAG Q (Gln)	AAG K (Lys)	GAG E (Glu)
UGU C (Cys)	CGU R (Arg)	AGU S (Ser)	GGU G (Gly)
UGC C (Cys)	CGC R (Arg)	AGC S (Ser)	GGC G (Gly)
UGA STOP	CGA R (Arg)	AGA R (Arg)	GGA G (Gly)
UGG W (Trp)	CGG R (Arg)	AGG R (Arg)	GGG G (Gly)

Codons are given in the RNA form (A adenine; C cytosine; G guanine; U uracil); in DNA U is replaced by T (thymine). Aminoacids are given in one-letter codes and three-letter abbreviations (Ala alanine; Arg arginine; Asn asparagine; Asp aspartic acid; Cys cysteine; Gln glutamine; Glu glutamic acid; Gly glycine; His histidine; Ile isoleucine; Leu leucine; Lys lysine; Met methionine; Phe phenylalanine; Pro proline; Ser serine; Thr threonine; Trp tryptophan; Tyr tyrosine; Val valine). AUG serves both as a codon for methionine and as a start codon.

Transcription

Transcription is a highly selective process. Only about 10% of the DNA in a human is ever transcribed, and in any given cell type the proportion is much lower. Even those sequences that are transcribed are transcribed at lower or higher levels, and turned on and off according to the requirements of the cell. Transcriptional control is the key to genetic programming of cells, and we understand only the very broad outlines of how it works. The key step is association of RNA polymerase (the enzyme that makes mRNA) with a particular point on the chromosomal DNA. Once correctly bound, the polymerase can move along the DNA, transcribing it until a stop signal is encountered. Only certain sequences (promoters) in the DNA can bind RNA polymerase, and these sequences mark the upstream ends of genes. Promoters are asymmetrical, so that only one strand of the double helix (the template strand) is selected to be transcribed.

RNA polymerase does not simply bind in a one-to-one interaction with the promoter. A large multi-protein complex must be assembled on the promoter to initiate transcription, and the other proteins in the complex modulate the whole process, turning it on or off and regulating the level of transcription. These *transcription factors* are crucial components of the cellular machinery, and are the subject of intense research. Abnormalities in transcription factors can have major effects on the genetic programme of the cell. The genes mutated in Waardenburg syndrome (Chapter 16) encode transcription factors.

Exons and introns

Genes of *eukaryotic* organisms (those with nucleated cells, i.e. everything above bacteria) have a curious and unexpected feature that has far reaching consequences for genetic research. The coding sequence is usually split into several sections (*exons*), interrupted by non-coding sequences (*introns*). This happens along an uninterrupted DNA double helix, like an audio tape carrying a series of successive songs. Initially the entire gene, exons and introns, is transcribed, then the mRNA is processed to remove the introns. This requires a complicated (and fallible) piece of cellular machinery, able to read the RNA transcript, detect splice signals, cut out the introns and splice together the exons.

Numbers, locations and sizes of introns vary enormously between different genes. A few genes have no introns; some have a few modest sized introns; at the extreme, the gene encoding the muscle protein dystrophin has 14,000 base pairs of coding sequence split into 79 exons scattered over 2,300,000 base pairs of genomic DNA. Despite much theorising, there is no convincing explanation for any of these features, and no way of predicting the exon-intron structure of a gene. However, this structure is crucially important for two reasons. First, it underlies the contrast between *genomic* DNA and cDNA (see below), and second, it explains the molecular pathology of many mutations.

Genomic DNA and cDNA

The difference between genomic DNA and complementary DNA (cDNA) must be appreciated in order to understand the research strategies described in the following chapters. Genomic DNA is the DNA as it occurs in the cell nucleus, complete with all the introns and the non-coding DNA lying between genes (intergenic DNA). Genomic DNA is easy to isolate, clone and manipulate, but only 2 – 3% of it comprises coding sequences, and there is no simple or foolproof way of identifying those sequences. cDNA is an artificially produced DNA copy of a mature mRNA (that is, mRNA with the introns removed). cDNA is made using a special enzyme, reverse transcriptase. It contains no nonsense, only the coding sequence; however, a particular cDNA can be made only if the corresponding mRNA is available. No single cell contains all mRNAs. Whereas genomic DNA is the same in every cell and tissue, the repertoire of mRNAs depends on the cell, the tissue, the stage of development and so on. Thus cDNAs important for hearing research are sought in mRNA preparations of the organ of Corti, or specifically of hair cells (see Chapter 4), but the resulting cDNA libraries are always incomplete. Additionally, cDNAs do not contain the promoter sequences (see above) that are so crucial for regulating gene activity; these can be studied only in genomic DNA.

How DNA is studied

A human cell contains 6×10^9 base pairs (6 million kilobases (kb) or 6,000 megabases (Mb)) of DNA. Thus the central problem in studying human DNA is how to recognise the one sequence of interest against a huge background of irrelevant but chemically identical DNA. Essentially there are two ways of doing this: hybridising the sequence of interest to a labelled probe, or cloning it.

DNA hybridisation and Southern blotting

DNA exists naturally as the famous Watson-Crick double helix. This is formed by two complementary strands, with A base-paired to T and G to C. The base-pairing can be disrupted by boiling (*denaturing*) the DNA. If complementary single strands are mixed, they will *hybridise* to form a double helix. If we add a Watson strand to a complex mixture of single stranded DNA, it will search out any matching Crick strand and hybridise to it. The Southern blot technique uses this to test for the presence and size of strands matching a *probe* strand. Thus foetal DNA can be sexed by testing for hybridisation to a probe made of Y chromosome specific DNA; or a cDNA can be used to find the corresponding sequence in genomic DNA (and vice versa). The probe is labelled, either radioactively with ^{32}P or ^{35}S, or by attaching a fluorescent dye, or by attaching a group such as biotin that can be detected by its binding to streptavidin. The test DNA is bound to a solid support such as a nylon membrane, and this is bathed in a solution containing the labelled probe. After removal and rinsing, we test for label stuck to the membrane. Presence of bound label means that the probe has found a matching sequence in the test DNA bound to the membrane.

A refinement of the basic assay arranges fragments of the test DNA on the membrane according to length. This is done by fragmenting the test DNA using special enzymes (restriction enzymes) and then running it through an electrophoretic gel. In agarose gels, DNA fragments migrate at a rate depending on their size, but not significantly on their sequence. Small fragments move fast and large ones move slowly. Hybridisation with the labelled probe is not technically feasible within the gel, so the fragments spread down the lanes of the gel are transferred, without altering their positions, to a nylon membrane. The trick for doing this was developed by E M Southern, hence the name Southern blot. Later variants were named Northern, Western etc. blots as a joke. On the membrane, the presence of bound probe signals the presence of a matching sequence in the test DNA, and its position reveals its size by showing how far it travelled through the agarose gel during electrophoresis.

Hybridisation is not an all-or-nothing process. Short or imperfectly matched sequences will hybridise at low temperatures, but dissociate at higher temperatures at which longer or more perfectly matched sequences remain hybridised. Manipulating the *stringency of hybridisation* is a useful tool. Short probes (typically 20 bases) can be made that stick only to a perfectly matched partner, and these can be used to distinguish test DNA molecules differing by only a single base. This allows detection of single base mutations in disease genes. Longer probes (a few hundred bases) will hybridise despite a few mismatches. They can be used to identify a particular gene in any person, even though there may be small individual differences in the sequence; or to look for sequences related, but not identical, to a known gene.

Cloning *in vivo* – genomic and complementary DNA libraries

If a DNA fragment of interest can be inserted into a living cell, then when the cell proliferates the inserted DNA may proliferate with it. This can produce an unlimited supply of the pure fragment. Usually *E. coli* bacteria are used for this purpose, though sometimes yeast or other cells may be needed. The key to understanding cloning is to appreciate the necessity for a *vector*. A fragment of DNA simply injected into a cell will not be replicated. In order to be replicated and stably propagated, the DNA must be provided with various functions recognised by the host cell, particularly replication initiation sequences. DNA fragments are cloned as recombinant molecules covalently linked (inserted) into a vector molecule that provides these functions (this is the origin of the term recombinant DNA). Additionally the vector must provide some feature enabling cells containing recombinant molecules to be recognised and selected. Much genetic engineering has gone into developing vectors optimised for different cloning strategies. An important decision is how large a DNA fragment one wishes to clone, because each type of vector has a maximum size of insert (Table 2.2).

Table 2.2 Examples of cloning vectors.

Vector	Cloning capacity	Host	Uses
Plasmid	5 kb	*E coli*	cDNA cloning
λ phage	20 kb	*E coli*	Cloning small genomic fragments; some versions adapted for gene expression
M13 phage	5 kb	*E coli*	Producing single stranded DNA for sequencing
Cosmid	45 kb	*E coli*	Cloning genomic DNA
P1 phage, Bac, Pac	100 kb	*E coli*	Cloning large genomic DNA fragments
YAC (yeast artificial chromosome)	1000 kb	Yeast	Cloning complete genes; building contigs

As well as cloning capacity (the largest piece of DNA that can be cloned using that vector), ease of manipulation, copy number per host cell and stability are important considerations.

The initial result of a cloning experiment is usually a large collection of independent clones, representing either a collection of cDNAs from some cell type or multiple fragments produced by breaking up genomic DNA. These clone collections are called *libraries*, but the term is seriously misleading. In a library the books are arranged in order, with a catalogue to enable any desired book to be quickly retrieved. Clone libraries would better be called haystacks, that may or may not include the desired needle. Clone libraries must be screened to find any desired clone, which may or may not be present. Libraries are screened using hybridisation assays, or by PCR as described below.

Cloning *in vitro* – the polymerase chain reaction (PCR)

Polymerase chain reaction (PCR) enables any short DNA sequence to be replicated specifically and to an unlimited degree, even starting from a single molecule, and with very quick and simple manipulations. Not surprisingly, the invention of PCR has revolutionised molecular biology.

PCR depends on a quirk in the way DNA is replicated. The DNA polymerase enzymes that replicate DNA assemble a new strand out of mononucleotides lined up on a template strand. But they cannot start with a bare template; they can only extend an existing *primer* which forms a short double-stranded region. In a complex mixture of single stranded DNA it is possible to control which DNA sequences are replicated by supplying only certain primers. In PCR this selectivity is used to start a chain reaction in which just the chosen sequence is replicated *ad libitum*. This requires two primers bracketing the selected region. To carry out a PCR, the input DNA, primers, monomers and DNA polymerase are mixed and put through cycles of temperature changes that control the various phases of the reaction. Each cycle takes about 1 – 2 minutes and theoretically doubles the quantity of the selected sequence whilst ignoring all others. Thus an hour or two of temperature cycling in an automated heating block will create an overwhelming preponderance of the selected sequence.

PCR has two main limitations. Specific primers must be designed, and this requires knowledge of the DNA sequence to which they must hybridise. An unknown sequence can be amplified, but only if it is flanked by known sequences. Secondly, only relatively short lengths of DNA can be amplified in this way. Until very recently the practical upper limit was about 2kb; now amplification of 20kb is possible, but this is still small compared with the size of a chromosome, of many genes, and of some clones. Molecular geneticists use innumerable technical tricks and dodges to circumvent these two limitations.

The strategy for discovering disease genes

Genes responsible for hearing loss (or any other disease) could in principle be identified in three ways:

1. Through studying affected cells, identifying an altered protein, working out the aminoacid sequence of the protein, and using this sequence, with reverse genetic coding, to design a probe to isolate the gene encoding that protein (the *functional approach*).
2. Through guessing that a previously characterised gene might be responsible, and showing that mutations in that gene are found in people with hearing loss (the *candidate gene approach*).

3. Through mapping the chromosomal location of the gene and then identifying genes at that location and testing them for mutations in affected people (the *positional cloning approach*).

Hearing loss research has relied on various combinations of the candidate gene and positional cloning approaches. Identification of the myosin VIIa gene in Usher syndrome (Chapter 14) is an example of pure positional cloning; identification of the collagen IV genes in Alport syndrome (Chapter 17) exemplifies a candidate gene approach, whilst identification of the *PAX3* and *MITF* genes in Waardenburg syndrome (Chapter 16) illustrates a common combination (positional candidate approach), where the gene is mapped to a chromosomal region, which then suggests a known gene as a candidate.

The methods are briefly outlined here, and described in more detail in Chapter 3 and in individual disease chapters.

Genetic mapping

Suppose a man inherits dominant hearing loss from his mother, caused by a gene on chromosome 1. Suppose further that he has 10 children, five of whom inherit his hearing loss. Those five children should inherit the chromosome 1 that he received from his mother, while the five unaffected children should inherit his other copy of chromosome 1. All his other chromosomes would segregate randomly. Thus we could discover which chromosome carried a disease gene by following each chromosome through a sufficiently large family where the disease is segregating, and seeing which chromosome tracks with the disease. This would be an example of *linkage analysis*, which is the principal means of *genetic mapping*.

Chromosomes are recognised and tracked by using *genetic markers*. A genetic marker is any character that is inherited in a simple Mendelian way and that is polymorphic, i.e. exists in variant forms in the population so that we can distinguish different forms as they segregate through the family. The argument of the preceding paragraph implied that one would need only 22 different markers, one for each autosome (i.e. non-sex chromosome). However, that argument ignored recombination. During meiosis, pairs of chromosomes line up and exchange segments. Each individual chromosome of a child is a mosaic of segments from the corresponding chromosome pair in each parent. The consequence for genetic mapping is that we must follow a specific chromosomal region, rather than a whole chromosome, through the pedigree. Such regions, identified by linkage analysis, are measured in centimorgans (cM). These units do not precisely measure DNA length, but on average loci 1 cM apart are separated by 1 megabase of DNA. About 400 highly polymorphic markers, spaced out across the genome, are needed to be reasonably confident of detecting linkage of a marker to a disease in a collection of families.

Genetic markers for linkage analysis

Blood groups, electrophoretic variants of serum proteins and tissue types have all been used as genetic markers, but all these have been superseded by DNA polymorphisms. DNA polymorphisms have several important advantages. There are so many different DNA polymorphisms that any region of any chromosome is bound to carry several, if they can be discovered. They can all be studied by the same methods, and the methods can be automated, so that laboratories can study large numbers of different DNA polymorphisms quickly. DNA is easy to isolate from blood, hair roots, mouthwashes and many other accessible tissues, and is easily stored and transported once isolated. Finally, several techniques (see Chapter 3) allow the chromosomal location of a DNA polymorphism to be determined easily, so that we can always know which chromosomal region a given polymorphism is tracking.

The human genome shows an enormous amount of DNA sequence variation. On average one nucleotide in 200 is significantly polymorphic (that is, more than one variant is frequent in the population). Most of this variability occurs in intergenic DNA (the DNA lying between genes that is not transcribed or translated), and has no obvious phenotypic effect. Two general types of DNA polymorphism are used in linkage analysis: restriction fragment length polymorphisms (RFLPs) and variable number tandem repeats (VNTRs). The bases of these variants are described in Chapter 3. Nowadays most linkage mapping uses a particular class of VNTR markers called microsatellites, which are easy to use and highly informative. One of the main achievements of the Human Genome Project in its first five years has been to generate, characterise and map over 5,000 microsatellite polymorphisms. Because of this effort, it is now relatively straightforward, though still laborious, to find a marker that cosegregates with any given Mendelian disease, provided suitable families are available for study.

Lod scores

We need a statistic for deciding whether a marker really does track with a disease, and the favoured measure is the lod score (see Chapter 3). Lod means logarithm of the odds (of linkage versus no linkage). Positive lod scores favour linkage, negative scores are evidence against linkage. A lod score of +3.0 corresponds to the conventional p=0.05 threshold of significance, whilst a lod score of −2.0 is significant evidence against linkage. Lod scores larger than −2.0 but smaller than +3.0 are not considered significant. Lod scores are logarithmic to the base 10, so a lod score of 4.0 is ten times as convincing as a lod score of 3.0. Computer programs are available for calculating lod scores from pedigree and marker data.

Positional cloning

Once a gene has been mapped to a particular chromosomal location, it must be cloned – but this can be far from easy. The problems of searching for an unknown gene increase more than linearly with the size of the region to be searched, and become almost insuperable when the region is much over one million base pairs. The initial mapping is likely to locate the gene only to within 10 – 20 million base pairs (remember that each chromosome contains 50 – 150 million base pairs of DNA). Usually the next step is to refine the mapping by studying large collections of families, often assembled by international consortia (such as the Usher Consortium or the Waardenburg Consortium).

As the candidate region is narrowed down, other clues are sought. Sometimes additional clues can be obtained from individuals with chromosomal abnormalities, or from linkage disequilibrium. *Linkage disequilibrium* or *allelic association* is a phenomenon in which the frequencies of certain marker alleles among affected people diverge from the frequencies in the general population. This happens if most of the affected people in the population, although apparently unrelated, are actually part of one extended family. It is seen (if at all) only for markers located very close to the disease gene, so it can provide a valuable clue to the location of the disease gene. Checks are made on known genes in the region, and sometimes (as in Waardenburg syndrome) this reveals the disease gene without the labour of positional cloning.

If there is no such lucky break, the next stage is to identify a series of contiguous clones that cover the entire candidate region (a *contig*; see Chapter 3). This area is then searched for genes using a number of techniques such as screening cDNA libraries, cDNA selection, exon trapping and computer analysis of the DNA sequence. All these methods are difficult and fallible, so that positional cloning is not a task to be embarked upon lightly. Identification of the genes for Usher IB and Treacher Collins syndromes were major achievements requiring years of intensive work by world class teams.

How genes can go wrong

To make a candidate disease gene plausible, mutations must be demonstrated in affected people. Why should a mutation affect somebody's hearing? In principle there are two possibilities:

1. The mutated gene may lose its function and do nothing.

2. The mutated gene may gain a harmful function. This is unlikely to be a totally novel function, but might involve being expressed at the wrong time, at too high a level, in the wrong place or in response to the wrong signal.

As a very broad generalisation, loss of function mutations normally cause recessive phenotypes, because by and large cells can function on a half dose of the gene product. This is not always true – Waardenburg syndrome type I is caused by the inability of certain neural crest cells to function correctly with a half dose of the *PAX3* protein (*haploinsufficiency*). Mutant versions of proteins that function as part of multimeric assemblies may prevent any remaining normal versions from working (*dominant negative effect*). Nevertheless, it remains generally true that one looks for loss of function mutations to explain recessive phenotypes and gain of function mutations to explain dominant characters.

Genes are long stretches of DNA, and we have seen that gene expression is a complex process. There are correspondingly many ways of destroying the function of a gene. These include deletion of all or part of the gene, disruption of its structure (e.g. by a chromosomal translocation), mutations that inactivate the promoter and mutations that change the signals required for correct splicing of the exons during mRNA processing. *Frameshift mutations* are small insertions or deletions that change the way the continuous mRNA strand is read in triplet codons. For example, deletion of the second C would change CAU.CAU.CAU.CAU to CAU.AUC.AUC.AU... Within the coding sequence, single base substitutions may replace a codon for an aminoacid with one of the stop codons, UGA, UAA or UAG (*nonsense mutation*); or they may result in one aminoacid being replaced by another (*missense mutation*). Whether a missense mutation matters or not depends on whether that particular aminoacid plays an important part in the function of the protein. In general it is not easy to predict the effect of a missense mutation, either on the protein or on the patient. Increasingly these problems of molecular pathology are being investigated by creating mice carrying the specific mutation under investigation.

There are two ways of describing a mutation. One is to describe the aminoacid change, using the one letter or three letter abbreviations given in Table 2.1. Taking examples from Figure 16.1 (Chapter 16) G99D means replace the glycine at position 99 with aspartic acid; this could equally have been written as Gly99Asp. Stop codons are designated X or Stop, so W274X (or Trp274Stop) replaces the UGG codon for tryptophan 274 with a stop codon, presumably UAG or UGA in this case. The second method describes the DNA change, for example 358del(1) means delete a single nucleotide at nucleotide number 358. Increasingly, databases of mutations are being established, and eventually these may make it possible to predict the phenotypic effect of a given DNA sequence change. At present, however, molecular pathology is an inexact science. Thus discovering what gene is responsible for a given form of hearing loss is only the beginning of the trail – the eventual aim is to discover what the normal version of that gene does to make normal hearing possible.

Chapter 3
Methods of identifying hearing loss genes

BRUNO DALLAPICCOLA, RITA MINGARELLI and
ANDREW P READ

Introduction: the target genes

Epidemiological data suggest that congenital hearing loss occurs with a prevalence of one in 1,000 births, and in half of all cases has a genetic origin. Among hereditary examples, 30% are syndromal, associated with other anomalies. Progress in defining genes for Mendelian non-syndromal hearing loss is reviewed in Chapters 21 and 22. Most of the syndromal disorders are also inherited as Mendelian characters, although some are associated with chromosomal imbalance or mutations in the mitochondrial genome. In fact, about 10% of all currently known disease-associated human genes, when mutated, cause hearing impairment of some type (McKusick et al., 1994). In a comprehensive and up to date clinical review, Gorlin et al. (1995) have reviewed 402 conditions in which genetic hearing loss is not isolated, and these are briefly summarised in Table 3.1.

Although chromosomal syndromes are not primary targets for gene identification, it is worth noting that hearing loss is a common, albeit little investigated feature of many chromosomal syndromes. Mental retardation, which is a major complication of chromosomal imbalances, often distracts from proper appraisal of hearing loss in these patients. Regardless of the type of aneuploidy or structural anomaly, the spectrum of hearing impairment is rather limited, typically including conductive or sensorineural hearing loss with dysmorphic and malpositioned external ears, narrow external auditory canals, inner ear malformations and/or dysplastic auditory epithelium. However, chromosomal hearing loss is not always genetic in origin. There are also enviromental causes, including repeated middle ear infections. In addition, in those syndromes in which cleft palate is a common feature, hearing loss may be, at least in part, secondary to the middle ear sequelae of the cleft.

Table 3.1 A summary of genetic syndromes including hearing loss, all of which present targets for gene identification.

Associated anomalies	No. of conditions*	Examples
External ear abnormalities (ranging from anotia to large, simple and cupped auricles)	30	Treacher Collins syndrome (see Chapter 20) Postaxial acrofacial dysostosis (Miller syndrome) Goldenhar syndrome Branchio-oto-renal syndrome (see Chapter 19) CHARGE association DiGeorge/velo-cardio-facial syndrome
Eye abnormalities	40	Disorders with retinitis pigmentosa, e.g. Usher syndrome (see Chapter 14) Syndromes with optic atrophy Marshall syndrome (myopia, cataracts) Ehlers-Danlos syndrome type VI Syndromes with blepharophimosis (Ohdo, Michels) Fraser cryptophthalmos syndrome Norrie syndrome
Abnormalities of the musculoskeletal system	87	Acral-orofacial syndromes Chrondrodysplasias Craniosynostoses Craniotubular bone disorders Skeletal disorders
Kidney abnormalities	23	Alport syndrome (see Chapter 17) Winter syndrome (renal and genital abnormalities) Renal tubular acidoses
Abnormalities of the central nervous system	63	Many syndromes with ataxia Spastic paraplegia Motor and sensory neuropathies Mitochondrial encephalomyopathies (see Chapter 26)
Endocrine and metabolic abnormalities	51	Mucopolysaccharidoses Oligosaccharidoses Gangliosidoses Adrenoleukodystrophies Syndromes of diabetes mellitus with gonadal, parathyroid and/or thyroid abnormalities
Skin abnormalities	56	Waardenburg syndrome (see Chapter 16) Multiple lentigenes (LEOPARD) syndrome Focal dermal hypoplasia (Goltz-Gorlin syndrome) Syndromes of congenital ichthyosis, hyperkeratosis, alopecia and onychodystrophy.
Oral and dental abnormalities	8	Otodental syndrome Gingival fibromatosis with hearing loss
Miscellaneous non-chromosomal syndromes	35	Jervell and Lange-Nielsen (long QT) syndrome Neurofibromatosis type II (see Chapter 18)
Chromosomal abnormalities	12	

* Numbers listed by Gorlin et al. (1995). For a fuller listing and discussion, see the monograph by Gorlin et al. (1995).

As new molecular technologies have rapidly reduced the time needed to map and clone a disease gene, including those related to hearing loss, our understanding of the basic biological defects is improving. These advances have very quickly passed into preventive medicine. The long-term aim must be development of effective drug or gene therapies, but the timetable for this is much less predictable.

Mapping hearing loss genes

As explained in Chapter 2, the first step towards identifying the gene underlying a clinical phenotype is normally to map the gene. Maps are of two types. The physical map of gene loci gives their position and distance on individual chromosomes, expressed in base pairs (bp) or related to cytogenetic features of the chromosome such as the banding pattern (Chapter 2). The genetic map gives the relative position of gene loci as determined by the frequency of recombination, expressed in centimorgans (cM). One cM corresponds to a frequency of recombination of 1%. The female genetic map is about 40% longer than the male map, because recombination occurs almost twice as often in oocytes as in spermatocytes.

Physical mapping

Physical mapping includes chromosome mapping, where a gene or DNA sequence is assigned to a specific chromosome or subchromosomal region; and DNA mapping, using a finer level of analysis which provides mapping information at the DNA level, including the physical relationship between DNA sequence polymorphisms and the gene structure. Physical mapping is used to map DNA clones, or sometimes defined proteins, but it cannot be used directly to map clinical phenotypes. The main chromosome mapping techniques include:

Gene dosage studies

A decreased amount of gene product in an individual with a deletion, or an increased amount in a trisomic subject, suggests the assignment of a structural gene to the particular unbalanced chromosome.

Use of somatic cell hybrids

These are obtained by fusing cells taken from two species. Human-rodent hybrid cells preferentially lose human chromosomes, eventually producing more or less stable cell lines containing a full rodent genome but only one or a few human chromosomes. For chromosomal mapping, a panel of such somatic cell hybrid clones is selected that retain different human chromosomes. Hybrid cell mapping panels, for sub-chromosomal localisation of genes or markers, can be constructed by using human cells that have chromosomal deletions or translocations. Expressed proteins can be mapped by comparing the human chromosome content of hybrid cells that do and do not produce the protein, and cloned DNA segments can be mapped by using DNA hybridisation or PCR (see Chapter 2 and below) to establish which hybrid cells contain the sequence.

In situ hybridisation

Single stranded labelled DNA sequences are incubated with standard chromosome preparations so that they hybridise to the homologous DNA sequence. In the past, the probe was labelled radioactively, but for gene mapping this method has been superseded by fluorescence in situ hybridisation (FISH). The probe is labelled with a dye that fluoresces in ultraviolet light, so that its position on the chromosome can be seen directly under a fluorescence microscope. Several differently coloured probes can be used simultaneously to order clones along a chromosome. This is one of the most powerful and direct methods for physically mapping any cloned DNA sequence.

Genetic mapping

For initial mapping of genes causing hearing loss, or any other clinically defined phenotype, the method of choice is usually genetic mapping. As briefly described in Chapter 2, this relies on family studies using genetic markers.

Family linkage analysis (Figure 3.1)

Two genes are linked if their loci are physically close together on the same chromosome and their alleles tend to co-segregate (to pass together into each gamete). The chromosomal location of one by inference allows mapping of the other to the same chromosomal area. The first step in linkage analysis is to collect single large pedigrees or several small-sized pedigrees in which the disease of interest is segregating. This is more difficult for disorders which impair reproductive fitness. Affected and healthy family members are examined with several polymorphic *markers*, located in different chromosome regions, to either exclude or support an association with the disease.

Genetic markers

As explained in Chapter 2, genetic mapping nowadays relies almost exclusively on using as markers DNA polymorphisms of two types,

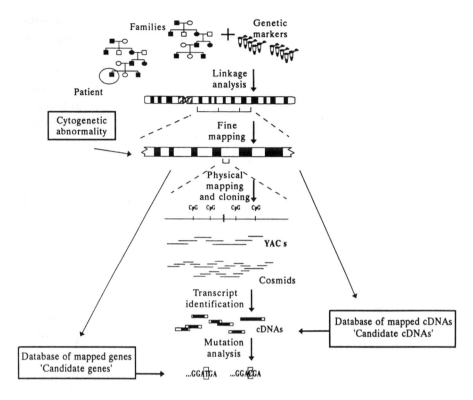

Figure 3.1 Positional cloning strategy. Starting with families and genetic markers (top), the strategy uses linkage analysis and fine mapping to establish a chromosomal location, the candidate region is cloned as a YAC or cosmid contig, transcripts originating from this region are characterised, and the disease gene identified by demonstrating mutations in affected patients. Treacher Collins syndrome (Chapter 20) is a good example of how this strategy is used.

restriction fragment length polymorphisms (RFLPs) and variable number tandem repeats (VNTRs) (see Botstein et al., 1980 for one of the original articles describing the concept of linked RFLPs).

The first DNA polymorphisms to be discovered and used were RFLPs. Bacteria make special enzymes, known as restriction enzymes, that cleave DNA molecules in a predictable manner at every occurrence of a recognition sequence, which is usually 4 or 6 bp long. Several hundred different restriction enzymes are known, each with its own recognition site – for example the enzyme *EcoRI* recognises and cuts the sequence GAATTC. RFLPs are caused by changes occurring (by chance) within a restriction site. If one person has GAATTC where another has GAAGTC, *EcoRI* would cut the DNA of one person but not the other at that point. The restriction fragments produced by cleavage will be of different length in different individuals, and so will migrate differently on gel electrophoresis. They can be observed after Southern blotting (see

Chapter 2) and hybridisation to a labelled probe that recognises just the appropriate fragment. RFLPs are inherited in a Mendelian codominant manner and can be used as markers for linkage analysis.

For genetic mapping, RFLPs have been largely superseded by VNTR polymorphisms. The human genome contains innumerable hypervariable DNA sequences consisting of variable numbers of tandem repeats of a short DNA sequence. VNTRs are consistently more polymorphic than RFLPs (many different alleles are possible, whereas an RFLP has only two alleles, corresponding to cutting or not cutting at a given site). In addition they can be demonstrated using any restriction enzyme, provided it does not cleave within the sequence of the repeat unit. Different families of VNTRs are known. Genetic mapping largely depends on microsatellites, which are di, tri, tetra or penta nucleotide repeats present in some 50 – 100,000 blocks in the human genome. The number of these repeats at any one site is often highly polymorphic between individuals, and, being inherited in a Mendelian codominant manner, can be used in linkage studies. Genetic markers defined as mapped DNA segments are designated by an abbreviation, normally the letter D (for DNA), followed by the number of the chromosome, S for single copy, and the serial number of the marker, for example D2S125 is the 125th single-copy DNA marker characterised on chromosome 2. Over 5,000 of these markers have been cloned and finely mapped to all chromosomes at intervals of about 1cM. Microsatellite analysis can be performed using automated systems and the polymerase chain reaction (PCR) technique, and this will allow the localisation of every unmapped disease locus.

These genetic markers, together with other non-polymorphic ones called STS (sequence-tagged site) markers, are also used for characterising and identifying individual DNA clones during positional cloning campaigns (Green et al., 1995).

Recombinant and non-recombinant offspring

For the sake of simplicity, we will consider the segregation in a multigenerational family of just two loci, a disease and a polymorphic marker of known chromosome position. All family members are examined to assess their disease status (affected or non-affected) and typed for the marker. Non-recombinant offspring inherit the same combination of disease and marker alleles from a parent as that parent inherited from the grandparent, while recombinant offspring inherit a different combination.

If the disease and the marker loci are on separate chromosomes, they will be found as often together as apart in the gametes, and therefore in the offspring. Recombinants and non-recombinants will be equally frequent. This is independent assortment. However, if the disease and marker loci lie on the same chromosome (that is, if they are syntenic), they will be inherited together in each offspring unless they are separated by crossing over at meiosis. Recombinant gametes for syntenic loci are the result of a crossover separating the disease and marker alleles. If the disease and marker loci lie far apart on the chromosome they are very likely to be separated; on the other hand, if they lie very close they will seldom be separated. The chance of crossing over and the proportion of recombinants decreases as the distance between the disease and maker loci decreases. The recombination fraction (Θ) is always in the range of zero (tight linkage) to 50% (independent assortment). For distant loci, on average the number of recombinants equals the number of non-recombinants and Θ is 50%, mimicking independent assortment.

On average about 52 crossovers occur per meiosis in males, and rather more in females, distributed over the 23 pairs of chromosomes. Thus chromosomal segments smaller than about one quarter of a chromosome tend to be transmitted intact through one meiotic division. A marker on the same one tenth of a chromosome as a disease might be expected to show linkage in a large multigeneration pedigree. In practice, linkage analysis involves the study of disease segregation in large pedigrees using 10 – 20 polymorphic markers from each chromosome.

Lod scores

Conceptually, linkage mapping is simple: all that is required is to scan the entire genome with a dense collection of genetic markers, calculate an appropriate linkage statistic at each position along each chromosome, and identify the regions in which the statistic shows a significant deviation from what would be expected under independent assortment. However, precise protocols and clear guidelines are needed for the interpretation of linkage results to avoid a flood of false positive claims. The mathematical interpretation of linkage analysis is complex, in particular when several physically close markers are used, as in multipoint linkage analysis.

The underlying principle involves the use of logarithms of likelihood ratios, known as lod scores or Z values. These allow the addition and cumulative analysis of results obtained in different families with the same disease. From family data showing the segregation of alleles at two possibly linked loci, a series of likelihood ratios is calculated for different values of Θ (ranging from 0 to 0.5). The likelihood ratio at a given value of Θ equals the likelihood of the observed data if the loci are linked at recombination value Θ, divided by the likelihood of the observed data if the loci are not linked ($\Theta = 0.5$). The lod score (Z) is the logarithm to the base 10 of this ratio. Lod score values of $+3.0$ or greater are considered confirmatory of linkage, corresponding to an odds ratio of 1,000:1. This may seem an over stringent threshold, but it is chosen because the prior probability of observing linkage between a randomly chosen pair of human loci is only about 1:50. Combining a

1:50 prior probability with an odds ratio of 1,000:1 gives overall odds of 20:1, corresponding to the conventional p=0.05 threshold of significance. A Z value of 4 at Θ of 0.05 means that in the pedigree(s) examined it is 10,000 (10^4) times more likely that the disease and marker loci are closely linked than unlinked.

Narrowing down the candidate region

When linkage and lod score analysis support an association, the region is then narrowed down further by examining other markers located in the relevant chromosome region. However, linkage analysis can seldom define a candidate region much smaller than several million base pairs. Therefore, for finer scale localisation of a gene a number of other techniques are used. Usually the first step is to isolate the whole of the candidate region in a series of physically mapped overlapping clones (a *contig*). The larger the clones, the fewer are required to form a contig, so large-insert vectors such as yeast artificial chromosomes (YACs, see Chapter 2, Table 2.2) are favoured for initial contig construction. Subsequent manipulations however are often best conducted using smaller clones such as cosmids. These may be obtained by subcloning the inserts of YACs.

YAC contigs are constructed by screening pre-existing publicly available YAC clone libraries to find YACs that contain markers known to map to the candidate region. Increasingly, such contigs are being defined as part of the ongoing work of the Human Genome Project, so if the investigator is lucky, he may find a ready-made contig for his region of interest. Otherwise YACs must be assembled by *chromosome walking*. This entails isolating and characterising the two ends of a YAC that maps to the region of interest, and then screening a YAC library for clones that contain these end sequences. Hopefully this will reveal one or more clones whose inserts overlap the first YAC, so giving some contiguous sequence. A further round of walking is then done by isolating the ends of the second YAC, and so on until the whole candidate region is covered in contiguous overlapping clones.

Pulsed field gel electrophoresis (PFGE) is used to establish a set of physical landmarks along individual YACs or contigs. PFGE is a variant method of gel electrophoresis that can resolve large DNA fragments, up to 2 million base pairs in size. Suitably large fragments are produced by digestion of DNA (for example a YAC insert) with special restriction enzymes whose restriction sites occur infrequently in genomic DNA (rare-cutter restriction enzymes). PFGE, combined with Southern blotting and hybridisation with suitable probes, allows reconstruction of a map of the rare-cutter restriction sites of large DNA stretches. This provides a set of landmarks that are used to identify and physically locate subclones etc.

Chromosome jumping or linking is a technique used to move in long steps across a region. Before the development of YAC cloning, chromosome walking was a desperately slow and laborious procedure, done using cosmids, and chromosome jumping sometimes allowed faster progress. For example, it was used to great advantage in the quest for the cystic fibrosis gene. Rare-cutter restriction enzymes are used to produce large starting fragments, which are then circularised. In this way segments far apart are brought together. A marker sequence capable of identifying recombinant clones is incorporated and intermediate segments are cut out with standard restriction enzymes and removed. The fragments lying far apart in the human genome, which are together in the ring, are cloned in phages and used to establish a *jumping library* of overlapping fragments.

Chromosome abnormalities associated with Mendelian diseases can be useful pointers to the exact location of a disease gene, and can short-cut a search process based on linkage analysis. They may produce a phenotype by haploinsufficiency or perhaps dominant negative effects, as explained in Chapter 2. Sometimes an apparently balanced rearrangement conceals a significant deletion, but the most valuable clues are provided by rearrangements that disrupt a relevant gene with a single clean break. DNA clones spanning the rearranged chromosome region can be isolated, a high-resolution physical map constructed, and the breakpoint exactly localised. If a gene is inactivated by the rearrangement, usually the breakpoint will lie within the gene. Sometimes, however this is not so. Expression of some genes is controlled by a locus control region, a DNA sequence that exerts an ill-understood control over transcription in an adjacent large chromosomal domain, perhaps encompassing several genes. If a rearrangement separates a target gene from its locus control region, expression may be affected even though the gene is grossly intact. Position effects can also silence intact genes by placing them near to permanently condensed (heterochromatic) chromosome regions. Thus locating a breakpoint gives a powerful clue to the location of the gene, but not an infallible direct pointer.

Chromosomal deletions are less helpful for pinpointing genes. They can be discovered using standard or high resolution cytogenetic analysis, or by fluorescent in situ hybridisation (FISH). However, cytogenetically visible deletions will remove many genes, any one of which might be responsible for any associated phenotype, so that identifying the candidate gene may not be straightforward. Deletions cause phenotypes by haploinsufficiency for deleted genes; sometimes they produce a contiguous gene syndrome, due to the combined effect of a number of physically associated genes, especially in males with X-chromosome deletions.

Identifying genes within a candidate region

The rate-limiting step in DNA mapping using these approaches is the identification of gene sequences within the target chromosome region (Collins, 1992). Several methods are available for doing this. Conceptually the simplest methods test for expression, for example by Northern blotting or cDNA selection. However, a negative result may mean just that the gene is expressed at too low a level, or in a different tissue from the ones tested. Thus methods that do not require expression of a gene in the initial phase of identification provide distinct advantages over methods that use cDNA or mRNA.

Northern blotting

As mentioned in Chapter 2, Northern blots are made by isolating mRNA from a tissue, and subjecting it to gel electrophoresis and blotting similar to Southern blotting. If a Northern blot is made using mRNA from a series of different tissues or developmental stages, it can be probed with labelled cosmid or phage clones from the chromosomal region of interest to check for the presence of an expressed sequence.

cDNA selection

Various protocols allow cDNA libraries to be screened using genomic DNA clones as probes. These methods are often more sensitive than Northern blotting but, like Northern blotting, they depend on expression of the gene at a reasonable level in the cells from which the cDNA libraries were made.

CpG island selection

This and the following methods search for features in genomic DNA that signal the presence of a gene, without any requirement that it should be expressed in any particular tissue. Normal genomic DNA of man and other mammals is relatively depleted of CpG sequences, that is, sequences where a cytosine occurs immediately upstream of a guanine. The reason for this is connected with a side-effect of an enzyme system that attaches methyl groups to such CpG sequences as part of a proof - reading control in DNA replication and repair. However, small regions of genomic DNA relatively enriched in CpG are often found near the promoters of genes. These 'CpG islands' can be detected as clusters of cleavable sites for several different rare-cutter restriction enzymes whose recognition sites contain one or more CpG sequences. Testing genomic DNA clones for CpG islands provides a rapid means for assaying large DNA stretches in a relatively short time for possible expressed sequences.

Cross-species sequence homology

This analysis ('zoo blotting') involves Southern blot hybridisation of a candidate genomic DNA fragment to genomic DNAs from a variety of species. If the candidate fragment cross-hybridises across species, class, order, or phylum boundaries, then it is likely to contain a gene, because coding sequences are much more highly conserved between species than non-coding sequences.

Exon trapping

This cloning strategy looks for splice sites, the sequences that signal the cell to cut out the introns from the primary RNA transcript of a gene (see Chapter 2). Random genomic DNA fragments are cloned into a specially designed trapping vector. This contains transcription signals and a splice donor site. The recombinant constructs are transfected into mammalian cells, which transcribe the inserts and attempt to splice the transcripts. Splicing can succeed only if the insert contains a splice acceptor site. Trapping vectors are designed so that clones whose transcripts are successfully spliced can be recognised and selected. The inserts of these clones contain splice acceptor sites, and so are likely to contain exons of genes present in the original genomic DNA.

Computer analysis of genomic DNA sequence

Comprehensive databases allow sequence comparisons to be made both between and within species. Sequence conservation may indicate the presence of an exon. Additionally, recent computational advances have enabled computers to go some way towards reading the subtle signals used by cells to recognise exons in genomic DNA. Exons contain strings of codons for aminoacids, uninterrupted by stop codons (TAA, TAG, TGA, see Chapter 2, Table 2.1), and flanked by splice sites or transcription initiation or termination signals. Computer programs like GRAIL scan genomic DNA sequences to identify potential exons. Thus one approach to identifying genes within a candidate chromosomal region is through large scale automated sequencing, followed by computerised exon searching.

Testing a candidate gene

The gene hunting process terminates when sequence analysis detects consistent mutations within a candidate gene in patients affected by the disease. *Candidate genes* are those genes that map to a chromosomal region where a single gene disorder has been located. Suspicion that a particular gene is responsible for the disease may be strengthened by knowledge that its function or tissue-specific pattern of expression is relevant to the disease process.

As transcriptional maps become more and more dense, once an initial map location for a disease is known, it is becoming increasingly possible to identify candidate genes by listing from public databases all the genes known to map to that region. In addition to defined genes, over 250,000 partial human cDNA sequences (*expressed sequences tags or ESTs*), which represent potential human genes, are deposited in various databases. Thus a *positional candidate approach* (Collins, 1995) increasingly enables the right gene to be picked for mutation testing without the need for exhaustive physical mapping and cloning.

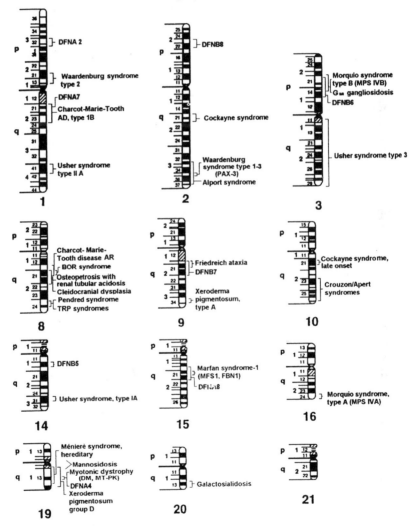

Figure 3.2 The human gene map of genetic disorders with hearing loss (October 1995). Approximate chromosomal locations are shown of genes responsible for syndromal and non-syndromal hearing loss.

Progress towards mapping and cloning hearing loss genes

The various methods of identifying human genes outlined above have been successfully applied to mapping and cloning a considerable number of hearing loss genes. Detailed mapping information is now available for about 100 of these genes (Figure 3.2).

For example, *linkage analysis* has been used to assign the Treacher Collins syndrome (TCS) locus to the long arm of chromosome 5, candidate genes identified by *exon trapping* and *cDNA selection*, and the correct gene identified by *mutation testing* (see Chapter 20). Linkage work

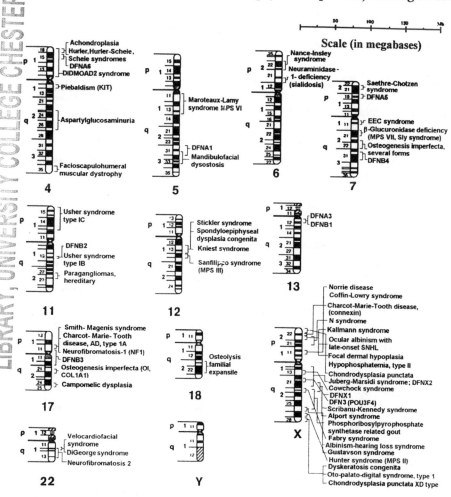

on Usher syndrome (*USH*) genes has confirmed the clinical heterogeneity and shown locus heterogeneity within clinical subtypes. At least six genes are involved in the disorder: three for USH type I (*USH1A* at 14q32, *USH1B* [myosin VII gene] at 11q13.5 and *USH1C* at 11p13-p15), two for USH type II (*USH2A* at 1q41, *USH2B* as yet unmapped), and one for USH type III (*USH3* at 3q) (see Chapter 14).

Gene hunting can be greatly helped by the serendipitous discovery of a *chromosome rearrangement* associated with a disease usually caused by a Mendelian mutation (Dallapiccola et al., 1995). A few genes responsible for syndromic hearing loss have been mapped using evidence of an association with a consistent cytogenetic anomaly. An illustrative example is the location of the branchio-oto-renal (BOR) syndrome gene to 8q21. This assignment was supported by the study of a large pedigree in which BOR and tricho-rhino-phalangeal syndrome type I were inherited together with a chromosomal inversion affecting the long arm of chromosome 8. This result was corroborated by linkage analysis in families with normal karyotype and isolated BOR syndrome, making available presymptomatic and prenatal molecular diagnosis in families at risk (see Chapter 19).

A remarkable example of *deletion mapping* is provided by DiGeorge/velo-cardio-facial syndrome (DGS/VCFS) in which del(22)(q11.21q11.23) occurs in 80 – 95% of the patients (Driscoll et al., 1992; Lindsay et al., 1995). The disorders caused by 22q11 hemizygosity, in addition to DGS and VCFS, also include conotruncal anomaly face syndrome, Opitz-Frias syndrome and isolated conotruncal cardiac defects. The main characteristics of these patients are now referred to by the acronym CATCH22, for Cardiac defect, Abnormal facies, Thymic hypoplasia, Cleft palate, Hypocalcaemia, and 22q11 deletions. However, the clinical spectrum in these patients can be wider, incorporating more than 30 features, including conductive hearing loss due to anomalies of middle ear development or secondary to frequents bouts of serous otitis media and cleft palate; sensorineural hearing loss; and small auricles with minor thickening of the helical rims (Goldberg et al., 1993). Budarf et al. (1995) (by cloning a translocation breakpoint) and Pizzuti et al. (1996) (by exon trapping) isolated a few genes from the common hemizygous region outside and within the shortest region of deletion overlap (SRO), supporting the theory that CATCH22 is a contiguous gene syndrome.

Disease gene tracking is often pursued using a combination of different approaches. The search for the gene causing X-linked progressive mixed hearing loss with perilymphatic gusher during stapes surgery (*DFN3*) is an interesting example. Although this disease is non-syndromal, in a number of patients it occurs in association with choroideraemia, mental retardation and hypogonadism. Linkage analysis mapped the *DFN3* gene to the long arm of the X chromosome, around Xq21. Some patients presenting with choroideraemia associated with complex syndromes have chromosome rearrangements at Xq21.1 (Cremers et al., 1990). Analysis of these patients allowed construction of a fine physical map of this region, from which the choroideraemia gene has been cloned; using this same map, microdeletions have been demonstrated in *DFN3* patients. The human homolog of the mouse *Brain 4* gene has been mapped to the same critical region. This gene, *POU3F4*, is deleted in a number of *DFN3* patients, indicating its causal relationship with *DFN3* (see Chapter 24).

The successful use of complementary techniques for gene mapping and cloning is also illustrated by Waardenburg syndrome (WS). Cytogenetic analysis provided the first clue to the location, when a de novo inversion of chromosome 2, inv(2)(q35;q37.3) was noted in a boy with de novo WS (Ishikiriyama et al., 1989). Linkage analysis confirmed this location (Foy et al., 1990). Further progress came via a mouse model. A few mutations associated with hypopigmentary changes were known in mice, one of which, *Splotch*, is located on mouse chromosome 1 in a region homologous to human chromosome 2q. A candidate gene, *Pax3*, was known to map in approximately the right position. Mutations were quickly identified within the *Pax3* gene in both the *Splotch* mouse and in WS type I (WS1) patients. More than forty different mutations have been identified within the human *PAX3* gene, which may account in part for the clinical variability found in different families. Finally, linkage analysis has shown that WS type II (WS2) is a genetically heterogeneous disorder. About 20% of families show linkage to 3p12-p14.1 (*MITF* gene), but other loci remain to be defined (see Chapter 16).

There are a number of hearing loss syndromes in which advances in genetic understanding are coming from mouse model studies (Brown and Steel, 1994 and Chapter 5). In addition to the *splotch* and *microphthalmia* mice, homologous to the human WS1 and WS2, an additional example is the *dominant spotting W* mouse, resulting from mutation in the gene encoding the *c-kit* growth factor receptor, which causes white spotting and hearing loss. Mutations of the homologous human *KIT* gene cause not less than 75% of forms of typical piebaldism (Ezoe et al.,1995) although not, apparently, hearing loss. An additional example is the *trembler* mouse mutant, which has abnormal auditory brainstem responses consistent with alterations of peripheral myelin, and shows mutations in the peripheral myelin protein 22 (*pmp-22*) gene. The corresponding human disease is Charcot-Marie-Tooth disease type Ia, which is usually caused by duplication of the *PMP-22* gene. Other mutations affecting the mouse auditory system are candidates for homology with human hearing loss and provide a valuable resource for comparative mapping of other human hearing loss genes.

Chapter 4
The use of gene libraries in the study of the molecular genetics of the auditory system

WILLIAM J KIMBERLING AND KIRK BEISEL

Introduction

Approximately 50% of all cases of hearing loss have a genetic aetiology. Many of the responsible genes can be localised roughly by standard linkage methods. However, the refined gene localisation that is needed to eventually clone the responsible gene will be difficult using standard approaches because of the great genetic heterogeneity in hearing loss defects. The standard process of positional cloning (see Chapter 3) first involves the localisation of a gene by family studies to as small a chromosomal segment as possible. When enough families are available, it is often possible to localise a gene to within 0.5 – 1 cM, which corresponds to about 500 to 1,000 kilobases of genetic material. This limits the search for the causative gene. However, when heterogeneity is present, localisation of a gene may not be as precise and the selection of potential genes by positional candidacy is less effective.

A second, and complementary approach, is to select candidates based on their function or pattern of tissue expression. One method used to identify candidate gene(s) based on pattern of tissue expression involves the construction of a cDNA library from the targeted organ or tissue. If one is interested in haematopoesis, then haematopoetic stem cell libraries are beneficial; retinal libraries are beneficial in vision research; the obvious organ of choice for hearing disorders is the cochlea. Identification of hearing loss genes provides a foundation for understanding the molecular mechanisms underlying inherited hearing disorders. The construction and characterisation of cochlear cDNA libraries from humans and other species provide an important resource for rapid identification of cochlear genes involved in hearing disorders (Wilcox, 1992; Ryan et al., 1993; Robertson et al., 1994).

A cochlear cDNA library will provide copies of the messenger RNA of most of the genes expressed in the cells of the cochlea. Many of these genes code for proteins that are needed by all cells in the body; these are called housekeeping genes. However, other genes code for proteins which give the organ its unique or tissue-specific properties. A cDNA library can be enriched for tissue-specific messages by subtraction hybridisation. This approach permits the enrichment of the tissue-specific genes found in the cochlea by the elimination of unwanted housekeeping genes. Selected cDNA clones from the cochlea-subtracted library can be examined individually to confirm that they are expressed only in the cochlea. Once their position in the genome is determined, they are logical candidates for any hearing loss disorders mapped to the same regions.

Subtraction cDNA libraries

Subtractive hybridisation permits the isolation of preferentially expressed mRNAs which are represented by cDNA clones, without requiring any prior knowledge about a gene or its product. Screening of cDNA libraries for rare mRNAs or mRNAs that occur in relatively low abundance (< 0.1%) is impeded by the fact that detection is dependent on abundance levels. Considering that, on average, there are $2 - 5 \times 10^5$ total mRNA transcripts present in a typical mammalian cell and probably $1 - 2 \times 10^4$ different mRNA species present per cell (Bishop et al., 1987; Lewin, 1987), there would have to be at least 100 polyadenylated transcripts per cell in order to detect a particular cDNA clone by the normal differential hybridisation procedure. Since the vast majority of tissue specific transcripts are not this abundant, a different procedure must be used to isolate these messages.

Enrichment of cDNA clones, representing mRNA expressed preferentially in certain cell types, was accomplished by subtraction hybridisation (Swaroop et al., 1991; Sive and St John, 1988; Rubenstein et al., 1990; Fargnoli et al., 1990; Brake et al., 1990). Subtraction of housekeeping genes and abundant transcripts eliminates or substantially reduces these clones from a cDNA library and enriches for tissue-specific, low abundance and rare messages. Using this approach, tissue and cell type specific cDNAs were identified for T cells (Hedrick et al., 1984), retina (Swaroop et al., 1991; Agarwal et al., 1991), cell cycle (Schneider et al., 1988), differentiation proteins (Mohn et al., 1991), tumour specific proteins (Schweinfest et al., 1990) and the cochlea (Robertson et al., 1994). Recent adaptations of the subtraction procedure using phagemid vectors and RNA labelled by biotinylation (Swaroop et al., 1991) have increased the sensitivity and efficiency of this technique and permitted use of lower amounts of mRNA. The development of strategies to make unidirectional cDNA libraries was essential to produce excess quantities of complementary biotinylated RNA by T3 RNA polymerase (Swaroop et al., 1991) to enhance the efficiency of the subtractive hybridisation step, since this approach uses single stranded recombinant phagemids.

Amplification of mRNA

Studies of the molecular genetics of the inner ear are hampered by its relative inaccessibility, by the limited numbers of cochlear and vestibular cells, and by our inability to maintain many of these cell types in long term cultures. The production of cDNA libraries from single cells or small cell populations is difficult with current conventional methods. These methods require 0.1 to 1 μg of polyA$^+$ mRNA (Gubler and Hoffman, 1983), but single cells have of the order of 0.1 to 1 ng of total RNA, only 1 – 5% of which is messenger RNA. PCR amplification of small RNA samples has been used, but suffers from error accumulation caused by infidelity of Taq polymerase during amplification, and from over representation of smaller mRNAs due to more efficient amplification of smaller templates.

A method for amplification of mRNA (van Gelder et al., 1990) was described that allows creation of a cDNA library from a single cell (Eberwine et al., 1992). The amplification of mRNA (amRNA) technique is becoming critically important to molecular studies of the inner ear, since it will free investigators from the sample constraints intrinsic to current methods. For example, amRNA should allow the construction of libraries specific to inner hair cells, outer hair cells, stria vascularis cells and afferent and efferent neurons. By overcoming the impediment of limited quantities of cochlear and vestibular tissue, it will allow characterisation of the genes expressed by specific cell types involved in hearing and balance. The amRNA technique can be combined with the patch microelectrode technique to study gene expression in individual cells important in the hearing mechanism.

Candidate genes for hearing defects

Increasingly, gene mapping studies are identifying the chromosomal locations of genes responsible for human genetic disorders in which hearing loss is observed (Leppert and Lewis, 1991). Such studies will soon be complemented by identification of candidate genes that reside within each chromosomal subregion. This is termed the positional candidate approach (Collins, 1995). Subtractive hybridisation techniques, along with the mRNA amplification techniques, can be used to develop cDNA libraries for use in identifying candidate genes for hearing loss. Suitable libraries will be specific for the target organ(s) and/or for the chromosome on which the defect gene is located. For example, the development of a cochlea/retina-specific cDNA library will be useful for the identification of the *USH1* and *USH2* genes. A chromosome 1p/cochlear cDNA library would be useful for the identification of the gene for *DFNA1*, the first dominantly inherited non-syndromal hearing loss gene to be localised.

Several rodent inner ear and cochlear cDNA libraries and a human foetal cochlear cDNA library have already been constructed (Wilcox and Fex, 1992; Ryan et al., 1993; Beisel and Kennedy, 1994; Robertson et al., 1994; Gibson et al., 1995). Human and rodent cochlea-subtracted cDNA libraries have a great significance for identifying genes controlling the development and maintenance of hearing. cDNA libraries constructed at different stages of development, and subtracted from each other, could be instrumental in identifying genes important at each stage of development of the cochlea. Libraries made from different tissues within an organ (e.g. inner versus outer hair cells) could be compared to identify genes that are needed for the differentiation of the cells into specific types. Clones from such cDNA libraries could be screened for candidate gene(s) for many different hearing loss disorders, such as Usher syndrome types Ia, Ic and IIa, Lawrence-Moon-Biedel syndrome, and others. In addition, these libraries have the potential of fostering the identification of other proteins unique to the cochlea and will contribute to the identification, characterisation, and functional analyses of these cochlea-specific proteins.

Once the candidate gene for a given type of hearing loss is cloned and decoded, the structure of its protein product can be determined. This will provide insights into the biochemical function of the gene product in normal cochlear tissue, and will show why the genetic mutations result in hearing loss. The validity of this approach is exemplified by the identification of the α-rhodopsin protein in dominant retinitis pigmentosa (Dryja, 1990), the dystrophin protein in Duchenne muscular dystrophy (Rowland, 1988), the cystic fibrosis transmembrane conductance regulator protein in cystic fibrosis (Rommens et al., 1989), the zinc finger protein in development of Wilms' tumour (Haber et al., 1990) and most recently by the identification of myosin VIIa in Usher type IB (Gibson et al., 1995; Weil et al. (1995). These discoveries have all led to a better understanding of their respective mechanisms of pathogenesis.

Useful gene libraries need not be solely of human origin; a murine cDNA library is of equal importance. From such a library, the murine equivalent of the human cochlear genes and their gene products can be identified. Alteration of the expression and/or structure of these proteins by site directed mutagenesis of the coding sequences will allow the structure-function relationship to be studied. In addition, through the use of homologous recombination and transgenic technology, *in vivo* mouse models of inner ear genetic disorders can be created.

Chapter 5
Mouse models for human hearing impairment

STEPHEN DM BROWN and KAREN P STEEL

Mouse genetics and the mouse gene map

The mouse is a pivotal organism in the study of mammalian genetics and biology (Brown, 1994). Outside of man, the mouse is the best characterised mammalian organism genetically. In addition, the mouse has long been employed as a tool for the dissection of numerous biochemical and physiological processes and developmental pathways. For these reasons, the mouse currently occupies a unique place as a model organism for improving our understanding of human disease processes and, in particular, human genetic disease (Brown, 1994). This is no less true for the study of the genetics of hearing impairment. The purpose of this chapter is to illustrate how work on mouse hearing loss mutations has contributed, and can contribute in the future, to the identification of genes underlying human genetic hearing loss and to the molecular dissection of auditory transduction mechanisms.

Mouse genetics and the mouse gene map – comparisons with human

The Human Genome Project has as its goal the determination of the complete sequence of the human genome and allied with that the localisation and determination of all the DNA sequences coding for the full gamut of genes. At the same time, a number of genomes of so-called model organisms are the focus of similar programmes. An extensive programme of work is under way to map the mouse genome (Brown, 1994) and to identify the bulk of coding sequences. Over 10,000 DNA markers have been mapped across the mouse genome (see for example Copeland et al., 1993; Dietrich et al., 1994). Many of these are gene sequences that are conserved between species, including genes conserved between mouse and human.

The availability of comparative maps of conserved coding sequences between mouse and human has a number of powerful uses that have been an important aid in the identification of mouse models for the study of human genetic disease (Copeland et al., 1993). Comparison of the genetic maps of mouse and human has identified a large number of regions between the mouse and human genomes in which gene content and gene order are conserved – the so-called conserved linkage groups or conserved ordered segments. The density of the comparative gene maps in mouse and human suggests that the bulk of these conserved linkage groups have now been identified (Copeland et al., 1993). Conserved linkage groups allow us to identify mutations mapped in the mouse that may be directly homologous to mutations mapped in man, and thus may represent new mouse models for human genetic disease (see also below). In addition, the availability of conserved linkage groups allows us to identify genes mapped in the mouse that may be candidates for human disease mutations, or alternatively, genes mapped in man that may be putative candidates for mouse mutations. Moreover, the availability of particularly rapid and powerful genetic techniques in the mouse for the localisation and identification of the genes underlying mouse mutations (Brown, 1994; Gibson et al., 1995, and see below) means that if a mouse mutation is identified as being a likely homologue for a human genetic disease, then it may prove easier to clone the relevant gene via the mouse. All these considerations dictate that for any biological system, the mouse represents a powerful experimental model for human disease processes – including the comparative analysis of mouse and human hearing loss mutations (Brown and Steel, 1994).

Mouse hearing impairment – mouse hearing loss mutations

Recent catalogues of mouse mutations (Lyon et al., 1995; Steel, 1995) document over 100 genes having effects on the inner ear, either on its development or its function. Mouse mutations causing hearing impairment demonstrate a range of pathologies similar to that catalogued in humans. As in the human, mouse mutations can be divided into the following three main classes according to the nature of the underlying pathology (Steel and Brown, 1994).

1. Morphogenetic abnormalities. Morphogenetic abnormalities correspond to, for example, Mondoni and Michel abnormalities in humans. Morphogenetic abnormalitites represent malformations of the labyrinth arising through defects in its proper development. Mouse mutations showing a morphogenetic abnormality of the inner ear might be classed as a syndromal hearing loss if the mutation were to be present in the human population. Examples of mouse mutations that fall into this category are given in Table 5.1.

Table 5.1 A summary of Morphogenetic, Cochleosaccular and Neuroepithelial defects in which the mouse and human hearing loss mutations have been confirmed as homologous and where the underlying gene has been identified.

Locus/Disease	Gene	Protein	Mutant Phenotype
A: Morphogenetic Defects			
Sp, splotch	*Pax3*	Paired box transcription factor	Homozygotes – inner ear malformation, prenatal lethal
	PAX3	Paired box transcription factor	1 homozygote reported – white skin and deaf
Xt, extra toes	*Gli3*	Zinc finger transcription factor	Homozygotes – inner ear malformation; prenatal lethal; hearing not studied in heterozygote
Grieg cephalopolysyndactyly syndrome (GCPS)	*GLI3*	Zinc finger transcription factor	No homozygotes reported. Heterozygotes (Grieg syndrome) – no hearing loss
B: Cochleosaccular Abnormalities			
W, dominant spotting	*kit*	Protein tyrosine kinase receptor	Homozygotes – white spotting and deafness; Heterozygotes – white spotting, no deafness
Piebald trait	*KIT*	Protein tyrosine kinase receptor	1 homozygote reported – white spotting and deafness; Heterozygote – piebald trait – white spotting and no deafness
mi, microphthalmia	*mi*	bHLH-ZIP transcription factor	Homozygotes – white spotting and deafness. Heterozygotes – white spotting and deafnes s in some alleles
Waardenburg syndrome type II, WS2	*MITF*	bHLH-ZIP transcription factor	No homozygotes reported. Heterozygotes – WS2 – white spotting and deafness
Sp, splotch	*Pax3*	Paired box transcription factor	Homozygotes (see above). Heterozygotes – white spotting, NO deafness
Waardenburg syndrome type I, WS1	*PAX3*	Paired box transcription factor	Homozygote (see above). Heterozygotes – WS1 – white spotting and deafness
C: Neuroepithelial Abnormalities			
sh1, shaker-1	*my7*	Myosin type VII	Deafness, vestibular dysfunction, NO retinitis pigmentosa
Usher type IB	*USH1B*	Myosin type VII	Deafness, vestibular dysfunction, retinitis pigmentosa

2. Cochleosaccular defects. Cochleosaccular defects represent a class of hearing impairment arising from disturbances in the stria vascularis, and are usually associated with pigmentation defects. The stria vascularis is responsible for maintaining the ionic composition of the endolymph within the cochlea. Melanocytes are known to populate the stria vascularis and are thought to play a role in its function (Steel et al., 1992) – hence the often-observed link between hearing impairment and pigmentation defects in many mammals. A number of cochleosaccular defects have been identified in both human and mouse. Some examples of mouse mutations demonstrating cochleosaccular abnormalities are provided in Table 5.1. The cochleosaccular abnormalities, in which the genetic basis is understood, are classified as syndromal hearing loss because of the association with pigmentation defects.

3. Neuroepithelial defects. A primary defect of the sensory neuroepithelia – including the organ of Corti – will lead to uncomplicated hearing loss or non-syndromal hearing loss. Indeed, non-syndromal hearing loss, the bulk demonstrating autosomal recessive inheritance, accounts for most of the genetic hearing loss in the human population – around two thirds (Fraser, 1976). As with the other classes of hearing impairment, mouse models for neuroepithelial genetic hearing loss have also been identified. Many of the mouse mutations demonstrating neuroepithelial type hearing loss may also exhibit shaker-waltzer type behaviour characterised by hyperactivity, head tossing and circling (Steel, 1991). However, these are presumed to result from associated vestibular abnormalities affecting balance and, indeed, it is recognised that many deaf individuals have vestibular dysfunction although they show no overt balance problems.

Comparative studies in mouse and man of morphogenetic and cochleosaccular defects are well developed. As indicated above, a number of mouse mutations have been identified in each class which are powerful models for the study of the developmental and epithelial inner ear lesions involved and, in a number of instances, the underlying genes have been identified (see Table 5.1). Nevertheless, until recently, nothing was known of the genes underlying the third and largest class of mutations – the neuroepithelial defects. Although autosomal recessive nonsyndromal hearing loss represents by far the biggest class of inherited hearing loss, little progress had been made in mapping the underlying genes. It is known that a large number of genetic loci are responsible for this class of hearing loss and this makes their mapping and ultimately their isolation difficult – although in the past two years, making particular use of isolated, inbred families, a number of loci have been mapped (see Table 5.2).

Table 5.2 A summary of recessive and dominant non-syndromal hearing loss loci that have been mapped to date in humans, along with their known map locations.

Locus	Chromosome Assignment	Mouse Chromosome Location/Homologous Mouse Locus	Reference
DFNA1	5q31	11 (27-30); 18 (29-35)	Leon et al., 1992
DFNA2	1p32	4 (48-53)	Coucke et al., 1994
DFNA3	13q12	5 (89-92)	Chaib et al., 1994
DFNA4	19q13	7 (2-23) - qv (**15**), quivering?; 9 (5-7); 10 (62)	Chen et al., 1995
DFNA5	7p15	6 (22-26); 13 (10)	van Camp et al., 1995
DFNA6	4p16.3	5 (19-41) - tlt (28), tilted?	Lesperance et al., 1995
DFNA7	1q21-23	1 (85-99)	Tranebjaerg et al., 1995
DFNA8	15q1	2 (64-67); 7 (28-29) - twt (28), twister?	Kirschhofer et al., 1995
DFNA9	14q12-q13	12 (27); 14 (19-21)	Manolis et al., 1996
DFNA10	6q22-q23	10 (6-27)	O'Neil et al., 1996
DFNB1	13q12	5 (89-92)	Guilford et al., 1994
DFNB2	11q13.5	7 (48) - sb1 (48), shaker-1?	Guilford et al., 1994
DFNB3	17p11.2-q12	11 (33-46) - sh2 (32/33), shaker-2?	Friedman et al., 1995
DFNB4	7q31	6 (6-7)	Baldwin et al., 1995
DFNB5	14q12	14 (19-21)	Fukushima et al., 1995
DFNB6	3p14-p21	9 (59-71) - sr (64), spinner?; 14 (2,8); 6 (42)	Fukushima et al., 1995
DFNB7	9q13-q21	19 (12-18) - dn, deafness?; 13 (22)	Jain, 1995
DFNB8	21q22.3	16 (69-70)	Veske et al., 1996
DFNB9	2p22-p23	12 (0-4); 17 (44-49)	Cahib et al., 1995
DFNB10	10q21-q22	10 (27-34) - v (28), waltzer?; Jc (30), jackson circler?; av (34), Ames waltzer?	C. Petit (pers. comm.)

The Table indicates the possible chromosomal locations of homologous mouse genes taking into account the known conserved linkage groups between man and mouse (see main text) – the figures in parentheses indicate the likely position on the relevant mouse chromosome. In some cases potential homologous mouse mutations lie in the identified regions and these are listed, though any homology they may have to the mapped human mutations is purely speculative and based only at this stage on homologous map position.

Until very recently, no genes underlying neuroepithelial-type hearing loss had been identified in any mammal. However, the availability of a large number of mouse mutations carrying neuroepithelial defects has had a profound impact on our progress towards identifying neuroepithelial genes. It is pertinent therefore first to consider the use of comparative models for morphogenetic and cochleosaccular abnormalities and the underlying genes involved, and then subsequently to consider how the use of mouse models for neuroepithelial-type hearing loss is beginning to uncover the genes determining the primary auditory transduction pathways in the neuroepithelia in the organ of Corti.

Mouse and human mutations for syndromal type hearing loss

Morphogenetic and cochleosaccular abnormalities

A number of homologous mutations have been identified in man and mouse that lead to either morphogenetic or cochleosaccular abnormalities. Those examples of morphogenetic and cochleosaccular abnormalities in which the mouse and human mutations have been confirmed as homologous and the underlying gene identified are listed in Table 5.1. For a more comprehensive listing and treatment of morphogenetic or cochleosaccular abnormalities in either human or mouse, along with the underlying gene identified, the reader is referred to Steel and Brown (1994). In many cases, a mouse homologue for the human mutation (or vice versa – a human homologue for the mouse mutation) has not yet been confirmed or identified.

Amongst the morphogenetic defects, the most notable findings include the identification of the mouse *Splotch* (*Sp*) mutation as a homologue for Waardenburg syndrome type I (WS1) (Epstein et al., 1991; Foy et al., 1990; Tassabehji et al., 1992; see Chapter 16). *Sp* heterozygotes have a white belly-spot of variable size, whilst homozygotes have severe neural tube defects and inner ear malformations. WS1 heterozygotes demonstrate developmental abnormalities associated with neural crest defects and often show hearing impairment. For some time, the map positions of *Sp* and WS1 had suggested that they might be homologous mutations (Foy et al., 1990), a conclusion that was supported by the fact that both showed pigmentary disturbances. This was confirmed when the *Pax3* gene was shown to encode *Sp* in mice (Epstein et al., 1991), and shortly afterwards the human homologue *PAX3* (or *HuP2*) was shown to be mutated in WS1 (Tassabehji et al., 1992; Baldwin et al., 1992). The pigmentary disturbances arise from defects in melanocyte migration and survival, which presumably result in strial dysfunction leading to the hearing loss observed in WS1. For this reason, WS1 and *Splotch* might be classed as both morphogenetic and cochleosaccular in origin (see Table 5.1). However, bizarrely, in *Sp* heterozygotes there is little evidence of hearing impairment (Steel and Smith, 1992.). Moreover in the single unambiguously documented case of a WS1 homozygote, unexpectedly mild defects were reported, with no neural tube defect (Zlotogora et al., 1995). It is important to note that, apart from dystopia canthorum, no feature of WS1 is fully penetrant and observed in every patient. It may be that genetic background effects have an important role to play in the development of hearing impairment arising from *Pax3* mutations.

A number of cochleosaccular mutations are well characterised in the mouse where spotting and hearing loss are associated. Genes underlying three mouse cochleosaccular abnormalities have been identified, and in two of these cases mutations have been identified in the homologous human gene (see Table 5.1). The mouse *dominant spotting* mutation, *W*, is encoded by *c-kit*, a growth factor receptor (Chabot et al., 1988) while the *Steel* mutation, *Sl*, is encoded by its ligand (Geissler et al., 1988). *Microphthalmia* (*mi*) encodes a novel transcription factor (Hodgkinson et al., 1993). The mouse *W* mutation is homologous to Piebald trait in humans, which is also encoded by *KIT*, a growth factor receptor and the homologous gene to *c-kit* in the mouse.

Perhaps the most interesting examples of homologous cochleosaccular abnormalities in mouse and human are the *mi* and Waardenburg syndrome type II (WS2) loci. Their study represents another example of the usefulness of mouse models in aiding the identification of genes underlying human hearing impairment (see Chapter 16). Both *mi* and WS2 show pigmentary disturbances associated with hearing loss. Following the identification of the gene encoding a transcription factor underlying the *mi* mutation, the homologous human microphthalmia gene (*MITF*) was shown to map to human chromosome 3p (Tachibana et al., 1994). Subsequently, it was found that some WS2 families carried mutations that mapped to this chromosome (Hughes et al., 1994; Tassabehji et al., 1995). Screening of a large number of WS2 families has shown that the *MITF* gene is involved in about 20% of families with WS2 (Tassabehji et al., 1995). However, it is clear that there are other genes involved.

Finally, it is worth noting that a number of syndromes are recognised in both human and mouse in which hearing loss often develops as an inconsistent or late onset feature. For many of these syndromes, the gene has been identified and the reader is referred to Steel and Brown (1994) for a more detailed discussion of this area. Although this particular area has not benefited to any great extent from the use of mouse models as an aid to gene identification, the availability of these mouse models for late onset hearing loss, along with the knowledge of the identity of the underlying genes, is likely to prove pivotal in understanding the genes and genetic interactions involved with the polygenic nature of much of the late onset hearing loss in the human population.

Neuroepithelial abnormalities

As discussed above, the bulk of genetic hearing loss in the human population can be accounted for by defects in genes affecting the neuro-epithelia of the inner ear and leading to autosomal recessive non-syndromal hearing loss. A much smaller proportion of non-syndromal hearing loss can be accounted for by dominant mutations. A large number of genes are involved with both recessive and dominant non-syndromal hearing loss, and this has confounded the mapping and identification of the loci involved. However, a number of loci have been mapped to date and are summarised in Table 5.2.

Most loci have been localised by mapping studies in a single large extended family in which a single mutation can be assumed to be segregating. Nevertheless, there are clearly limitations to the mapping power of an individual family, however large, and it may not be feasible to employ standard strategies of positional cloning, i.e. it may not be possible using the available family resources to localise the mutation to a sufficiently small region of a chromosome in order to have a realistic chance of identifying the underlying gene. For these reasons, until recently, no gene had been identified for a non-syndromal hearing loss locus. Clearly, identifying genes involved with the neuroepithelia of the inner ear provides a powerful route for identifying the critical pathways involved with auditory transduction. The use of a mouse model was an important route towards the cloning of the first gene for neuroepithelial hearing loss and a first step towards defining the structure of the primary neuroepithelial auditory transduction pathway.

The mouse shaker-1 mutation

Mice homozygous for the recessive *shaker-1* (*sh1*) mutation show typical neuroepithelial-type defects involving dysfunction and degeneration of the organ of Corti (Steel and Harvey, 1992) along with the shaker-waltzer type behaviour that is so typical of many mouse deaf mutants and results from vestibular defects. This mutation thus represents an excellent model for non-syndromal hearing loss in the human population. In order to identify the gene encoding the *sh1* mutation, a positional cloning strategy was employed. The strategy took particular advantage of the fact that large numbers of mice can be bred segregating the hearing loss mutation of interest, allowing as a first step the genetic localisation of the mutation to a very small chromosomal region (see Figure 5.1).

*Localising the mouse shaker-1 mutation on mouse chromosome 7
and mapping its human homologue*

The *sh1* mutation was already known to map to mouse chromosome 7 in the vicinity of the β-globin (*Hbb*) and tyrosinase (*Tyr*) loci. Over 1,000 mouse progeny were derived from a back-cross segregating the *sh1* mutation, and analysed for DNA markers from this region of chromosome 7 (Brown et al., 1992). One marker – the Olfactory marker protein (*Omp*) gene was demonstrated to be very closely linked to the *sh1* mutation (Brown et al., 1992) and acted as a start point for the construction of a physical map in the region of the *sh1* mutation (see below and Figure 5.1). The physical map would provide access to all of the genes in that region and allow us to isolate and assess potential candidate genes for *sh1*.

At the same time, the Olfactory marker protein gene was mapped in man. Given the close linkage of *Omp* to *sh1*, the map position of the

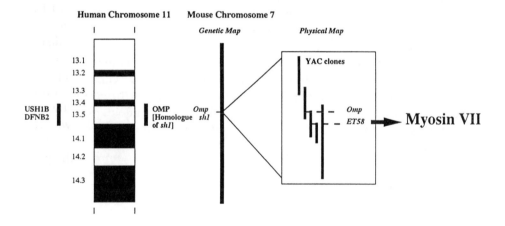

Figure 5.1 Positional cloning of the mouse *shaker-1* (*sh1*) hearing loss gene. *sh1* was shown genetically to lie very close to the *Omp* gene on mouse chromosome 7. The *Omp* gene was used as a start point to generate a physical map of overlapping YAC clones - a YAC contig - that encompassed the *sh1* locus. A variety of methods were used to identify potential candidate genes for *sh1* within the YAC contig. Exon trapping (see Gibson et al., 1995) identified an exon (ET58) from an unconventional myosin gene, a myosin VII, that was subsequently shown to encode *sh1*. *OMP* in the human genome was shown to map to 11q13.5 (Evans et al., 1993). Around the same time, it was shown that the *USH1B* and *DFNB2* loci mapped to the same region, indicating that either or both of these mutant loci represented potential homologues to the mouse *sh1* gene. It was subsequently confirmed (Weil et al., 1995) that *USH1B* is also encoded by the myosin VII gene that underlies *sh1*.

human homologue (*OMP*) would be likely to identify the map position of the human hearing loss gene homologous to *sh1*. *OMP* in man mapped to 11q13 (Evans et al., 1993), and in the vicinity of one of three loci underlying Usher syndrome type I – the Usher type IB locus, *USH1B* (Kimberling et al., 1992). Usher syndrome type I is a deaf-blind syndrome demonstrating severe congenital hearing impairment, vestibular defects and a slowly progressive retinitis pigmentosa (see Chapter 14). In addition, a locus for autosomal recessive non-syndromal hearing loss (*DFNB2*) also maps to 11q13 (Guilford et al., 1994; see chapter 21).

A physical map encompassing the mouse shaker-1 locus – identifying the mouse shaker-1 gene

The *Omp* gene was used to construct an overlapping array (or contig) of YAC (yeast artificial chromosome) clones encompassing 1.5 Mb of mouse DNA around the *sh1* locus (Gibson et al., 1995). Analysis of these clones by a variety of techniques allowed the identification of a number of different genes from this region. One gene (*ET58* – see Figure 5.1) that encoded a myosin-like protein was expressed in the inner ear and was pursued further. The gene was shown to code for a myosin VII – a poorly characterised class of myosins whose function was unknown. Confirmation that this was indeed the *shaker-1* gene was helped by the availability of seven different *shaker-1* mutant alleles (Gibson et al., 1995). Analysis of the available coding sequence from the motor head region of the myosin molecule in all seven mutant alleles uncovered mutations for three of the alleles, confirming that the myosin VII was indeed the *sh1* gene.

Myosin VII and Usher type IB

Myosin VII was subsequently examined as a potential candidate for Usher type IB. Screening of a number of Usher type IB families identified several mutations in the head region coding sequence of human myosin VII, confirming that Usher type IB was encoded by the same gene that leads to the *shaker-1* phenotype in the mouse (Weil et al., 1995). It is still unknown whether the myosin VII encodes the *DFNB2* mutation which maps to the same region as *USH1B* (see above and Figure 5.1). Resolution of this point awaits the complete characterisation of the very large myosin VII coding sequence.

The function of myosin VII in the neuroepithelium of the inner ear

The identification of the first neuroepithelial hearing loss gene represents an important step towards a better molecular picture of hair cell function. Nevertheless, for the moment the function of myosin VII in the inner ear remains enigmatic. However, progress is rapid. It is now known that myosin VII expression in the inner ear is confined to the sensory hair cells in the organ of Corti and in the vestibule (Steel and Brown, unpublished data). In addition, the aberrant development of stereocilia on the surface of hair cells in some of the *sh1* mutants suggests that one function of the myosin VII is in stereocilia development. However, the normal development of stereocilia in one *sh1* mutant suggests that myosin VII has additional functions within hair cells.

Myosin VII is also expressed in the retina in both mouse and human (Weil et al., 1995) and this observation presumably underlies the progressive retinitis pigmentosa that develops in Usher type I. However, *sh1* mice never appear to develop any retinopathy, even when older (KP Steel, unpublished data), and the reasons for the differing phenotypes between mouse and human resulting from similar mutations in the homologous gene remain to be clearly established.

Conclusions

The mouse has proved a valuable model in the identification of genes for both syndromal and non-syndromal hearing loss. Indeed, the use of a mouse model – the *shaker-1* mutant – has led to the identification of the first gene for neuroepithelial-type hearing loss. It is likely that the many other mouse mutants of the shaker-waltzer type that demonstrate neuroepithelial defects and are currently under study will reveal their causative genes before long. It is to be hoped that these studies will provide a fuller picture of the critical proteins involved in hair cell development and function and the auditory transduction pathway. It is also likely that many of the identified genes will be found to underlie autosomal recessive and dominant non-syndromal hearing loss in the human population.

Chapter 6
Gene linkage in genetic hearing loss: Where are we now?

COR WRJ CREMERS[1]

Introduction

Research into hereditary hearing loss began in the second half of the nineteenth century with studies by William Wilde (1853) in Dublin, Uchermann (1869) in Oslo and Arthur Hartmann (1880) in Berlin. The concept of heredity as a cause of hearing impairment came to be accepted in the last quarter of the nineteenth century. In his textbook on otology, Politzer (1882) stated 'The most frequent causes of congenital hearing loss are: heredity, including the direct transmission from the parents as well as the indirect transmission from forefathers and marriage between blood relations ....' Mendel's Laws (1865) did not become widely known until the beginning of the twentieth century.

Background

The first reports of a number of fairly common hereditary syndromes with hearing loss as one of the characteristic symptoms appeared in the second half of the nineteenth century. The German ophthalmologist Albrecht von Graefe in Berlin (1858) was the first to describe the occurrence of retinitis pigmentosa and congenital hearing loss in three affected brothers. This autosomally recessively inherited Usher syndrome, named after the ophthalmologist Charles Usher from Aberdeen, proved later to be the most frequent genetic cause of combined hearing loss and blindness. Mandibulofacial dysostosis, or Treacher Collins syndrome, was described for the first time, incompletely, by Thomson in 1846, and later by Berry in 1889 and by Edward Treacher Collins in

[1]Edited by CWRJ Cremers, and based on a review by Cremers, Brown, Steel, Brunner, Reed and Kimberling (1995), with permission of the publishers.

1900. The first complete and extensive report of this syndrome was published in 1949 by Adolphe Franceschetti and David Klein from Geneva. The description of the branchio-oto-renal syndrome, initially based on a case report by Heusinger in 1864, was subsequently reported by James Paget in two generations of a family (1878).

In the first half of the twentieth century, studies on the causes of hearing loss continued on a large scale and several impressively large isolates were published in detail, demonstrating autosomal recessive hereditary hearing loss. Knowledge of the syndromal and non-syndromal forms of hereditary hearing loss has greatly increased over the last fifty years. During this period the first overviews appeared of the many and ever increasing number of hereditary syndromes (nowadays about 350) with hearing loss as one of the symptoms. Attention was given to the degree of penetrance of the syndrome and the degree of expression of the separate symptoms.

Where we are now

In the field of human genetics we are no longer satisfied simply to show that a certain disease is inherited and in an autosomal or sex-linked recessive or dominant pattern. We want to know the gene product of the mutated gene, and the mechanism by which it causes the pathological syndrome. Possible preventive and/or therapeutic approaches depend very much on knowledge of the gene products (Waelsch, 1991). In this last quarter of the twentieth century, we have seen a world-wide effort to identify and sequence, or read, the code of the human genome which is the complete set of instructions or genes for a human. Already many hereditary diseases with hearing loss as a feature have been mapped and, in some cases, the genes identified (Table 6.1).

In the application of linkage analysis and other tools of modern genetics to hearing loss, the main obstacle to progress has been the fact that different genetic conditions result in identical clinical findings in patients with non-syndromal hearing loss. This explains why no gene linkage for any of these types of congenital hearing loss was found until 1994. In the modern industrialised world a third of cases of children with congenital hearing loss are caused by recessive genes. Now isolates with non-syndromal congenital hearing loss are being studied using the most recent genetic markers and the first genes are starting to be mapped. Recently Guilford et al. (1994) showed linkage to chromosomes 13 and 11 for a non-syndromal congenital hearing loss in a Tunisian isolate.

To progress from the genetic localisation on a given chromosome to the identification of the defective gene still requires a major effort. Cloning genes for hearing loss, including non-syndromal autosomal recessive hearing loss, is a more feasible goal in mice because numbers

Table 6.1 Chromosomal location of genes causing inherited diseases with hearing loss.

A: Autosomal Dominant	Linkage	MIM#	Gene cloned	References
Neurofibromatosis type I	17q	162200	+	Wallace et al., 1990
Neurofibromatosis type II	22q	101000	+	Rouleau et al., 1993
Branchio-oto-renal syndrome	8q	113650	-	Kumar et al.,1992
				Smith et al., 1992
Stickler syndrome	12q	120140	+	Knowlton et al., 1989
Stickler syndrome	6p	108300	+	Brunner et al., 1994
Crouzon syndrome	10q25-26	123500	+	Reardon et al., 1994
Saethre-Chotzen	7p	101400	-	Rose et al., 1994
Osteogenesis imperfecta	17q	120150	+	McKusick, 1992
Osteogenesis imperfecta	7q	120160	+	McKusick, 1992
Treacher Collins syndrome	5q31.3-32	154500	-	Dixon et al., 1994
Facioscapulohumeral muscular dystrophy	4q	158900	-	Wijmenga et al., 1992
Piebald trait	4q	172800	+	Spritz et al, 1993
Rieger syndrome	4q	180500	-	Shiang et al., 1987
Waardenburg syndrome type I	2q3-7	193500	+	Foy et al., 1990
Waardenburg syndrome type II	3p12-14		+	Hughes et al., 1994
Waardenburg syndrome type IV (Hirschsprung)	13q22	277580	-	Puffenberger et al., 1994 van Camp et al., 1994
Non syndromal:				
DFNA1	5q31	124900	-	Leon et al., 1992
DFNA2	1p32	124800	-	Coucke et al., 1994
DFNA3	13q12			Chaib et al., 1994
DFNA4	19q13			Chen et al., 1995
DFNA5	7p15			van Camp et al., 1995
DFNA6	4p16.3		-	Lesperance et al., 1995
DFNA7	1q21-23			Tranjeberg et al., 1995
DFNA8	15q15-21			Kirschofer et al., 1995
DFNA9	14q12-13			Manolis et al., 1996
DFNA10	6q22-23			O'Neil et al., 1996

B: Autosomal Recessive				
Hurler syndrome	4p	252800	+	Scott et al., 1990
Usher syndrome type IA	14q32	276900	-	Kaplan et al., 1991
Usher syndrome type IB	11q14		+	Kimberling et al., 1992
Usher syndrome type IC	11p14-15			Smith et al, 1992
Usher syndrome type IIA	1q41	276901	-	Kimberling et al., 1990
Usher syndrome type III	3q		-	Sankila et al., 1994
Wolfram (didmoad) syndrome	4q	222300	-	Polymeropoulos et al., 1994
Alport syndrome	2q	203780	+	Mochizuki et al., 1994
Thyroid hormone resistance and deaf-mutism*	3q		+	Takeda et al., 1992

Table 6.1 Contd.

	Linkage	MIM#	Gene cloned	References
Non syndromal:				
DFNB1	13q12	220700	-	Guilford et al., 1994a
DFNB2	11q13.5	220800	-	Guilford et al., 1994b
DFNB3	17p11.2		-	Friedman et al., 1995
DFNB4	7q31			Baldwin et al., 1995
DFNB5	14q12			Fukushima et al., 1995a
DFNB6	.3p21-14			Fukushima et al., 1995b
DFNB7	.9q13-21			Jain et al., 1995
DFNB8	2p22-23			Chaib et al., 1995
C: X-linked				
Albinism-hearing loss syndrome	Xq26.3-27	300700	-	Shiloh et al., 1990
Alport syndrome	Xq21-22	303630	+	Barker et al., 1990
Hearing loss, conductive, with stapes fixation (and stapes gusher)	Xq21	304400	+	Brunner et al., 1988 Cremers, 1989
Encephalopathy-hearing loss-blindness-mental retardation	Xq22	304700	-	Tranebjaerg, 1994
Hunter syndrome	Xq27-28	309900	+	Le Guern et al., 1990
Norrie disease	Xp11-3	310600	+	Berger et al., 1992 Chen et al., 1992
Otopalatodigital syndrome type I	Xq28	311300	-	Biancalana et al., 1991
Pelizaeus-Merzbacher disease	Xq	312080	+	Raskind et al., 1991

*Hearing loss is only a feature in autosomal recessive GRTH, in which the *while* gene is deleted, and is not seen in autosomal dominant GRTH.

of back-crosses can be arranged which would give a high density of recombination break points around the gene of interest. There is an abundance of mouse mutants available and many are either known to affect the inner ear or have been identified as candidate genes for hearing loss. The similarities between the features of hereditary hearing loss in humans and mice suggest that mice are likely to be useful for understanding human hereditary hearing loss. The mouse *shaker-1* (*sh1*) is one of those important genetic models for autosomal recessive non-syndromal genetic hearing loss in the human population, because it shares several features with the human Usher syndrome.

Several forms of autosomal dominantly inherited hearing loss genes have been localised by linkage analysis. Examples include Waardenburg syndrome type I (2q35), Treacher Collins syndrome (5q32-q33.2) branchio-oto-renal syndrome (8q) and a non-syndromal progressive hearing loss (5q31). Linkage analysis for autosomal dominant inherited traits requires a collection of families in which the transmission of the disease gene can be correlated with the transmission of a genetic marker on at least 10 occasions, preferably 20 – 30. These should preferably be all in one family, but for well-defined syndromes several families can be combined. Up to 200 different markers may have to be tested in order to find linkage. It is highly desirable to define a candidate region rather than search the entire genome.

Candidate regions may be defined by homologies with mapped mouse genes or through rare individuals who show the syndrome in conjunction with a chromosomal abnormality. Linkage analysis may define a candidate region of 10 million base pairs of DNA. Identifying the actual gene often depends on knowing a candidate gene or finding chromosomal abnormalities such as translocation or small deletion in an affected person. A good example of the use of biochemical information in the process of disease gene identification is Alport syndrome, an X-linked dominant (sometimes autosomal recessively inherited) nephropathy with progressive sensorineural hearing loss. Biochemical evidence implicated type IV collagen, which is expressed in basement membranes of the eye, kidney and inner ear. When the gene encoding the fifth chain of type IV collagen was assigned to Xq22 this provided researchers with a logical candidate gene. The detection of mutations in the *Col4A5* gene in Alport syndrome patients duly confirmed this hypothesis. The association of a collagen abnormality with a high tone progressive sensorineural hearing loss may be more widespread than originally realised. Defects in collagen type I are seen in type I osteogenesis imperfecta, defects in collagen type II in Stickler syndrome and defects in type IV collagen in a variant of Stickler syndrome. Each of these syndromes also has a high frequency sensorineural component to their hearing loss.

Compared with X-linked and autosomal dominant disorders, autosomal recessive inherited disorders are difficult subjects for analysis. Usher syndrome is an autosomal recessive disorder and the cause of most cases of genetically determined combined hearing loss and blindness. Phenotypically at least two types of Usher syndrome can be distinguished: type I associated with a profound hearing loss and absent vestibular responses, and type II with a mild sloping to profound hearing loss and normal vestibular responses. Type III shows normal vestibular responses and a progressive sensorineural hearing loss. At least six different genes have been implicated through linkage analysis in Usher syndrome. Three loci have been identified for type I (IA on 14q32, IB on

11q13, IC on 11p13 and one unlinked to these regions) and two loci for type II (IIA on 1q32, IIB unlinked). Type III has been linked to 3q (Sankila et al., 1995). Type IB and IIA are the most common. Another type I gene is believed to be unlinked to any of these regions.

The identification and analysis of mouse and human mutants for hearing loss are expected to improve our understanding of the normal function of the gene product, of how that function is affected by the mutation and of how anomalies in the affected cell types influence auditory function and structure. Studies of genetic hearing loss in the wider context of the human genome project will thus provide important new knowledge for understanding the physiology of hearing and the pathophysiology of hearing loss.

Part II
Audiology

Chapter 7
Epidemiology of genetic hearing impairment

Background

During the second half of the nineteenth century concepts of heredity were introduced into the field of hearing disorders, and in the last quarter of the nineteenth century heredity was accepted as a cause of hearing impairment (for historical reviews see: Stephens, 1985; Ruben, 1991; Reardon, 1992). Since then substantial knowledge has been accumulated on genetic and phenotypic heterogeneity and the various modes of transmission of the numerous mutant genes involved in genetic hearing impairment. This knowledge has resulted in several systems of classification, such as: according to age at onset and/or site of lesion and/or often subdividing genetic hearing impairment into disorders without (i.e. non-syndromal) and with (syndromal) additional clinical manifestations of the mutant gene in question (see e.g. Fraser, 1976; Königsmark and Gorlin, 1976; McKusick, 1992; Jacobson, 1995; Cohen and Gorlin, 1995).

The last few decades have seen a rapid development of knowledge within the field of genetics concerning the structure and function of chromosomes, resulting in the localisation and isolation of several thousand genes causing diseases, including some involving the auditory system (see e.g. Annas and Elias, 1992; Smith, 1995). With the continuous mapping and future completion of the human genome project the scientific community may be provided with an invaluable resource for the diagnosis and prevention of almost any genetic disease (Cox et al., 1994). This may also account for very rare human diseases, which are often characterised by complex traits, for which highly polymorphic gene markers have resulted in both mapping and positional cloning of the genes (Lander and Schork, 1994; Davis et al., 1995). New techniques for the tracking of disease genes and their expression also seem promising for the future amelioration and prevention of genetic hearing impairment (Ryan et al., 1993; Althous, 1994; Rosenthal, 1994; Smith, 1995).

This contribution on the epidemiology of genetic hearing impairment will concentrate mainly on figures in childhood and describe some of the difficulties in obtaining appropriate epidemiological data, arising from lack of uniform clinical terminology and criteria for inherited hearing impairment. In adult populations the information on the prevalence of genetic hearing impairment is scarce, mainly due to the lack of large scale epidemiological studies within the framework of medical services, and thus the section on inherited hearing impairment in adults will be brief.

Permanent hearing impairment in childhood

Overall the prevalence of permanent hearing impairment in childhood is low – depending on the age and gender of the targeted childhood population, the audiometric criteria used, the age at onset, and the classification – according to site of lesion – of the hearing impairment (Davidson et al., 1988; Davis and Wood, 1992; Mauk, 1993; Parving, 1993a). There is also considerable variability in the sources of the data, which are often based on clinical samples poorly defined from an epidemiological perspective (Morton, 1991; Parving, 1995). Thus the estimated prevalence of permanent hearing impairment in childhood varies considerably, ranging from 0.5 – 4.2/1,000 according to Davidson et al. (1988), which can be attributed to true differences in the prevalence between countries, and to a lack of uniform definitions and criteria. Some appropriate prevalence estimates have been obtained from identical birth cohorts (1983 – 88) from England and Denmark, estimating the prevalence of bilateral hearing impairment of sensorineural or mixed type $\geq$ 40 dB for the average across the audiometric frequencies 0.5 – 4 kHz. Based on the combined data an estimated prevalence of 127 per 100,000 (CI:113 – 143/100,000) was found, with no significant differences between countries. However, significant differences in the severity of the hearing impairment were found, the proportion of children with severe to profound hearing impairment being significantly higher in Denmark than in England in the birth cohorts studied.

Although a direct comparison between the two countries concerning the factors causing the permanent hearing impairment could not be addressed, significantly more children in Denmark had a family history of hearing impairment, whereas significantly more children in England had passed through neonatal intensive care units. This may imply that genetic hearing impairment is more prevalent in Denmark than in England, at least within the local areas evaluated (Davis and Parving, 1994).

Genetic factors causing permanent hearing impairment

In numerous surveys throughout the world, the proportion of genetic causes of hearing impairment in childhood varies from 9 – 54%, as shown in Table 7.1. In the survey performed in 1977 on 2,988 subjects living in the member countries of the European Community and born in 1969, genetic factors accounted for 9% of the hearing impairment. Although the survey was limited according to geography and birth cohort, and the criterion for hearing level strictly defined (i.e. ≥ 50 dB

Table 7.1 Extent of genetic causes of hearing loss.

	Birth Cohort	N	HL (dB)	G %	Unknown cause %
Martin et al., 1981 (EU)	1969	2 988	≥ 50	9	42
Kankkunen, 1982 (Sweden)	1970 – 79	179	≥ 50	42	16
Newton, 1985 (England)	1977 – 80	111	≥ 25	30	39
Parving, 1988 (Denmark)	1970 – 80	138	≥ 25	48	17
Upfold, 1988 (Australia)	not defined	1 158	≥ 25	19	42
Hirsch, 1988 (Sweden)	1976 – 80	251	≥ 50	45	35
Lenzi and Zaghis, 1988 (Italy)	not defined	1 568	severe/profound	25	32
van Rijn, 1989 (Holland)	1960 – 75	162	≥ 35	40	34
Dias and Andrea, 1990 (Portugal)	not defined	1,024	severe/profound	20	27
Arnos et al., 1992 (USA)	not defined	659	deaf	54	33
Parving, 1993(b) (Denmark)	1980 – 90	181	≥ 25	46	20
Vanniasegeram et al., 1993 (England)	not defined	101	≥ 50	40	29
Liu et al., 1993 (China)	not defined	236	deaf	43	20
France and Stephens, 1995 (Wales)	1975 – 79	90	≥ 50	50	31

The table shows data from published surveys, indicating the birth cohorts (when defined), size of the sample (N), the hearing level (dB), the proportion of genetic hearing impairment (G), and the proportion of unknown cause.

in the better hearing ear, averaged across the audiometric frequencies of 500, 1,000, and 2,000 Hz), a high proportion of 42% of unknown causes of the hearing impairment favours the argument of a true higher proportion of inherited hearing impairment. This is supported by more recent European studies, demonstrating a higher proportion of genetic hearing impairment and somewhat lower proportion of unknown causes (Table 7.1). The wide range in the inclusion criteria, definition of samples, age of the children (some including adults) and the definition of hearing level between the studies does not allow a direct comparative analysis, nor is it possible to aggregate data in order to obtain more valid figures on the prevalence of inherited hearing impairment. However, it may be anticipated that the proportion of inherited hearing impairment is substantially higher, considering that the proportion with unknown causes of the permanent hearing impairment varies from 16 – 42% in the subjects studied.

It is likely that the wide variation in the proportion of genetic hearing impairment reflects true differences in the genetic expression within the various target populations, and some support for a true variation in the prevalence of genetic hearing impairment was found by Davis and Parving (1994). However, some preliminary data comparing the proportion of genetic hearing impairment in two identically defined birth cohorts from 1975 – 79 living in Wales and Denmark, respectively, demonstrated both a similar prevalence of permanent hearing impairment and an identical proportion of inherited hearing impairment comprising 51 – 52% in the two samples (Parving et al., 1996).

Mode of transmission

It has been noted that the most common forms of genetic hearing impairment are the autosomal recessive forms accounting for about 80% of cases, autosomal dominant forms accounting for about 15%, and X-linked inheritance for 2 – 3% of cases (Fraser, 1976; Rose et al., 1977; Newton, 1985; Morton, 1991). In addition to the classical Mendelian traits (monogenic inheritance), abnormalities on both the autosomal and X-linked chromosomes may result in hearing impairment (chromosomal inheritance) (Liu et al., 1993; Diefendorf et al., 1995; Cohen and Gorlin, 1995), and evidence for the role of mitochondrial inheritance and mitochondrially determined pre-disposition to hearing impairment inducing environmental agents is increasing (Gold and Rapin, 1994; Reardon and Harding, 1995; Strasnick and Jacobson, 1995).

From the clinical perspective the estimated proportions of the Mendelian traits seem difficult to confirm. Thus a proportion ranging from 13 – 45% of hereditary hearing impairment could be ascribed to recessive inheritance, whereas a proportion of 7 – 44% could be ascribed to dominant traits and 1 – 5% to X-linked inheritance (Ruben and Rozycki, 1971; Newton, 1985, van Rijn and Cremers, 1991; Morton,

1991; Parving, 1993b). A Chinese study has indicated a proportion of 92% of recessive inherited hearing impairment, whereas only 5% was caused by dominant traits. Genetic hearing impairment in cases with mitochondrial and polygenic inheritance has been reported, but understanding of the epidemiology in different populations concerning these modes of transmitting mutant genes is unknown.

The previously estimated frequencies of the transmission mode of the genes causing hearing impairment may be fairly close to the truth, despite the lack of documentation from the clinical field. The lack of a firm relationship between the audiometric configuration and the mode of transmission presents a major problem in the clinical field, as does the lack of sensitive methods for revealing a carrier state in recessive inheritance. Although it has been claimed that dominantly inherited hearing impairment is milder than recessive (van Rijn and Cremers, 1991; Liu and Xu, 1994) the finding has been contradicted in other samples (Parving, 1993b). Thus, for the clinician, not only does the unknown group of hearing impairment represent a major diagnostic challenge, but also the mode of transmission presents a problem. It can be anticipated that at least some recessive and incompletely penetrant dominantly inherited hearing impairment can be identified if the clinical audiological methods are improved, and in combination with linkage analysis and gene mapping such a development will have implications for genetic counselling (Coucke et al., 1994; Cohen and Gorlin, 1995).

Non-syndromal/syndromal genetic hearing impairment

Although many different genetic syndromes affecting hearing sensitivity have been described (Fraser, 1976; Konigsmark and Gorlin, 1976; Gorlin et al., 1990), the overall prevalence of syndromal genetic hearing impairment is very low. The few estimates on the prevalence of specific syndromes, such as shown in Table 7.2 (see also other chapters in this book), have been based on limited numbers of subjects, and the wide range in estimates may reflect both true variations between populations in the prevalence of the specific syndromes and also differences in diagnostic criteria, clinical activity and the systematic approach used when performing aetiological evaluation.

Table 7.2 Estimated population prevalences for some more common genetic syndromes with hearing loss.

Syndrome	N/100,000
Branchio-oto-renal	2.5
Mandibulofacial dysostosis	1.0 – 2.5
Pendred	0.8 – 7.5
Usher	2.5 – 4.5

(from Marres et al., 1995; Gorlin et al., 1995)

It has been noted that syndromal inherited hearing impairment accounts for more than ⅓ of all hereditary hearing impairment (Konigsmark and Gorlin, 1976; Gorlin et al., 1990). Although a valid estimate of the prevalence of syndromal genetic hearing impairment does not exist, some information on the proportion can be obtained from previous ascertainment studies, as shown in Table 7.3. The proportion of syndromal genetic hearing impairment among the children recognised as having inherited hearing impairment varies from 6 – 30%. It is, however, likely that these figures represent an underestimate due to unrecognised syndromes, as the ages of many of the children in the samples do not permit sophisticated aetiological evaluation due to lack of co-operation in various examination procedures. Thus in a cohort of children with permanent hearing impairment born 1980 – 90, of the 46% (N = 84/181) categorised as having a genetic aetiology at the time of data collection (January, 1992), only 5% had recognised syndromes, which is significantly lower than the 24% found in an identically defined birth cohort from 1970 – 80 within the same area. Although the proportion of non-syndromal and syndromal genetic hearing impairment may have changed, it is likely that more syndromes will be recognised in the clinic with increasing age of the sample.

Table 7.3 The proportion of non-syndromal/syndromal genetic hearing impairment in some studies.

	van Rijn and Cremers (1991)	Newton (1985)	Parving (1988)	Arnos et al. (1992)	France and Stephens (1995)
	N = 64/162	N = 33/111	N = 66/138	N = 353/659	N = 45/90
Overall heredity	40%	30%	48%	54%	50%
Non-syndromal	78%	94%	76%	70%	76%
Syndromal	22%	6%	24%	30%	24%

Some social and longitudinal aspects

Throughout the history of genetic hearing impairment, it has been learned that prelingual hearing loss affects both marriage and reproduction rates, and that marriages between deaf persons are frequent (Ruben, 1991; Christiansen, 1991; Dolnick, 1993). The historical surveys, however, include only profoundly hearing-impaired individuals, and limit the interpretation from an epidemiological perspective.

It has been shown that a higher prevalence rate of 2.6/1,000 of profound hearing impairment is present in Asian children compared with the prevalence rate of 0.7/1,000 in non-Asian children, and that 68% of Asian mothers attending a maternity unit gave a history of marriages between cousins (Lumb, 1981). An epidemiological study demonstrated a prevalence of hearing impairment among consanguineous marriages of 12.9/1,000, whereas the prevalence in non-consanguineous marriages in the same area was 3.1/1,000 (Al Shihabi, 1994). Thus it can be stated that the prevalence of inherited hearing impairment depends on both the social-cultural practice and the genotypic expression in the target population, and that the increasing heterogeneity within many populations arising from an extensive global exchange of people may result in national and even local changes in the prevalence of permanent hearing impairment. This assumption is supported by a significant increase from 35% to 46% in genetic factors causing hearing impairment in a longitudinal study based on two 10-year birth cohorts (Parving, 1993b). Other birth cohorts living in the same area also demonstrated an increase in the proportion of children with inherited hearing impairment from 20% to 37% (Parving and Christensen, 1995), and in the school for the deaf a change from 29% to 43% in inherited hearing impairment over 40 years has been found (Parving and Hauch, 1994). The documented increase in the proportion of recognised genetic hearing impairment in these cohorts may reflect a concomitant increase from 5.1% to 8.6% in the proportion of immigrants in the local area with different ethnic and religious backgrounds, where marriages between relatives are frequent (Københavns Statistiske Årbog, 1975; 1993). Conversely, data from Israel showed a decline in the prevalence of childhood hearing loss, which could be ascribed to a decline in the rate of consanguineous marriages, most evident within those of non-Ashkenazi ethnic origin (Feinmesser et al., 1990). These changes in genetic hearing impairment found within local areas may be in part ascribed to improved diagnostic evaluation, but also emphasise the need for continuous local epidemiological studies.

Epidemiology of genetic hearing impairment

The proportions of children with genetic hearing impairment indicated in the literature should always be considered as underestimates, and it can be argued that valid epidemiological data on the prevalence of genetic hearing impairment in childhood do not exist. An estimate of 50 per 100,000 of genetic hearing impairment has been suggested, which is somewhat lower than the prevalence of 88 per 100,000 reported in the first decade of life in an age-matched population-based study (Parving, 1993b). Although the implementation of appropriate protocols aimed towards aetiological evaluation has been useful (Parving, 1984; France and Stephens, 1995), genetic hearing impairment may remain unrecognised due to poor specificity and low sensitivity of clinical methods for revealing carriers of genes causing permanent hearing impairment (Anderson and Wedenberg, 1968; Parving, 1978; Parving and Schwartz, 1991; Meredith, 1991). Lack of interest in the aetiology or lack of co-operation from patients and relatives in families in which genetic hearing impairment is suspected, and in addition ignorance among professionals and non-professionals about factors causing permanent hearing impairment, reflect the problems facing the clinician when ascertaining the aetiology of hearing impairment in children.

Genetic hearing impairment in adults

Recent population-based surveys on hearing have reported an overall prevalence of 15 – 20% of hearing impairment (i.e. > 25 dB HL for the average across 0.5 – 4 kHz in the better ear) with an increasing prevalence as a function of increasing age affecting approximately 50% of the population by age 80 (Davis, 1989, 1994; Pedersen, 1990; Parving et al., 1983, 1993).

Although these surveys offer important epidemiological information concerning prevalence figures as a function of age, gender, hearing level, and social class, only limited figures on the factors causing the hearing impairment have been reported. Thus virtually no epidemiological information exists on the prevalence of genetic hearing impairment in adult populations. However, genetically determined hearing impairment may develop at any age throughout life, either as the sole manifestation of the mutant gene such as in otosclerosis – affecting 5 – 10% of the adult population – and in inherited low-frequency hearing loss, or as part of an inherited syndrome, such as e.g. in neurofibromatosis, Alport, Ahlström, and Refsum disorders (Reardon, 1992; Jacobson, 1995). In addition, genetic factors – both karyotic and mitochondrial – interact with exogenous factors, such as noise, ototoxic drugs and middle ear infections, resulting in a higher susceptibility to these environmental factors. Thus maternally transmitted non-syndromal hearing impairment has been described in families with susceptibility to aminoglycoside ototoxicity caused by a mutation in the mitochondrial DNA (Prezant et al., 1993; Hutchin and Cortopassi, 1995), and pigmentation as a factor affecting the susceptibility to noise has been discussed for many years (review: see Borg et al., 1995).

Major similarities between genetic hearing impairment in humans and mice have been described (Steel, 1991), and valuable information has been obtained also from other animal studies on the degenerative processes developing in the auditory system as a function of age. The role of genetic factors in the development of age-related hearing loss in humans is not yet known. However, it is likely that the rapid development of molecular genetics based on appropriate animal models will clarify this matter.

Conclusions

As the prevalence of permanent hearing impairment in childhood is low – and hearing impairment caused by genetic factors even rarer – national and international collaboration within the framework of health services may provide more appropriate information on the epidemiology of genetic hearing impairment, when based on well-defined target population studies and protocols including an interdisciplinary approach.

In order to aggregate data on the epidemiology of genetic hearing impairment throughout life, protocols based on uniform terminology, description and criteria (Parving and Newton, 1995) for the diagnosis of genetic hearing impairment should be implemented, and the specificity and sensitivity of current and new audiometric methods for the recognition of a genetic carrier state should be evaluated.

Chapter 8
The audiological approach to genetic hearing impairment in children

EDOARDO ARSLAN and EVA ORZAN

Introduction

Epidemiologically, at least one third of all hearing losses are of genetic origin; moreover, about one half of children with profound hearing loss have an inherited type of hearing loss. According to Gorlin et al. (1995) there are over 400 types of genetic hearing loss, amongst which 22 are recognised as being transmitted without any accompanying symptoms, the rest being syndromal. In such a context, an accurate clinical assessment in paediatric audiology should always consider a genetic aetiology. The number of genetic causes already delineated offers a possibility of aetiological diagnosis and, consequently, better patient care. Associated organ anomalies in syndromal hearing loss, together with progression of the hearing loss, can have a considerable effect on the treatment and rehabilitative programmes.

The family of an affected child will ultimately benefit from accurate assessment and counselling. Clear information, upon which they may base the often difficult process of acceptance of the hearing loss, will help in psychological terms, especially when it helps to eliminate the fear of a more serious underlying cause. The possibility of a progressive hearing loss and other organ involvement will furthermore, not come as a surprise.

At the present time the correct paediatric audiological evaluation should comprise a flexible but targeted protocol. This starts with the definition of the sensory deficit, the auditory threshold and the clinical features. It is the baseline with which subsequent evaluation can be compared, particularly when monitoring the stability of the hearing impairment. An audiological evaluation can be considered complete only when accurate and reliable responses from 250 to 8000 Hz for each ear have been obtained (Table 8.1).

Table 8.1 Clinical description of hearing loss (after Parving and Newton, 1994).

Severity	• Normal: ≤ 20 dB for better ear hearing level
	• Mild: 21 – 40 dB
	• Moderate: 41 – 60 dB
	• Moderately severe: 61 – 80 dB
	• Severe: 81 – 100 dB
	• Profound/deaf: > 100 dB
Age of onset	• Congenital
	• Early onset, i.e. 1st decade
	• Onset 2nd to 5th decade
	• Late onset, 5th+ decade
Type of hearing loss	• Conductive
	• Sensorineural, i.e. cochlear-retrocochlear
	• Mixed sensorineural and conductive
Frequencies involved	• Low frequencies: i.e. 250, 500 Hz
	• Mid frequencies: i.e. 1,000, 2,000 Hz
	• High frequencies: i.e. 3,000, 4,000, 6,000, 8,000 Hz
	• All frequencies: 250 – 8,000 Hz
Configuration of audiogram	• U-shaped/saucer i.e. ≥ 15 dB difference between the better hearing thresholds and the poorer hearing threshold(s)
	• Low frequencies i.e. ≥ 15 dB from the better to the poorer hearing threshold at the low frequencies to the mid frequencies
	• Flat i.e. <15 dB difference from 250 – 8,000 Hz
	• Sloping i.e. >15 dB between 1,000 and 4,000 Hz
	• None of the above configurations
Unilateral/bilateral involvement	• Right/left ear
	• Symmetrical/asymmetrical (i.e. ≤ 10 dB difference between ears in at least 2 frequencies)
Steady/progressive	• Progressive: i.e. >15 dB HL in at least 2
	• frequencies or >10 dB HL for average of 4 frequencies (e.g. 0.5 – 4 kHz)

While the audiogram is not the only, or even the best, predictor of outcome, an early and accurate auditory assessment of an infant's hearing allows intervention plans to be formulated and initiated. This leads to the most important paediatric audiological activity, which aims to obtain functional information about the child's use of his/her hearing. The assessment should comprise a quick definition of the auditory response, a prompt and optimal correction of the sensory deficit across the speech frequency range, the constant use of the amplification device together with frequent monitoring of the effects of the intervention strategy. Every step should furthermore meet the physiological stages of child development.

Due to the diagnostic urgency and the age of the patient, it is necessary to choose the simplest strategy which will give the desired and quickest response. The clinician should therefore have a good knowledge of current procedures (see Appendix and Table 8.2) and their efficiency. A battery of tests, with cross-checking of test results, is important for the confirmation of hearing levels. Consistency across the procedures must be monitored. Corroboration of results should finally be sought using information gained from the case history, parental comments, observation of behaviour, otoscopy and imaging of middle and inner ear structures.

Table 8.2 Stimuli and dB reference levels in different threshold measurement techniques.

Threshold Measurement Technique	Evoking Stimuli	dB Measurement
ABR	Click (headphone)	dB nHL or dB pe SPL
ECochG	Click (loudspeaker)	dB nHL or dB pe SPL
VRA	Warble tone narrow band noise (loudspeaker)	dB SPL dB nHL
Play Audiometry	Pure tone (insert earphone, headphone, air conduction stimulator)	dB HL

Measurement of auditory sensitivity

During the first few months of life it is difficult to implement any formal behavioural test technique to obtain information regarding thresholds. *Behavioural hearing tests* for assessment of hearing sensitivity at this age are therefore generally qualitative and not quantitative, based on skilled observation of changes in the baby's behaviour in response to auditory stimulation. More sophisticated and reliable responses such as localisation responses can be expected to develop in normal infants by six months of age. Formal test procedures available from this age, such as distraction tests (McCormick, 1993) or visual reinforced audiometry (VRA – Bamford and McSporran, 1993) generally give information in a sound field setting with the sound delivered by loudspeakers. Frequency-specific signals can and should be used and most clinicians use electronically generated signals such as narrow band noise or warble tones to control and specify the relevant stimulus parameters (intensity and frequency). The most obvious limitations of sound-field audiometry are the impossibility of obtaining thresholds from each ear separately and of obtaining bone-conduction thresholds. Another drawback can also be the failure to obtain responses from young children who have severe or profound hearing losses, because of the output limitation when the sound is presented over loudspeakers. Typical audiometers generally provide a maximum output of about 100 dB HL for mid-high frequencies (1,000 – 4,000 Hz) at 1 m from the loudspeaker.

The testing of young children can be a difficult and challenging task, requiring experience and skill in child handling and interaction. Small children can require long periods of conditioning before giving accurate and repeatable responses: serial evaluations are often important to confirm and extend the initial impression. Moreover, behavioural techniques cannot be applied reliably in children with mental and physical disabilities. Interpretation of test results should take into account the fact that progressive improvement in behavioural response sensitivity is observed as a function of increasing age in the first year of life (Northern and Downs, 1991). This has not been closely examined in hearing impaired children and it is therefore not correct to think in terms of threshold, in the normal sense of the term used for pure tone audiometry, before 12 to 18 months of age and before several assessments.

At around 12 – 18 months of age, the child should be able to understand simple verbal instructions permitting more informative responses through play audiometry. The technique may be employed in a sound field condition, with insert earphones, headphones or bone conduction vibrator. Air and bone conduction thresholds may, therefore, be obtained giving ear-specific air and bone conduction assessments.

It is unlikely that future methods will completely replace the need for behavioural tests because of the wealth of information they provide about the child's actual use of their hearing (McCormick, 1994). This functional aspect makes behavioural responses invaluable in audiological management and monitoring hearing aid effectiveness. As hearing threshold descriptors, they gain more value after the first year of developmental age, when behavioural procedures can lead to the estimation of ear-specific sensitivity threshold across the whole frequency range.

Objective techniques for measuring auditory sensitivity are the *auditory evoked responses*, classified in terms of the latency at which the response occurs after the auditory stimulus: early, middle or late responses. Because of the influence of sleep condition, sedation and anaesthesia on middle and late responses, the more reliable methods for auditory assessment of children are the auditory brainstem responses (ABR) and electrocochleography (ECochG). Typical examples of ECochG and ABR in Figure 8.1 show the principal features and differences between the recordings. Both techniques give very stable and highly repeatable ear-specific responses regardless of a child's age (Weber, 1982) and show good agreement with psychoacoustical thresholds at the test frequencies (Hyde et al., 1990; Arslan, Conti and Prosser, 1986). ECochG is limited by the need for an intratympanic electrode and consequent general anaesthesia of the child. The ABR technique has, therefore, come to have a leading role in the assessment of children's hearing.

Objective techniques are highly useful clinical procedures when behavioural audiometry is not suitable or when the results of such testing are inconclusive (Weber, 1994). Comparing the two electrophysiological techniques, ABR represents the test of choice, giving high accuracy and permitting outpatient testing. It is, none the less, important to note that there are rare but important situations in which ABR gives unreliable results. After excluding recognisable errors such as those due to the child moving or due to muscle activity artefacts, the most important factor which can influence ABR findings is disrupted central neural activity. Immature central auditory pathways or a lesion of the neural structures of the brainstem can influence the generation of this response, altering its main parameters or abolishing it altogether (Garruba et al., 1991; Kraus et al., 1984; Lenardt, 1981). Even if rare, this mechanism can sometimes lead to serious errors in audiometric evaluation and inappropriate hearing aid fitting (Arslan et al., 1995).

In cases with suspected central nervous system pathology, the ECochG recording is a valuable test for use after ABR to confirm a diagnosis, since it permits evaluation of peripheral auditory function uninfluenced by the anatomical and functional conditions of the brainstem (Arslan et al., 1986).

A significant limitation of both ABR and ECochG techniques is the limited range of stimuli that can be used to elicit the responses, requiring transient stimuli with poor frequency specificity and with the energy concentrated at high frequencies. Thus, ABR and ECochG testing with click stimuli provides information only about peripheral hearing status in the upper portion of the speech range (2,000 – 4,000 Hz). The most serious clinical error in paediatric hearing aid fitting is, in fact, to overestimate the hearing loss severity when based on the ABR results alone. Efforts to develop an effective evoked potential technique such as ABR or ECochG with more frequency-specific stimulation (e.g. tone-burst, click-masking techniques) to obtain information about low frequencies has not yet led to good practical solutions compatible with the needs of brevity and simplicity of testing. Distortion product otoacoustic emissions at low frequencies are probably the most promising future technique in this context. At the present time sensitive behavioural hearing tests should be performed as soon as the child is capable of responding reliably.

Techniques for definition of the nature of the hearing loss

The latency-intensity function shape for wave V in the ABR and the AP in ECochG can provide information as to the localisation and configuration

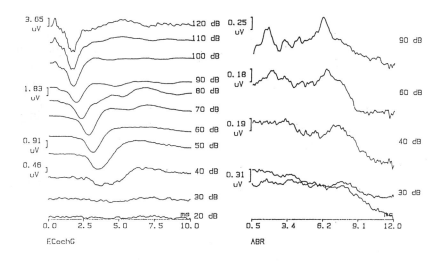

Figure 8.1 The compound action potential (AP) is a high amplitude and easily recognisable response which makes any repetition of the stimulation unnecessary for its validation, even at threshold level. The ABR is much weaker with a less favourable S/N ratio; the presence of wave V must be validated by its repetition in subsequent traces. The threshold values are given by the lowest trace on which the AP and wave V appear.

of the hearing loss. The effect of conductive hearing loss on the ABR waveform is to prolong the latencies of all components, including wave V. The effect of cochlear hearing loss is rather more complex, and can be summarised as an invariance of wave V latency with stimulus intensity. Fortunately, retrocochlear pathology, associated with an unpredictable waveform picture, is rare in children.

Otoadmittance has a considerable diagnostic potential in exploring the middle ear function in children. The amount of information to be gained from otoscopy alone is, in fact, dependent on the skill and experience of the clinician. Behavioural audiological tests provide information about air conduction thresholds only. Comparison of air and bone conduction thresholds in conventional pure tone audiometry provides only inferential information about the state of the middle ear and the origin of conductive hearing loss. All of these methods are, furthermore, subjective. Tympanometry and middle ear measurement provide, however, a rapid method for obtaining objective information about the pathological state of the middle ear such as the presence of fluid in the middle ear, the integrity of the ossicular chain and Eustachian tube function. The accurate application of admittance measurement in the test battery approach (Table 8.3) can provide meaningful information on the nature of the hearing loss and assistance in diagnosing the site of the auditory lesion.

Table 8.3 Audiometric and admittance measurements in paediatric audiological assessment.

Threshold Level (dB HL)	Tympanogram Type (Jerger 1970)	Contralateral Acoustic Reflex	Ipsilateral Acoustic Reflex	Hearing Loss Type	Further Diagnostic Procedure
0 – 20	A	Normal	Normal	Normal	Stop
20 – 40	B/C	Absent/increased threshold	Absent	Conductive hearing loss (OME)	Stop
20 – 40	A	Absent/increased threshold	Absent	Conductive hearing loss (tympanossicular pathology)	Stop
> 40	A	Normal/increased threshold/ absent	Normal/increased threshold/ absent	Sensorineural loss	Stop
> 40	B/C	Increased threshold/ absent	Absent	Mixed hearing loss	Repeat tests after therapy

Threshold levels are referred to behavioural or auditory evoked potential measurement (after Maurizi et al., 1992).

Because of its objective nature, the measurement of otoadmittance at the tympanic membrane can be most valuable in the assessment of young children, but does have some diagnostic limitations: there are poor correlations between tympanometry and the actual condition of the middle ear below the age of 7 months (Keith, 1973). In small children, body and head movement and hyperactivity may lead to movement of the probe, causing misleading peaks on the tympanogram or making it impossible to maintain an airtight seal with the probe tip.

Diagnosis of middle ear disease can, in conclusion, rarely be made on the basis of tympanometry alone. The test has a high sensitivity but it is not uncommon to see abnormal patterns in normal ears, so resulting in poor specificity (van Camp et al., 1986). The converse may also occur (Muchnik et al., 1989). The value of tympanometry lies in its objective nature, its ease of performance and its confirmation of other measures as part of a clinical battery (Table 8.3).

New techniques

There is now agreement that *otoacoustic emissions* (OAEs) are the result of a cochlear mechanical response to acoustical stimulation and therefore have the potential to provide an indirect but non-invasive objective measure of active cochlear mechanical function. Given a healthy middle ear, OAEs appear to be almost always present if the threshold is better than 20 dB HL and almost always absent if the threshold is worse than about 50 dB HL. This technique does not provide sufficient information to predict audiometric thresholds. At the present time the most promising application of OAEs is for hearing screening in infants and difficult to test patients (Norton, 1994). There is general agreement that the presence of OAEs effectively predicts the presence of normal cochlear function. The presence of either transient evoked oto-acoustic emissions (TEOAEs) or distortion product otoacoustic emissions (DPOAEs) indicates normal cochlear status or, at worst, mild hearing loss at the frequencies comprising the evoking stimulus (Balkany et al., 1994).

More than any other diagnostic auditory test, OAEs are sensitive to peripheral pathologies affecting the external and middle ears (Lonsbury-Martin et al., 1994). Thus it is important to accurately rule out the presence of a middle ear disorder before OAE results can be interpreted. The greatest potential of OAEs, after screening, can be found in their use to confirm pathology of cochlear origin and provide information on cochlear status, and as part of a diagnostic test battery. The particular cellular pathology cannot yet be differentiated by currently available OAE measures.

It is unlikely that OAE measures will replace traditional audiometry (Gorga et al., 1994) but they should be viewed as additional, objective, non-invasive audiological tools of potential clinical value. Many questions remain to be answered regarding measurement and interpretation, but the use of OAEs has been advocated as a potential tool in screening peripheral auditory system dysfunction in babies and difficult to test patients; separating the cochlear and neural components of sensorineural hearing loss; monitoring the effects of cochleotoxic agents and assessing fluctuant hearing loss (Lonsbury-Martin et al., 1995).

Progression of hearing loss

Genetic disorders are among the most likely causes of hearing loss to result in a progressive increase in thresholds. A progressive hearing loss is not easy to detect in infancy. Clinical observations are unreliable in small children and a variation of the hearing threshold can also be a reflection of behavioural, methodological and even instrument bias. At least three conditions should be met before expressing a reasonable suspicion of progression:

1. The presence of any conductive component should be excluded using tympanometry.

2. The threshold comparison should be made utilising the same audiometric technique.
3. The threshold should show > 15 dB shift for at least two frequencies
   or > 10 dB HL for an average of four frequencies (e.g. 0.5 – 4 kHz).

Because of their high variability, behavioural techniques are not the
best techniques to assess the stability of the hearing loss. Responses
should always be supported by observation of the child's behaviour. It
is important to observe the progression in the three frequency zones
(low, middle and high) of the audiogram and thus reduce some measurement variability. Objective threshold techniques, such as ABR, give
better reliability despite their other limitations.

Conclusions

An effort must be made to use uniform terminology and description of
hearing loss in order to facilitate delineation of specific genetic disorders and assure better patient care (Parving and Newton, 1994).
Children require special clinical experience and skill in their management. A good knowledge of current audiological procedures is necessary and their efficacy in assessing different aspects of a genetic hearing
loss should be well understood. Finally, particular attention should be
given to the frequent association with physical, mental and sensory
deficits. The selection of appropriate audiological techniques and cross
checking of test results is particularly important.

Appendix: current instrumental procedures available in paediatric audiology

Behavioural hearing tests aim to record the quietest level at which the
child consistently responds to a specific acoustic stimulus. The choice of
the appropriate response and consequently the formal test technique
(distraction test, visual response audiometry, play audiometry) is based
on the developmental rather than on the chronological age of the child.

Auditory brainstem response (ABR) is the electrical activity evoked in
the cochlear nerve and brainstem pathways recorded by far-field surface
electrodes. It comprises five or more waves which occur within 10 ms of
a click or a brief tone-burst stimulus. The presence of ABR waves and the
measurement of their latency and amplitude provide information on
hearing sensitivity and integrity of brainstem auditory pathway.

Electrocochleography (ECochG) refers to the method of measuring the
stimulus-related electrophysiological potentials of the most peripheral

portions of the auditory system, the cochlea and the cochlear nerve. ECochG picks up the signal by means of a needle electrode resting on the promontory and therefore has to be performed in children under general anaesthesia. The stimulus-related electrical potentials recorded are the cochlear microphonic (CM), the summating potential (SP) and the compound action potential (AP).

Otoadmittance provides a measure of the efficiency of the middle ear system in receiving and transmitting sound energy. Measurements that commonly make up the basic acoustic admittance battery are tympanometry and the acoustic reflex thresholds. Tympanometry is the measurement of the acoustic admittance when air pressure in the external canal is varied. Alterations in the middle ear system or function will change the normal tympanometric results. The acoustic reflex refers to the contraction of stapedius muscle (which causes a decrease in admittance) to an acoustical signal of sufficient intensity and duration. Abnormality in the middle ear system, afferent and efferent neuronal systems of the stapedius reflex arc may reflect in abnormalities in the acoustic reflex measurement.

Otoacoustic emissions are sounds generated within the normal cochlea, either spontaneously or in response to acoustical stimulation. Spontaneous otoacoustic emissions (SOAEs) occur in the absence of external stimulation and are present in approximately 30 – 60% of normal ears. Evoked otoacoustic emissions (EOAEs) occur during or after external acoustical stimulation and are present in the vast majority of all normal ears. Evoked OAEs can be divided into subclasses based primarily on the stimuli used to evoke them: transient evoked otoacoustic emissions, distortion product otoacoustic emissions and stimulus frequency emissions.

Chapter 9
Audiometric patterns of genetic hearing loss

ALESSANDRO MARTINI and SILVANO PROSSER

Introduction

It is common to be asked by a patient with a hearing loss about the cause of the impairment and its possible progression. Despite thorough investigation with current techniques and an accurate medical history, a considerable number of patients have no identifiable exogenous causative factors. As the prevalence of genetic causes is high, both within congenital and early childhood and within late onset hearing loss cases (Morton, 1991; Sill et al., 1992; Marazita et al., 1993), counselling of hearing impaired individuals presents a special challenge not only for the geneticist but also for the clinical audiologist and otologist.

Recognition, interpretation and classification of cases with associated abnormalities are discussed in other parts of this book. However, 70% of genetically determined hearing impairments occur in non-syndromal forms (Gorlin et al., 1994) and it is often very difficult to distinguish a 'non-syndromal' genetic hearing loss from other causes of hearing loss. Non-syndromal sensorineural hearing loss (NSSNHL) represents the most common form of genetic hearing impairment (Kimberling, 1993). While phenotypic expression is very similar, a high degree of genetic heterogeneity has been recognized. Discriminating between the different forms of hereditary NSSNHL usually focuses on the mode of inheritance, the type and severity of hearing loss, and vestibular function.

Two main issues arise from a clinical point of view. The first is whether it is possible to distinguish between a genetic and a non-genetic hearing loss; the second is whether the audiometric pattern can differentiate different genotypes. Albrecht (1922) observed that the recessive forms of hearing loss are profound or total, congenital and non-progressive, whereas the dominant forms are usually less severe, postnatal and variably progressive. Langenbeck (1935) was probably the first to report that the 'symmetry of hearing function is by itself a probable indicator of heredity' and only a few cases have been reported of unilateral SNHL due to genetic causes (e.g. Smith, 1939; Everberg, 1957). Knowledge about syndromal and non-syndromal forms of genetic hearing impairment has greatly increased over the past half century, while during the last few years a worldwide research effort has been casting a new light on the genetic mechanisms of hearing loss (Cremers et al., 1995).

It is well known that the fundamental processes involved in the mechanism of hearing are controlled by hundreds of genes (Nance, 1980). Recently the action of some of them has been identified in normally hearing (Ernfors, 1995; Hasson,1995) and deaf humans as well as in animals (Weil et al., 1995; Steel,1995; Gibson et al., 1995).

The rationale for a classification based on pure-tone audiometric results, stems from the fact that differences in threshold profile and degree of hearing loss correspond to differences in the spatial and quantitative distribution of hair cell and/or ganglion cell damage within the cochlea. As a first hypothesis, these may be thought of as a direct effect of different genes or different genetic expression.

Recent developments

The majority of authors report that it is impossible to subclassify autosomal recessive SNHL (ARSNHL) by audiometric criteria as there is extreme heterogeneity (and phenotypic variability) in the audiometric profile (Smith et al., 1995). Fukushima et al. (1995), by examining consanguineous nuclear families with ARSNHL, identified a recessive locus on chromosome 14q (*DFNB5*) in 10 families, while one family showed probable linkage to *DFNB2*. This last family, however, differs in age of onset of the hearing loss from the original family used to map *DFNB2* (Guilford et al., 1994b), suggesting that characteristics of hearing impairment are not valid criteria by which families can be pooled for linkage analysis (Fukushima et al., 1995). Other genes which so far are known to be involved in ARSNHL are:

- *DFNB1* (13q12, Guilford et al., 1994b), hearing loss was profound, prelingual, fully penetrant, in two kindreds.
- *DFNB3* (17p11.2, Friedman et al., 1995) profound, congenital, at all frequencies, in many kindreds in an isolated Balinese village.
- *DFNB4* (7q31, Baldwin et al., 1995) profound congenital in a Druze family.
- *DFNB6* (3p14-21, Fukushima et al., 1995)
- *DFNB7* (9q11-13, Jain et al., 1995)
- *DFNB8* (21q22, Veske et al., 1996)
- *DFNB9* (2p22-23, Chaib et al., 1996)

The picture is different for autosomal dominant SNHL, probably due to the wide range of audiometric patterns which the affected individuals may exhibit. At the time of writing, eight different genes (*DFNA 1 – 8*) have been identified and the possible relationship between genotype and audiometric features is considered below.

Two large and well documented multigenerational pedigrees have been reported as showing *low frequency hearing loss*, which led to the identification of two different genes: *DFNA1* localized to chromosome 5q31 (Leon et al., 1992) and *DFNA6* localized on chromosome 4p16.3 (Lesperance et al., 1995). Although the audiometric patterns and ages of onset (about age 10 years) appear similar, the progression is different in the two families. It is very rapid in the large kindred from Costa Rica in which SNHL progresses to severe hearing loss across the entire frequency range by the age of 30, leading to profound flat hearing loss at approximately 40 years of age (Leon et al., 1992). It is, however, slow in the Vanderbilt kindred, where hearing loss progresses to a flat audiogram of about 50 dB HL by the age of 50 years (Hall et al., 1995).

Four genes involved in *high frequency* SNHL have been localized. *DFNA2* (1p32, Coucke et al., 1994) causes high tone hearing loss and progresses at a highly variable rate to affect all frequencies. The current results involve four large kindreds from different continents (van Camp et al., 1995). In the large Indonesian kindred the SNHL starts in the second to third decade, usually preceded by tinnitus: the audiograms vary markedly, ranging from curves showing a normal threshold up to 2,000 Hz with a drop at higher frequencies, to relatively flat severe SNHL. In the American kindred the SNHL is more severe and of early onset: a hearing loss of at least 60 dB was diagnosed in several of the affected members by the age of 6 years. Most of the cases presented with a sloping configuration above 1 kHz. Tinnitus was reported by some of the affected members. Belgian and Dutch families showed a similarly progressive high frequency SNHL.

DFNA3 (13q12, Chaib et al., 1994) causes moderate to severe SNHL predominantly in the high frequencies (sloping or residual), prelingual, within the first 4 years of life, not progressive or, in a few cases, worsening slightly through life; no vertigo has been reported.

DFNA5 (7p15, van Camp et al., 1995) causes SNHL at high frequencies, starts between 5 and 15 years of age and in the fifth decade the hearing loss becomes severe, involving low frequencies; vestibular function remains normal and there is no tinnitus.

DFNA7 (1q21-23, Tranebjaerg et al., 1995); causes high frequency, slightly progressive SNHL.

As regards *mid-frequency* or *flat hearing loss*, the audiometric profiles of a family described by Chen (Chen et al., 1995) in which *DFNA4* was localized on chromosome 19q13 and of a family reported by

Kirschhofer (Kirschhofer et al., 1995) in which *DFNA8* was localized on chromosome 15q15, are similar: moderate to severe SNHL involving all the frequencies of about 60 – 70 dB HL. However, in the first kindred, the hearing impairment was fluctuant and progressive, leading to a severe to profound SNHL; in the second family the threshold was stable over time. So far, only two genes have been identified as responsible for X-linked SNHL, and only a few kindreds identified with NSSNHL due to mutation in mitochondrial genes.

According to Chen et al. (1995) in multigenerational kindreds, linkage mapping is relatively straightforward if there is a careful phenotypic characterization of the hearing loss in affected members, as it permits exclusion of environmental factors which can result in diagnostic errors (false positives).

The identification of patients exhibiting particular patterns of progression of hearing loss, or collecting families with common audiometric profiles could be useful in isolating homogenous groups. The availability of individuals with similar phenotypes is the basic condition for conducting a successful search for genetic loci responsible for SNHL, as was the case with syndromal forms such as Usher or Waardenburg syndromes (Kimberling et al.,1990; Read, 1990). However, there is no general agreement on the audiometric parameters required for the definition of a clinical classification. In addition, further questions arise when audiometric data are considered in relation to the subject's age, or the family generations. Is the threshold profile repeatable within a family? Is the hearing loss constant throughout the individual's life span, or susceptible to further deterioration with age? And, if the latter should be the case, what will be the effect of age-related hearing loss (AgeRHL) – simply additive and predictable on the basis of the 'normal population' data, or more adversely, inducing a severe or profound hearing loss at a relatively early age?

Audiometric parameters

At present, pedigree analysis and audiometric morphology are still the most useful means of attempting a subcategorization of the large number of isolated types of genetic hearing impairments. Two approaches have been employed. The first, proposed by Fisch (1955) and, with some modification by Liu, Xu and Newton (Liu et al., 1994), is a strictly quantitative classification of the shape of the audiogram which, according to the authors, allows some inferences to be made about the nature of the hearing loss. The second, is a more comprehensive nosology, resulting from the pioneering work of Konigsmark and Gorlin (1976), recently revised by Gorlin, Toriello and Cohen (1995).

In a previous investigation (Martini et al., 1996a in press), we have made a reappraisal and a comparison of the morphometric analysis of audiograms and the Konigsmark and Gorlin classification. The families, assigned to the autosomal dominant or autosomal recessive groups as shown by pedigree analysis, were classified after Konigsmark and Gorlin on the basis of the whole family data. Notwithstanding the differences in recruitment of cases, and considering the classification criteria adopted, our figures resembled those obtained by Liu et al. (1994) in 28 families studied. In both studies most subjects were characterized by milder and/or non-congenital forms of hearing loss compared with the majority of reports (Fraser, 1976). Furthermore ADSNHL was more common and less severe than ARSNHL inherited forms. Profound hearing loss is almost, if not exclusively represented by ARSNHL; in our opinion this observation should be taken in account in genetic counselling.

Variations of audiometric pattern in respect of transmission and age

It is important to evaluate the consistency of the genetically transmitted audiometric configuration and hearing loss across family members. If a specific audiometric pattern has a high probability of transmission from parents to children, then such a phenotypic pattern could correspond to a specific genotype. However this hypothesis is complicated by the fact that many forms of hereditary hearing loss are progressive from an early age, other forms may be progressive in the elderly, mimicking a presbyacusic effect, and others can be stable throughout adulthood. In spite of such limitations, we have attempted to evaluate, at least descriptively, the persistence of a given audiometric profile and hearing loss across the generations (Martini et al., in press, 1996b).

To determine whether the AD hearing loss is age dependent, a regression analysis was performed using as a dependent variable the mean thresholds at 2 and 4 kHz ($PTA_{2,4 \text{ kHz}}$). These frequencies are typically involved in age-dependent hearing deterioration (presbyacusis). The $PTA_{2,4 \text{ kHz}}$ and age appear to be significantly correlated ($p < 0.001$). Since the slope of the PTA-age function is similar (0.645 vs. 0.690) to that predicted for the normal population (ISO 729,1984), it is plausible that the hereditary hearing loss increases with age due to the effect of the same age-dependent factor responsible for the presbyacusis in the normal population, which simply adds to an inherited loss from early age (Figure 9.1).

However, this hypothesis seems to be contradicted by the results of a regression analysis using as dependent variables the mean hearing loss at 0.5 and 1 kHz ($PTA_{0.5,1 \text{ kHz}}$), a frequency range which is only marginally involved in the presbyacusis (Figure 9.2). This analysis also demonstrated

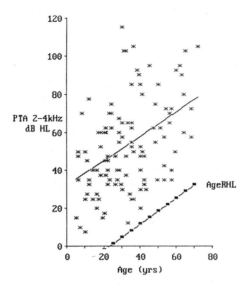

Figure 9.1 Regression analysis: mean threshold at 2 and 4 kHz vs age. Dotted line represents prediction of the normal population.

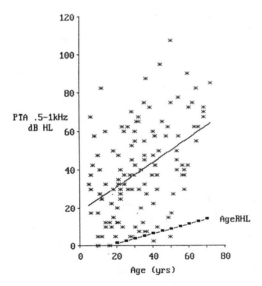

Figure 9.2 Regression analysis: mean threshold at 0.5 and 1 kHz vs age. Dotted line represents prediction of the normal population.

a significant dependency of the PTA$_{0.5,1\,kHz}$ with age. If the progression of the hereditary hearing loss could be mainly explained by the additive effect of presbyacusis, involving the high frequencies, the hearing in the low to mid frequencies should be relatively unchanged throughout the adult life. Although such an analysis does not exclude the possibility that in some subjects the high frequency loss can be due to a presbyacusis effect, in general the age-dependent increase of hereditary hearing loss can be attributed to a mechanism inherent in cochlear damage developed at an early age.

In the attempt to evaluate the progression of hearing loss within the affected members of a family, a methodology similar to the approach used in the estimate of long term effects of acoustic trauma was adopted, in which the hearing loss at the time of the observation can be considered as the product of two factors, one that depends on age and is estimated from a 'normal database' (AgeRHL), and another that is very unpredictable and depends on noise exposure (NoiseRHL) (ISO 729, 1984).

A sample of cases was selected, belonging to 11 families with 3 or more affected subjects covering a sufficiently wide age span. For each family the $PTA_{2,4\ kHz}$ and the $PTA_{0.5,1\ kHz}$ of the single members were analysed by a linear correlation. By comparing the PTA functions to those of the AgeRHL at the corresponding frequencies, four different patterns were identified:

1. A pattern represented by a $PTA_{2,4\ kHz}$ and a $PTA_{0.5,1\ kHz}$ function with a slope similar to the respective AgeRHL functions. In this case the progression of the hearing loss could be attributed to an additive effect of presbyacusis on a relatively stable inherited loss.
2. A pattern represented by a $PTA_{2,4\ kHz}$ function with a slope similar to the corresponding AgeRHL, and a $PTA_{0.5,1\ kHz}$ function with a growth rate higher than that predicted by the corresponding AgeRHL. In this case it is likely that the progression of hearing loss was mainly caused by factors associated with the inherited cochlear lesions, with an adverse effect extended to a wide frequency range.
3. A pattern represented by relatively flat $PTA_{2,4\ kHz}$ and $PTA_{0.5,1\ kHz}$ functions. In this case the hereditary hearing loss seemed to be resistant to the effect of AgeRHL. A similar picture for hearing loss occurring at a young age has often been described, which seems to be relatively unaffected by presbyacusis.
4. A pattern represented by $PTA_{2,4\ kHz}$ and $PTA_{0.5,1\ kHz}$ parallel functions, much steeper than the corresponding AgeRHL functions. In this case the deterioration of hearing loss is probably attributable to factors associated with the inherited character, involving a rapid and extended degeneration of the cochlear elements, relatively independent of AgeRHL.

Conclusions

Non-syndromal SNHL, in a congenital sporadic or familial presentation, still remains a great challenge for the audiologist and the geneticist. In the congenital sporadic cases, differentiation between a genetic or environmental aetiology is usually based on the exclusion of the latter, so genetic counselling is given on a probabilistic basis. Also in the familial cases, it is often difficult to make firm statements about the inheritance of the condition and its possible progression. Even ruling out a syndromal hearing loss may take several years of monitoring.

NSSNHL is almost exclusively monogenic and highly genetically heterogeneous, with the number of involved genes estimated to be over one hundred (Chaib et al. 1995). At the present time, pedigree analysis and audiometric morphology are still the most popular means of attempting a subcategorization of the isolated types of genetic hearing loss. However, whether or not the information associated with pure tone audiometry can reliably separate homogeneous subgroups within a multifamilial cohort of affected subjects appears questionable. Our case studies have indicated that hearing loss and threshold profiles fail to show a clear replication from parents to children, with the exception of a few cases with ascending and U-shaped threshold profiles (Martini et al., in press, 1996b). Hearing loss may deteriorate with age, and consequently the threshold profile may change. It is known that many forms of hereditary hearing loss are progressive. However, the adverse effect due to heredity proved to be not easily separable from that typical of presbyacusis in a normal population. A combination of both these factors accounts for the significant relationship between age and hearing loss as revealed in our data. A better knowledge of hearing loss progression is needed to achieve a better discrimination between classes than that obtained by inspection of the audiogram.

Should this kind of result be confirmed by further investigations of affected subjects, either within and across families or by longitudinal case observation, the different ways in which hearing loss increases with age may assist in separating classes of individuals who could differ for specific genotypes responsible for the development of cochlear damage.

The audiometric features which have to be taken in account seem to be not only the audiogram shape, but also the nature of the progression of the HL, the presence of tinnitus and vestibular function, and the thorough evaluation of a kindred for its correct classification. It may happen that a family previously classified as NSSNHL, shows on more extensive evaluation that the hearing impairment is part of a more complex syndrome (Mohr and Mageroy, 1960; Tranebjaerg et al., 1995).

Chapter 10
The detection of carriers of genetic hearing loss

DAFYDD STEPHENS and MARY FRANCIS

Introduction

In a clinical situation, information about carrier status in relatives of individuals with recessive and X-linked hearing loss has an important role in the counselling of the patient and his/her family. It is also potentially useful in a research context in defining individuals who could be investigated in terms of DNA studies and gene identification. In an isolated non-syndromal case of hearing loss testing the proband's parents and siblings could be used to define the likelihood that such a condition is recessive.

These three roles of carrier identification impose different constraints on the tests used for the identification of carriers. Thus for determination of the carriers in a well defined family (e.g. Usher syndrome type II), a test with high sensitivity but relatively low specificity may be adequate. To help the selection of patients for DNA studies, high specificity is of more importance than the sensitivity of the test.

In the determination of evidence that we are dealing with a case of non-syndromal recessive hearing loss (NSRHL) we are faced with something of a dilemma. We obviously require a test or tests which have high sensitivity. However, we are dealing with a large number of different genes (see Chapter 21) causing a similar hearing loss, so that we cannot realistically expect them all to be expressed in the same way in carriers. We may therefore be looking for a limited test battery including several procedures which between them should have high sensitivity across the various recessive conditions, with the individual tests having high specificity within a particular family. Thus if we have four tests (a,b,c,d), ideally we would like to expect that one or more of these would be abnormal in all carriers of NSARHL, but that both parents and 2/3 of hearing siblings of a proband in one family would show an abnormality in test (a), whereas in the family with the hearing loss due to a different gene, such relatives would show an abnormality in test (c) etc.

These are the ideal conditions, and in many families the results will be obscured by concomitant acquired hearing losses in carriers which will render many of the sensitive measures proposed invalid. Furthermore, in a proportion of individuals, there may be uncertain paternity and, with or without this, some studies have found a higher proportion of 'carrier-related' abnormalities in female than in male first degree relatives (e.g. Anderson and Wedenberg, 1968; Stephens et al., 1995). We are also faced with the problem that with genes for NSARHL being common in the population, many individuals may be carrying more than one such gene.

Within this chapter we shall be obliged to admit that we are far from defining any ideal test in terms of either sensitivity or specificity. Perhaps the closest approximation so far comes in the sensitivity of the Audioscan in the detection of Usher II syndrome (Meredith et al., 1991) but even these results need replication and support from DNA studies.

This chapter will therefore concentrate on results which have so far been obtained and consider these by the type of procedure used, to provide possible pointers for future developments. We shall start by briefly considering the expression by heterozygote carriers of other recessive conditions. The chapter will be restricted to a consideration of carrier status in autosomal recessive conditions and, to a lesser extent, in X-linked conditions. It must be borne in mind in the latter conditions that Lyonization occurs, and results in very variable findings in the X-linked dominant conditions such as Alport syndrome and perilymph gusher, which will be considered briefly. In the past there have been problems and confusion of results with inclusion of patients with autosomal dominant hearing loss of variable expressivity, for which some of the sensitive measures may be useful, but which are outside the scope of this chapter. Finally there are no data available on mothers of children with mitochondrial hearing loss, an area which merits investigation.

Heterozygote expression in other conditions

In autosomal recessive conditions in which only a single copy of the gene is functioning, the principle of a gene dosage effect is most commonly employed. This rests on the knowledge of the biochemical defect where the protein product is known and assayed. One might expect obligate carriers to have roughly half the level of enzyme found in the affected homozygotes. This is indeed the case in some conditions such as Refsum disease, where an isolated deficiency of phytanic acid exists and assay of the enzyme alpha-oxidase accurately predicts carrier status (Herdon et al., 1969). In mucopolysaccharidoses (Neufeld and Muenzer, 1995) and in Gaucher's disease (Beutler and Grabowski, 1995), overlap in enzyme levels occurs between the two groups leading to interpretation difficulties. Scoring systems have been devised to help overcome this problem in amenable conditions, of which I-cell disease (Ben-Yoseph et al., 1984) and hereditary orotic aciduria (Fox et al., 1973) provide examples. The decreased enzyme level is combined with either an increased level of a precursor substrate or an abnormal metabolite generated in the metabolic pathway prior to the enzymatic block.

Other limitations are imposed by this method which relate either to technical difficulties of the assay in question or to extraction of the specific enzyme from tissue culture. Thus it follows that not all heterozygous carriers will be identified. Nonetheless, it has met with considerable success in selective population screening in Tay-Sachs disease (Kaback et al., 1977) and remains the currently most reliable method of carrier detection in congenital adrenal hyperplasia (New et al., 1983).

An alternative complementary approach to heterozygote expression is careful clinical scrutiny to detect the effect of an enzyme deficiency in a target organ. This also relies, to some extent, on a knowledge of the biochemical defect in question and also the ease with which a target organ may be examined. In oculo-cutaneous albinism, the effects of tyrosinase deficiency on the skin and eye may be readily studied. Giant melanin granules found on microscopic examination of melanocytes in skin biopsies allowed Winship et al. (1984) to assign carrier status in this condition. The same task was accomplished by Nyhan and Sakati (1987) based on the finding of areas of depigmentation in the fundus and iris upon eye examination. Similarly, there are documented cases in the literature on Niemann-Pick type C disease, where parents were found to have some changes in skin biopsies (Ceuterick et al., 1986) and in bone marrow examinations (Frank and Lasson, 1985) typically associated with the homozygous state.

Morton (1991) argued that heterozygote expression may be more readily identified in X-linked rather than autosomal recessive transmission, given the random inactivation of one copy of the X-chromosome that occurs in all cells. Indeed, as mentioned above, this is supported when two populations of cells are cloned from cells of an individual with an X-linked condition. In testicular feminization syndrome, for example, where a deficiency of a receptor for dehydrotestosterone exists, cells with normal androgen receptors and cells with deficient receptors may be demonstrated by culture in heterozygous females (Meyer et al., 1975). Carriers of ectodermal dysplasia likewise have patches of normal skin and patches which lack sweat glands, and carriers of glucose-6-phosphate dehydrogenase deficiency show a mixture of normal and deficient red blood cells (Read, 1989). However, Read argued that where a carrier test involved a diffusible product, it is less reliable and other statistical tests are employed to estimate the ultimate risk of a carrier state. This is the case in haemophilia A and B where heterozygotes may have lowered Factor VIII or IX levels. Likewise, raised serum creatinine kinase levels due to diseased muscle cells are often found in heterozygote carriers of Duchenne muscular dystrophy, and immunostaining of muscle cells will show dystrophin positive and negative patches indicative of the carrier state.

These examples indicate that it would not be unreasonable to expect some subclinical abnormalities in carriers of recessive hearing loss, although these may not be invariably present.

Standard pure tone audiometry

Pure tone audiometry dates back to 1919 – 20, and its first application to carriers of genetic disorders came with the study of Tinkle (1933) using a Western Electric 2A Audiometer, one of the earliest portable machines. He studied presumed heterozygous parents and siblings of deaf children, but Meredith (1991) has argued that close examination of his subjects suggests that none were carriers of autosomal recessive hearing loss.

In the 1940s and 50s, a variety of studies by Lidenov (1945), Johnsen (1954) and by Stevenson and Cheeseman (1956) failed to find any significant abnormalities in carriers, using pure tone audiometry. Wildervank (1957), in a more carefully documented study, likewise reported null results, but close examination of his results indicates a number of parents of deaf children with mild mid-frequency hearing losses.

Kloepfer, Laguaite and McLaurin (1966), studying Usher syndrome carriers, argued that their hearing was slightly worse across the range than control subjects, although it is not clear how well age matched the controls were. More recently Wagenaar et al. (1995) and van Aarem et al. (1995) have examined audiometric thresholds of carriers of Usher syndrome type I and type IIA respectively. The latter study used ISO 7029 data to control for age and sex effects and found significantly elevated thresholds at 250 and 500 Hz. However, the validity of using ISO 7029 has recently been questioned. Re-analysis of the results of van Aarem et al. using age group, sex and ear matched population data from the National Study of Hearing (Davis, 1995) indicates that the Usher type II carriers had significantly better hearing at 1,000, 2,000 and 4,000 Hz than the normal population (Table 10.1).

Table 10.1 Comparison of pure tone thresholds of carriers for Usher type IIA.

Frequency Hz	250	500	1000	2000	4000	8000
Mean threshold Usher type IIA	18.7	15.5	8.7	12.7	20.0	30.5
Mean threshold NSH	16.8	15.1	14.7	18.0	28.3	35.8
t	0.95	0.18	2.9	2.34	3.05	1.01
p	NS	NS	0.008	0.03	0.007	NS

(van Aarem et al., 1995) with normative data from the National Study of Hearing (Davis, 1995).

The data for Usher type I syndrome (Wagenaar et al., 1995) were also compared with ISO 7029 and showed a divergence from the ISO 7029 data that increased with increasing frequency. However, the raw data were not presented so that they cannot be considered further. Like van Aarem et al. (1995), these authors argued that the results were too variable to be useful in the detection of carriers.

Parving (1985) examined the configuration of the hearing of carriers of Norrie syndrome (an X-linked recessive condition) and found a mid-frequency dip in 3/5 of obligate carriers and 1/20 individuals with a 50% risk of being carriers. Békésy audiometry (see below) showed notches in the same proportion of obligate carriers but 3/20 of the possible carriers.

Finally, studies on females carrying the X-linked dominant genes for Alport syndrome (Sirimanna et al., 1995) and perilymph gusher (Reardon et al., 1992) show very variable results attributable to the Lyonization process.

Sweep frequency testing

This approach provides more details of the individual's hearing using either 'sweep frequency' Békésy audiometry (Békésy, 1947) or the more recent Audioscan technique (Meyer-Bisch, 1990). Békésy audiometry was first introduced in this field by Anderson and Wedenberg (1968, 1976). They reported mid-frequency dips over 1 octave wide and 25 dB deep in the frequency range 500 Hz to 3 kHz to be more common among carriers of recessive hearing loss than among control subjects. They did not test above 3 kHz to avoid possible effects of noise.

Subsequent studies by Taylor et al. (1975) and Marres and Cremers (1989) failed to support these findings, but the former used a sweep rate of 2 octaves/s and the latter was restricted to a single large Dutch family. Parving (1978) tested carriers of Norrie's syndrome and found more notches than in controls, although a follow-up using different stimulus parameters was less encouraging (Parving and Schwartz, 1991).

One of the problems with Békésy audiometry is that its excursions, and their size in certain individuals, can mask discontinuities in the threshold reflected in narrow notches. This can be overcome using the Audioscan technique with which Meredith (1991) found that of 30 subjects shown to have audiometric notches (including carriers, possible carriers and controls), 29 had notches on Audioscan testing but only 6 on Békésy testing. He found that, with Békésy notches, the sensitivity for the detection of carriers was 22% and the specificity 100%, whereas the Audioscan had a sensitivity of 78%, and a specificity of 87%. Examples of notches produced by the two techniques using the same subject are shown in Figure 10.1.

Meredith examined different stimulus parameters and found a sweep rate of 30 s/octave over the frequency range 500 – 3,000 Hz taking a notch size of 15 dB or more gave the optimal results. With this stimulus paradigm, 106 controls from 3 separate studies showed a 14.2% occurrence of notches. Adding the further data from 30 adults obtained by Cohen et al. (1996) increases the figure to 15.4%.

When the test was administered to obligate carriers of Usher syndrome type II (Meredith et al., 1992; Sirimanna et al., 1992) 100% of obligate carriers were found to have notches, as were 57% of possible carriers (Table 10.2). These results are remarkable and merit repetition, and comparison with DNA results.

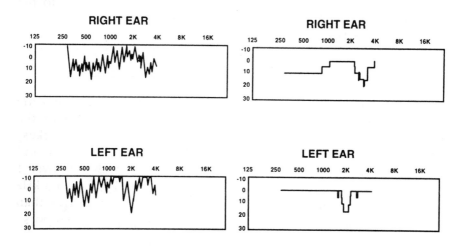

Figure 10.1 Békésy (left) and Audioscan (right) traces from the same obligate carrier of a non-syndromal autosomal recessive hearing loss.

Table 10.2 Usher syndrome type II with Audioscan notches.

	Tested	Notches	% Notches
Controls	106	15	14.2
Obligate carriers	9	9	100
Possible carriers	23	13	56.5

(from Sirimanna et al., 1992)

A recent study by Wagenaar et al. (in preparation) failed to replicate these findings in patients with Usher syndrome type I. However, there were differences in the stimulus parameters and criteria used in this study, but it seems possible that there is a real difference between carriers of Usher type I and Usher type II syndromes.

Not surprisingly, with non-syndromal autosomal recessive hearing loss the situation is less clear, as many different genes may be involved. However, taking the data from three studies (Stephens et al., 1995; Janjua (personal communication) based on consanguineous Pakistani families; Cohen et al., 1996), we obtain the data shown in Table 10.3, in which the findings for parents and siblings are amalgamated and compared with a combination of the three control groups from Stephens et al. (1995) and the two control groups for Cohen et al. (1996). The differences here again were, however, highly significant and encouraging for further studies in that some 39% of all subjects tested showed notches, despite coming from an heterogenous group of subjects, compared with 18.7% of the control subjects.

Table 10.3 Non-syndromal autosomal hearing loss obligate and possible carriers with Audioscan notches.

	Tested	Notches	% Notches
Controls	160	30	18.7
Stephens et al. (1995)	42	22	52.3
Janjua (personal communication)	35	11	31.4
Cohen et al. (1996)	32	12	37.5

Sirimanna, France and Stephens (1995) have also studied obligate (female) carriers of Alport syndrome. They found that, of 8 tested, 4 had hearing losses and the other 4 had notches on the Audioscan. Similarly among 15 possible female carriers, 3 had hearing losses, 5 showed notches on Audioscan and 7 had normal hearing.

Thus the Audioscan, at present, seems a promising test. It must, however, be borne in mind that some 14 – 19% of control subjects show notches whether due to unknown carrier status or artefact. It is, furthermore, a test which requires attention and concentration from the subject, and so should be performed early in the test protocol. These data apply only to testing using the stimulus parameters defined above; including higher frequencies considerably alters the picture by introducing consequences of noise exposure and trauma.

Acoustic reflex thresholds (ARTs)

Anderson and Wedenberg (1968, 1976) also found significantly elevated ARTs in their obligate carriers. This is a somewhat non-specific finding which may be caused by a number of different factors. While Meredith (1991) found significantly more elevated ARTs in possible carriers than in control subjects, this finding was not replicated by Almqvist and Haugen (1992). Furthermore neither of these studies found a significant relationship between elevated ARTs and the presence of notches on testing with the Audioscan or Békésy audiometry.

In other studies, Marres and Cremers (1989) found no elevation of ARTs in their study on an extensive family with NSARHL, and both Wagenaar et al. (1995) in Usher type I syndrome and van Aarem et al. (1995) with Usher type IIA syndrome found normal ARTs.

Elevation of ARTs could theoretically be regarded as a potentially useful approach to an aspect of hearing loss different from that giving minor auditory threshold abnormalities. ARTs do, however, entail the normal functions of too many different anatomo-physiological structures to give precise results in this field, and can be influenced by long term consequences of common acquired conditions such as otitis media with effusion.

Other test procedures

Amongst those techniques investigated in different groups recently have been speech audiometry, auditory brainstem responses, evoked otoacoustic emissions and frequency resolution measures. Wagenaar et al. (1995) and van Aarem et al. (1995) have examined speech discrimination measures and ABRs in carriers of the Usher syndromes and found no significant abnormalities. Various evoked otoacoustic emission measures including transient evoked and distortion product otoacoustic emissions have been examined by several groups of workers but appear to show no consistent effects in carriers, although various minor abnormalities have been found. Wagenaar et al. (in preparation) failed to show any significant difference in transient evoked otoacoustic emission amplitudes between carriers of Usher syndrome type I and control subjects. This is, however, a domain which probably merits further attention.

This is also true of the application of balance tests, studied by Wagenaar et al. (1995) and van Aarem et al. (1985) in carriers of Usher syndrome types I and IIA, and which again showed no consistent abnormalities. These investigations included an extensive electronystagmographic battery and rotating chair tests.

Conclusions

The approach of the Nijmegen group (Wagenaar et al., 1995; van Aarem et al., 1995) in using a limited test battery approach to obligate carriers of specific conditions is likely to be the best way forward in this field, identifying tests which may be useful in specific syndromes. Problems arise in the group in which the tests are most needed, namely nonsyndromal autosomal recessive hearing loss, and it may be that the audiologists will have to follow the geneticists rather than lead them in this respect, concentrating initially on families in which the gene responsible has been identified. An intermediate step may be to concentrate on the carriers in large consanguineous families. Undoubtedly the future will be in the use of a small battery of carefully defined tests.

Chapter 11
Balance function and hearing loss

CLAES MÖLLER

Introduction

Approximately 50 – 75% of all cases of hearing loss with severe hearing impairment are due to a genetic condition. Most hereditary losses are inherited in a recessive manner. Because of this, small families and extensive genetic heterogeneity, the aetiology of hearing loss in many patients is difficult to establish.

When hearing loss occurs in a family it is often a traumatic experience which turns their world upside down. The child does not talk and several years may elapse before an alternative mode of communication, signing, is established. The child will get a late start in communication and discovering of the world. It is also common for deaf people to be 'clumsy', which often is treated as a trait of hearing loss and caused by the hearing loss in itself. It is often forgotten, even among physicians, that the inner ear consists of two parts of the 'same' organ, namely the cochlea and the labyrinth. Few studies of the deaf have, however, examined balance function in general and vestibular function in particular.

The task of keeping good balance is performed by three different systems:

1. The proprioceptive system.
2. The visual system.
3. The vestibular system.

Afferent signals from all three systems converge in the brainstem, pons and cerebellum where they are processed and then transmitted through efferent nerve fibres to maintain coordinated movements.

Man can live and have sufficient balance without vision and vestibular signals. The visual system performs its task during slow movements, while the vestibular system, through the vestibulo-ocular reflex, coordinates the head and eyes when performing rapid movements. As long as the vision is sufficient, a deaf person with vestibular loss can perform nearly normally. On the other hand, when in the dark or when walking on an uneven surface, the loss of a functional vestibular system can make the same person very clumsy and insecure.

This has been known for some years, although few studies have been undertaken which focus on balance function among deaf people. Shambaugh (1930) collected information from approximately 5,000 deaf students and concluded that 70% had normal balance function, with no difference between those with congenital and childhood onset hearing loss. He did not, however, perform any vestibular tests.

In 1955, Arnvig reported a study of nearly 500 children who were deaf or severely hard of hearing. He found approximately 40% to have abnormal caloric reactions. No distinction was made between congenital and childhood onset hearing loss, and the calorics did not meet current standards. Sandberg et al. (1965) presented the results from 57 children who underwent caloric irrigation according to present standards using the Dix-Hallpike technique. They found a fair parallelism between the degree of hearing loss and the loss of vestibular function with deficiencies in vestibular function in 80% of the deaf population. No attempt was made to distinguish between different aetiologies.

Usher syndrome

Hallgren (1959) and Möller et al. (1989) studied vestibular function in Usher syndrome and found it to be extremely important in explaining some behavioural patterns, and in the classification and diagnosis of the condition. In Usher syndrome, neither the degree of hearing loss nor the visual deficiency is enough to discriminate between type I and type II. Measures of the vestibular function have, however, proved to be reliable techniques to separate them.

- Usher type I (deaf + retinitis pigmentosa) – all cases which have been genetically linked have shown bilaterally absent vestibular function.
- Usher type II (hard of hearing + retinitis pigmentosa) – on the other hand have normal vestibular function bilaterally.
- Usher syndrome type III (USHIII) – which has recently been genetically linked, is characterised by progressive hearing loss and retinitis pigmentosa. The vestibular function in USHIII seems to follow the hearing loss with a gradual deterioration of the vestibular function.

Thus in order to study hearing disorders and to provide a better means of classification, vestibular function must be evaluated.

Means of assessment

One important issue is the assessment of early motor milestones. This is generally performed by retrospective evaluation, preferably by questioning the parents.

Early motor milestones are:

6 weeks	holding the head in the plane of the body
12 weeks	holding the head above the plane of the body
16 weeks	good head control
6 months	unsupported sitting
10 months	standing up with support
12 months	walking

The questions should be simple and very down to earth such as:

- At what age did the child sit unsupported?
- At what age did the child walk?
- Did the child experience difficulty in learning to ride a bicycle?
- Does the child have problems when walking in the dark and on an uneven surface?
- Does the child experience motion sickness?
- Does the child have problems in gymnastics and sporting activities?
- Is the child considered to be clumsy?

Balance assessment should include:

1. Ear, nose and throat examination.
2. Cranial nerve tests.
3. Romberg test, tandem feet with eyes open and closed.
4. Standing on one leg with eyes closed.
5. Electronystagmography (ENG) noting possible spontaneous and positional nystagmus. For recording of horizontal eye movements Ag/AgCl electrodes should be placed on the outer canthus of each eye and a ground electrode attached to the forehead. Vertical eye movements should be recorded by applying one electrode above and one below the eye. The electrode impedance is recorded before each test session. Calibration of eye movements before testing is essential, preferably using two light emitting diodes 20 degrees apart. Evaluation of possible gaze nystagmus with the subjects fixating on light emitting diodes 60 degrees apart can reveal possible CNS dysfunction. Eye movements are best recorded in darkness using the direct current (DC) electro-oculographic (EOG) technique. Smooth pursuit and saccade tests should, if possible, be performed in order to exclude central nervous oculomotor dysfunction.

6. Bithermal binaural calorics (250 ml 30°, 44°C) should be performed with eyes open in the dark. The velocity of the slow phase is the best parameter to assess. An inter-aural difference of > 20% is considered pathological and a total sum of the four irrigations of < 40°/sec is considered hypoactive. Our experience is that calorics can, after careful preparation, usually be performed in children from 4 to 5 years of age.

7. Ice-water calorics performed binaurally (50 ml 8°C) should be performed in those cases which do not show responses in normal caloric tests. This test cannot, however, be quantified, but is merely an indication of any vestibular function.

8. Sinusoidal rotatory chair tests are by far the best means of evaluating possible bilateral vestibular loss in small children. They can be performed using an EOG technique and/or with infrared TV monitoring. The tests should be performed in darkness, and if vestibular function is present, a resulting nystagmus will appear immediately. In some cases good EOG recording is not possible, and in those cases infrared TV monitoring focused on the eyes of both the child and of the parent, will immediately show the difference in response if a bilateral vestibular loss is present. This test is, however, difficult to quantify, and will not with certainty differentiate between a unilateral vestibular loss and bilateral normal function (Möller and Ödkvist, 1989).

9. Dynamic posturography, if available, will provide an assessment of functional aspects of posture. We have used the Equitest system. This system uses a movable force platform capable of quantifying sway and shear forces. A visual surrounding is also movable through tilting, thus creating six different tests (So 1–6) with different visual and surface support conditions (Cyr et al., 1988). Falling on tests So 5 and 6, when the surface and the visual surround is sway referenced, indicates bilateral vestibular loss. However, the test cannot be applied reliably before 6 years of age.

Clinical results

We have performed a balance study on 74 subjects suffering from severe or profound hearing loss. All 74 subjects received a questionnaire concerning their balance. Of those who answered, 32 subjects (62%) participated in extensive balance testing.

The subjects were divided into two groups; deaf and severe hearing loss. The deaf group could experience only vibrations, did not use hearing aids, communicated solely through sign language and had a hearing loss > 90 dB HL at 500 – 8,000 Hz. The group with severe hearing loss had some residual hearing, some used hearing aids, all communicated by sign language but some used oral communication as well. Their hearing loss was, at most frequencies, between 60 and 110 dB HL. The following is a summary of the results of our study:

- Walking age – more than 50% of all subjects first walked later than 18 months.
- Cycling – about 40% of subjects in both groups reported problems cycling, especially at night.
- Walking in darkness and on uneven surfaces – over 50% of the subjects had significant problems getting around in the dark, especially in wintertime.
- Sea and motion sickness – very few had experienced any motion sickness. None reported motion sickness during car rides.
- Gymnastics – a large majority (75%) remembered problems in sports and gymnastics. Many of the subjects reported spontaneously 'I never cared for it because I was so clumsy'.
- Romberg test with feet together and eyes closed – the overall falling rate was 63%.
- Calorics – a total of 35% of subjects displayed bilateral vestibular areflexia.
- Rotatory tests and dynamic posturography – in these tests, abnormalities suggesting bilateral vestibular loss were found in 35%.

The aetiology of hearing loss was uncertain in some cases. It is clear from other studies that at least 50% of hearing losses can be expected to be of hereditary origin, in most cases recessive (van Rijn, 1990). In our patients, a subgroup with congenital hearing loss accounted for 70%, and childhood onset hearing loss caused by meningitis for 30%. Hearing loss due to rubella accounted for 10% of our patients and the unknown group was 30%. It is reasonable to assume that the unknown group of congenital hearing loss was of genetic origin, thus together with the group with confirmed heredity (25%), a probability of 60% hereditary hearing loss is a reasonable estimate.

Conclusions

We have, in a previous study, shown that no child with absent vestibular responses can walk before 18 months (Möller et al., 1989). This was also demonstrated in this study. All the subjects who had absent vestibular responses in the caloric and rotatory tests reported a walking age later than 18 months.

Even deaf subjects with intact vestibular function could be considered a little late, which might be a result of the hearing loss in itself (lack of auditory response when crawling, walking etc.). Conversely, no child who walks significantly earlier than 18 months can be considered to have bilateral vestibular loss. Thus, in future studies, and by further subgrouping and with larger patient samples, differences in 'vestibular involvement' can be clarified.

From a genetic perspective, vestibular tests can discriminate hearing loss into two groups. It is likely that a phenotype reflects an underlying defect which is gene-specific. If so, hereditary hearing loss should be categorised according to whether the labyrinth is involved or not. If vestibular involvement is consistent within families, then hearing loss with or without vestibular symptoms represents two major clinical categories of hearing impairment. As we have shown in the case of Usher syndrome, it is already possible to use vestibular tests to subdivide the condition, as normal vestibular function in deaf children excludes them from having Usher syndrome type I (Möller et al., 1989). It is due time to start evaluating the 'other half of the organ ...'

Part III
Syndromal Conditions

Chapter 12
The diagnostic approach to syndromal hearing loss

ELISA CALZOLARI and ALBERTO SENSI

Introduction

The main role of the clinical geneticist in the management of hearing loss is attempting to recognize syndromal forms and provide appropriate counselling. Therefore a close collaboration between audiologists, otologists and clinical geneticists is essential for the evaluation of patients with hearing loss of hereditary or unknown origin.

The spectrum of hereditary hearing loss is broad and ranges from simple hearing loss without other abnormalities to conditions in which hearing loss is one of a number of clinically recognized signs. There are many factors that make syndromal diagnosis a difficult task. We shall briefly mention the main problems and some strategies generally adopted to overcome them:

- The *rarity* of most of these conditions precludes direct experience of the majority of them in the course of one's whole professional life.
- *Heterogeneity* – a single phenotype may be the consequence of different pathogenetic and aetiological events.
- *Pleiotropy* – a term meaning that a single gene may cause many different phenotypic effects, often apparently unrelated pathogenetically.
- *Non-specificity* of individual defects.
- Wide *variability* of clinical expression.
- *Absence* in most cases of a *unique specific and sensitive test*.

Of course, the rarity of many types of syndromal hearing loss can be addressed only by reference to authoritative texts (Jones, 1988; Buyse, 1990; Gorlin et al., 1995; Gorlin et al. 1990; Stevenson et al., 1993) and databases (Possum, London), while pleiotropy implies that a multidisciplinary approach is often needed to achieve a complete view of these complex clinical pictures.

With rare exceptions, a clinical diagnosis of the pattern of malformations cannot be made on the basis of a single defect and usually depends on the detection of the overall pattern of anomalies. Recognition of minor defects may be as helpful as that of major anomalies in this regard.

The variability of the clinical expression is so great in most syndromal hearing loss that the hearing impairment may constitute the main or apparently the only problem in some subjects, while the prominent involvement of other organs or systems may sometimes obscure hearing loss in others. Waardenburg syndrome type II is a good example of variability of expression; affected subjects may present with bilateral profound hearing loss with only minimal hypopigmentation, while relatives may show classic heterochromia iridium or white forelock, but normal audiometry or only minimal or unilateral hearing loss. In these cases, only by examination of the whole family can we establish the correct diagnosis (Sensi et al., 1994). Moreover, the complete expression of the syndromal phenotype may be age-dependent so that hearing loss may be detected well before other symptoms, such as retinitis pigmentosa in Usher syndromes or goitre in Pendred syndrome. In these cases, a careful systematic search for the early subclinical manifestations, repeated over the years, can lead to the specific diagnosis.

On the other hand, hearing loss may develop very late and sometimes is detected just because the syndrome is suspected. Indeed, it is common in Alport syndrome to find subjects in whom hearing loss becomes clinically apparent after the renal involvement has already led to renal failure. Similarly, in Vohwinkel syndrome (mutilating keratoderma), the palmoplantar keratosis is evident from the first months of life, while hearing loss may be mild even in adulthood (Sensi et al., 1994). In these cases involvement of other organs is apparent, but the relationship between the first disease and hearing loss may be missed. Thus, faced with the diagnosis of syndromal hearing loss, the clinician must not miss the syndromal nature of hearing loss when only subclinical involvement of other systems or subtle dysmorphological elements are recognizable, and must correctly diagnose complex clinical pictures.

For the first aim a systematic approach is needed with a standard screening procedure targeted at conditions with syndromal hearing loss. Obviously, the approach must be adapted to the age and the general condition of the patients and the suggestions made here are merely indicative.

Excluding the specific audiological and vestibular examinations dealt with elsewhere in the text (Chapter 8) we shall consider only the anamnestic, physical, laboratory and specialist evaluations which should be included as the screening procedure (Table 12.1).

Table 12.1 Standard Screening Procedure.

- Specific clinical history (with pregnancy serological documentation)
- Dysmorphologic evaluation
- Pedigree analysis (with audiometric examination of all the first degree relatives)
- Ophthalmologic examination
- Electrocardiogram
- TSH and fT4
- Creatinine and urea nitrogen
- Venous blood pH
- Electrolytes
- Urine standard analysis.

Diagnostic evaluation of hearing impaired patients

Family and medical history

A detailed family history including at least three generations of family members has to be obtained. It is worth noting that syndromal hearing loss may or may not be genetic (monogenic, polygenic, mitochondrial or chromosomal), and that negative pedigrees are commonly found in both cases. Consanguinity and even remote family history of early onset or late onset of hearing loss have to be sought, and significant medical or physical features in deaf individuals or relatives, such as pigmentary alteration, structural anomalies (ear, cardiovascular, skeletal) must be evaluated. Photographs of other affected relatives for whom personal examination is not possible may prove helpful.

A history of the pregnancy with particular emphasis on prenatal exposure, prenatal events and postnatal events must be obtained, and serological tests performed during pregnancy should be recorded.

Special diagnostic tests

An ECG for QT evaluation should be always obtained in order to rule out Jervell Lange Nielsen syndrome, an autosomal recessive condition characterized by possible fainting attacks during which the affected subjects may die. Although the most specific test for Pendred syndrome diagnosis is the perchlorate test, the TSH and thyroxine determination together with physical examination of the neck can be considered a satisfactory screening procedure for practical clinical purposes.

Specialist ophthalmological evaluation should be always performed with indirect fundoscopy for the retinal periphery and slit lamp examination. The examination is of relevance not only for the detection of retinitis pigmentosa or optic atrophy, but also for congenital infections that very often reveal themselves as peripheral chorioretinal reliquates or lens opacification. Cataracts also occur in many metabolic conditions.

Psychomotor and neurological evaluations can be approached at a non-specialist level in a screening schedule, although the difficulties in assessing mental retardation by a non-specialist may be relevant in deaf children. Moreover, possible delays in walking may raise suspicions of vestibular involvement.

Urine sediment, creatinine, blood pH and serum electrolyte anomalies indicate the subjects needing further evaluation for conditions associating renal disease with hearing loss. A specific cytogenetic examination may be required after the dysmorphologic evaluation. Special procedures or also a targeted re-examination may be requested after one or more specific diagnostic hypotheses have been made. Reference to authoritative databases or texts is mandatory in this case.

The dysmorphologic approach

A dysmorphological evaluation requires a good knowledge of 'normality' and its variations and specific information about embryological development and its aberrations. To provide such information is beyond the scope of this section; here we try only to suggest how to observe and describe a patient with birth defects, with particular regard to the elements most relevant to syndromal hearing loss. Many minor abnormalities or variants may be of relevance only in the overall context of a diagnostic hypothesis, taking into account the familial and racial characteristics; however the more precise the description, the better.

A more detailed description of physical examination in dysmorphology and tables of normal physical measurements can be found in specific texts (Jones, 1988; Aase, 1990; Hall et al., 1989).

Face

The overall appearance of the face is first observed. However, comments of very little value such as 'sui generis face' or 'dysmorphic face' should be abandoned for a more analytic description.

Facial symmetry must be first assessed. Here we mention only the importance of this element in the diagnosis of the oculo-auricolo-vertebral spectrum (OAV). The general shape can be described as 'triangular' as in Treacher Collins syndrome (Chapter 20), 'square' as in CHARGE association, 'elongated' as in BOR syndrome (Chapter 19) or 'round' as in Cornelia de Lange syndrome. These general definitions are of value for the dysmorphologic description and sometimes are also relevant for the diagnosis. However, the specific regions of the face must also be examined in detail.

Skull

The form and symmetry of the skull are simply investigated with lateral, frontal and overhead observations. Palpation is useful for ridging, detection of sutures (seen in craniosynostosis) and to assess patency of fontanelles in young infants. The calvarium (neurocranium) may be distorted in different ways when one or more sutures fuse prematurely (Figure 12.1). Hearing loss (generally conductive) is frequently found in many genetically determined craniosynostoses.

The most important measurement of the skull is the occipitofrontal circumference which can be measured with a tape measure positioned from just above the glabella to the most prominent part of the occiput (the measure should be repeated for accuracy). Both microcephaly and macrocephaly are associated with hearing loss in different syndromes. Hearing loss syndromes with microcephaly are generally associated with neurological and/or mental impairments and other specific dysmorphologic findings, while macrocephalic conditions are often associated with skeletal and metabolic diseases.

Ocular region

In this region the examination can start with the supraorbital ridges which may be prominent as in frontometaphyseal dysplasia or flat as in most craniosynostoses. The palpebral fissures should be assessed to determine whether they are normally orientated (Figure 12.2), with inner and outer canthi on the same line when the face is carefully positioned vertically, or slanting upwards (outer canthi higher) as in branchio-oculo-facial (BOF) syndrome, or slanting downwards as in Treacher Collins syndrome.

The shape of the palpebral fissures has to be noted; among the most relevant findings for syndromal hearing loss diagnosis are a coloboma of the lower lid, pathognomonic of Treacher Collins syndrome and a cleft of the upper lid in Goldenhar syndrome.

The inner canthi may be covered by a skin fold from the upper lid, a morphological variant termed the 'epicanthic fold', frequently found in newborns and only rarely persistent after 18 months (Figure 12.2). It can be found in several chromosomal abnormalities, in BOF syndrome, in foetal alcohol syndrome and in many other syndromes.

Special attention must be paid to the observation and measure of three fundamental distances; inner canthal, outer canthal and inter-pupillary (Figure 12.2). These measures can be obtained with a simple transparent ruler with the eyes wide open (tables of normal values are available – Hall et al., 1989). Without these measurements it is difficult to distinguish between a flat nasal bridge and a true broad nasal bridge

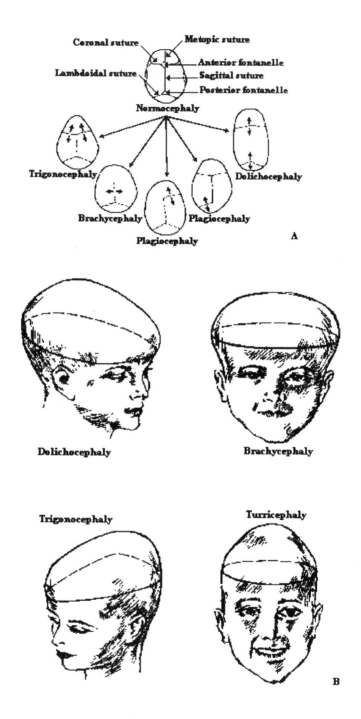

Figure 12.1 Craniosynostosis. A. Premature fusion of different cranial sutures and resulting skull growth (after Pruzansky, 1973). B. Cranial shapes in craniosynostoses (after Aase, 1990).

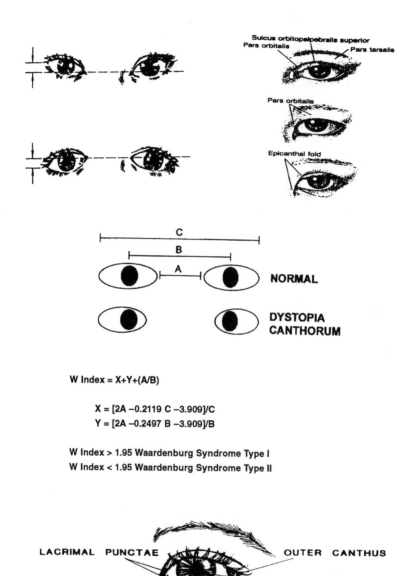

Figure 12.2 Elements of the ocular dysmorphology examination: Top left hand corner: upslanting ('mongoloid slant') and downslanting ('antimongoloid slant') palpebral fissures. Top right hand corner: normal eye, epicanthal fold (typically seen in orientals), epicanthal fold more frequent in Down' syndrome. Middle of page: dystopia canthorum assessment (see text). Bottom of the page: anatomical landmarks of the eye. (after Aase, 1990; Farrer et al., 1994; Goodman and Gorlin, 1977)

with hypertelorism. Hypertelorism and telecanthus must also be clearly differentiated; the former means that orbits are more distant than normal and both inner canthal and interpupillar distances are increased, the latter implies that only the inner canthi are laterally displaced, while the other measures are normal. These concepts are of particular relevance for Waardenburg syndrome type I (WS1) i.e. with telecanthus, and type II (WS2) i.e. with normal inner canthal distance. A special index (W index) was developed as an objective evaluation of dystopia canthorum. This W index (Figure 12.2), was calculated in WS1 (2.39± 0.32) as well as in unaffected (1.74±0.21) and WS2 individuals (1.66±0.30) (Farrer et al., 1992, 1994). Examination of the whole family is recommended for the correct diagnosis. As a screening procedure, it is useful to measure the inner canthal distance, easier to obtain and generally sufficient for raising suspicions.

The observation of the ocular globe can start with its protrusion, which can be influenced by the retrobulbar soft tissues or by the orbit conformation. Protruding eyes are seen in craniosynostoses because of shallow orbits; on the other hand deep set eyes may be noted in many conditions (Cockayne syndrome, for example).

Sclerae should be inspected for colour (blue in some osteogenesis imperfecta) and for presence of epibulbar dermoid (Goldenhar syndrome); irides should be very carefully observed for heterochromia and for colobomas. A complete specialist ophthalmological evaluation should be performed, as reported in the previous section.

Nose and midface

The nose plays a central role in giving the general impression of a face and should be observed carefully and accurately described. Thus the description should consider the nasal root, bridge and tip, the columella and alae nasi (Figure 12.3). The midfacial region includes the nose and the central part of the face, excluding the malar or zygomatic area.

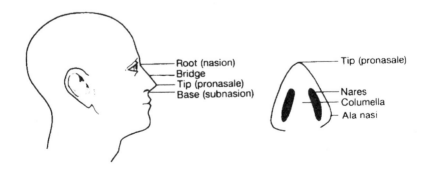

Figure 12.3 Anatomical landmarks of the nose.

A beaked nose is a hooked nose with a high nasal bridge, generally with a prominent columella and hypoplastic alae nasi, as is commonly seen in Crouzon, Saethre Chotzen and Johanson Blizzard syndromes.

A long tubular nose, with a prominent nasal bridge and hypoplastic alae nasi is typically seen in velocardiofacial syndrome. A long nose is commonly associated with a short philtrum; conversely a short nose is generally accompanied by a long philtrum and midfacial hypoplasia as in Apert syndrome. A broad nasal root, accompanied by hypertelorism, often with bifid nose and occult anterior encephalocele is seen in frontonasal malformation.

A nasal malformation of relevance for syndromal hearing loss is choanal atresia or choanal stenosis, seen in various conditions including Treacher Collins and CHARGE syndromes. Nasal pits or bulging of the nasal bridge should be carefully considered for their implication of an occult anterior encephalocele.

Malar area

Malar hypoplasia with flattening of zygomata is a common dysmorphism that should be distinguished from midfacial hypoplasia, although, obviously, the two elements are frequently associated. A flattened malar area is typically seen in Goldenhar syndrome (often asymmetrically), Treacher Collins syndrome and velocardiofacial syndrome.

Oral region and jaw

We omit the oral cavity which is obviously familiar to the ENT specialist. Cleft lip (midline or paramedian), cleft palate, the Pierre Robin sequence and jaw abnormalities are associated with many types of syndromal hearing loss. We shall outline only some specific minor elements that could be more easily overlooked.

Micro or retrognathia may imply microstoma, but in some conditions, such as Treacher Collins syndrome and OAV spectrum, they are frequently associated with true macrostoma and the presence of lateral clefts at the angles of the mouth.

The philtrum may be flattened as in foetal alcohol syndrome (in which hearing loss may be more frequent than in the general population), or deeply grooved as in Noonan syndrome or in BOF syndrome.

The mouth may be downturned, with a protruding lower lip (carp like) as in Apert syndrome. A protruding lower lip is seen in WS1, and thick lips may be one of the elements that gave the impression of a coarse face.

External ear.

Structural defects of the external ear are a part of more than 100 syndromes. Unfortunately, in most such conditions, these anomalies are non-specific, and their value in diagnosis is supportive rather than primary. Figure 12.4 shows the normal anatomy of the external ear and the position of the ear in relation to other facial structures.

Failure of complete migration of the ear angle leads to a low-set ear, whose position can lie anywhere between the original midline location and a point just slightly caudal to the normal site. Small ears, ears posteriorly rotated along their longitudinal axes or the appearance of low set ears is an illusion due to the head tilting or the shape of the cranium.

Ear length is measured by using a transparent ruler placed along the longest axis of the pinna. Inadequate neural crest and/or mesenchymal tissue in the proximal portion of the first and second branchial arches results in hypoplasia of the pinna or microtia. The severity of this anomaly ranges from a measurably small external ear with minimal structural abormality, to the ear with major structural alteration, or even to total absence of an ear. Anotia/microtia can be classified in four types; type I – a small auricle that retains most of the overall structure of the normal ear, type II – a longitudinal mass of cartilage that bears some resemblance to the pinna, type III – a rudimentary soft tissue with the auricle no longer similar to the normal pinna, type IV – no pinna tissue present at all. Types I–III are occasionally accompanied by a preauricular tag. Types II–IV are mostly (80%) associated with external auditory canal atresia; about 10% have ipsilateral facial nerve weakness; 14% are labelled as having hemifacial microsomia (Gorlin et al., 1990, 1995). Varying degrees of microtia are usually seen in syndromes involving developmental anomalies of the branchial arches, and the most important condition associated with microtia is the OAV spectrum. An association between microtia and cervical spine fusion (not as part of the OAV spectrum) is documented, suggesting that individuals with isolated microtia have to be investigated for the presence of cervical spine abnormalities. Even when the defect is unilateral (the right side is more frequently involved), hearing problems in the contralateral, normally formed, ear very frequently occur.

A subtle form of microtia is absence of the superior crus of the antelix, associated with at least a 15% incidence of ipsilateral hearing loss. Recognized environmental causes of microtia/anotia are isotretinoin and thalidomide embryopathies, foetal alcohol syndrome and maternal diabetes embryopathy.

Lop/cup ear is an anomaly of the auricle involving a downward folding and deficiency of the superior aspect of the helix, often associated with maldevelopment of the concha. Most of the syndromes that include microtia/anotia can also involve this milder auricular abnormality (BOR, Townes-Brocks and lacrimo-auricolo-dento-digital syndromes). Congenital external auditory canal atresia or stenosis without external ear malformation or microtia is uncommon (deletion 18q, trisomy 18, Rasmussen syndromes).

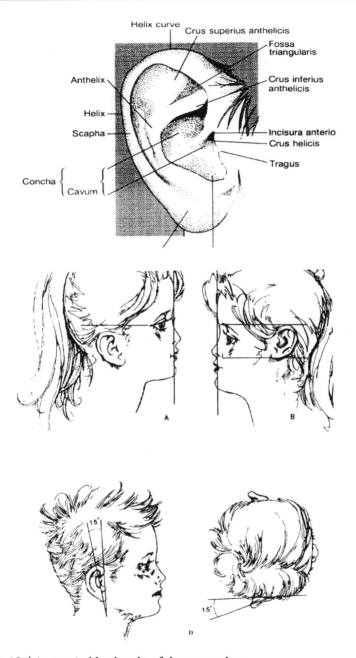

Figure 12.4 Anatomical landmarks of the external ear:
A. The line from the outer canthus should intersect the helix root (low set and posteriorly rotated ear).
B. The pinna should lie between the eyebrow and the base of the ala nasi as in this picture.
C. Orientation of the pinna should be about 15° posteriorly rotated.
D. Pinna also protrudes about 15° from the head.
(after Aase, 1990; Hall, 1989)

Preauricular appendages or tags (skin coloured, fleshy appendages represented as a nodule or skin protrusion) occur in about 0.5 – 1% of individuals. They are believed to represent remnants of early embryonic branchial cleft or arch structures and are located usually just in front of the auricle near the tragus. This defect varies in size from 1 – 2 mm to several centimetres, and can be pedunculate. The preauricular tags can extend down from just anterior to the tragus to the angle of the mouth; in this case the defect is frequently combined with other malformations (microtia) and is commonly seen in the OAV spectrum.

A pit depression (dimple) at the anterior margin of the ascending limb of the helix is associated with other malformations in 10% of individuals and is part of several syndromes (OAV spectrum, BOR syndrome).

Neck

The general inspection and palpation should be concentrated on the length of the neck, which may be reduced in vertebral abnormalities, such as Klippel Feil anomaly (seen in Wildervanck syndrome and MURCS association), or apparently shortened by the presence of lateral neck webbing as in Noonan syndrome. Abnormal masses should be detected, with special reference to the enlargement of the thyroid. Finally, branchial remnants should be carefully looked for. Their relevance for the diagnosis of BOR syndrome has been outlined elsewhere.

Chest and abdomen

The chest and abdomen should be included in any physical examination. Heart defects are a feature of many hearing loss syndromes, and of particular diagnostic significance in velocardiofacial syndrome. Special attention should be paid to observation of the abdomen for hepatosplenomegaly that could suggest a metabolic disease, and for megacolon seen in WS and in specific conditions associated with hearing loss.

Limbs

The recording of height, span (measure of the distance between the tips of the middle fingers of each hand when the upper limbs are placed horizontally) and lower segment length are generally sufficient to raise the suspicion of skeletal dysplasias that are associated with hearing loss (generally conductive). Reference tables have to be used (Hall et al., 1989).

A measure of total length of the hand together with the palm length should always be recorded and reference tables consulted. Polydactyly, syndactyly and brachydactyly are associated with syndromal hearing loss. Radial ray abnormalities are common features of Nager syndrome. When some impression of alteration of the normal proportions is raised, a metacarpophalangeal profile should be drawn from a suitable radiograph (Hall et al., 1989). The inspection of the hand should be completed taking note of the presence of abnormal lines. The single palmar crease is a non-specific finding, but can contribute to the definition of specific phenotypes as in chromosomal disorders, or in sequelae of intra-uterine environmental conditions.

Skin and adnexa

Pigmentary abnormalities of the skin and hair in WS have been discussed in the introduction to this chapter and in Chapter 16. Skin should be also inspected for café au lait spots which are a hallmark of neurofibromatosis. Multiple lentigenes should not be overlooked, as they are a component of LEOPARD syndrome. Disorders of keratinization are also associated with hearing loss. Nail examination should be recorded, because of the association between onychodystrophy and hearing loss.

Chapter 13
Auditory dysfunction in genetic disorders of the skeleton

PETER BEIGHTON

Introduction

Hearing impairment is a component of a large number of genetic disorders in which the skeleton is primarily involved. In many of these conditions the pathological processes leading to hearing loss are progressive and the impairment may eventually be profound. In some disorders of this type the auditory dysfunction is overshadowed by other syndromal features, while in others the hearing deficit is the major clinical problem. The main categories of genetic skeletal disorders in which involvement of the hearing mechanism is an important feature are:

- Sclerosing bone dysplasias.
- Dwarfing skeletal dysplasias.
- Osteogenesis imperfecta.
- Mucopolysaccharidoses.
- Craniofacial malformation syndromes.
- Miscellaneous skeletal disorders.

The fact that the auditory dysfunction is predominantly conductive in many of the genetic skeletal conditions, and sensorineural or mixed in others has important implications for treatment. Similarly, the mode of inheritance and the severity of the clinical manifestations are very relevant in the context of genetic management.

The terminology of the genetic disorders of the skeleton is complex but details can be found in the International Classification of Osteochondrodysplasias (Spranger et al., 1992; Beighton et al., 1992). Further information concerning the conditions mentioned in this chapter is provided in a number of reviews and monographs (Beighton 1988 a,b,

1990; Beighton and Sellars, 1982). The classical monograph Syndromes of the Head and Neck by Gorlin, Cohen and Levin (1990) is especially informative in this field.

Sclerosing bone dysplasias

The sclerosing bone dysplasias are a group of genetic disorders which are characterised by overgrowth and increased radiological density of the skeleton (Beighton and Cremin, 1980) (Figure 13.1). These conditions are differentiated by their clinical and radiological manifestations; at the mild end of the spectrum, the clinical stigmata are trivial (as in osteopetrosis), while at the severe end, the changes may be gross (as in sclerosteosis) (Figure 13.2). Although rare, the sclerosing bone dysplasias are given prominence here as severe auditory impairment is a consistent feature of many conditions in this group. The various sclerosing bone dysplasias in which auditory impairment is a feature are listed in Table 13.1. Hearing loss is progressive and predominantly the result of entrapment of the eighth cranial nerves due to bone overgrowth in the cranial foramina. In addition, to a lesser extent, the bony capsules of the middle and inner ears may be involved. Cranial nerve decompression, with or without additional surgical measures, is often helpful, as is the provision of a hearing aid. It is noteworthy, however, that surgical operation may be difficult due to the hyperostosis and the hard texture of the abnormal bone. A detailed account of the conditions in this category can be found in the monograph Sclerosing Bone Dysplasias (Beighton and Cremin, 1980).

Dwarfing skeletal dysplasias

Stunted stature is the major clinical feature of more than 100 heritable

Table 13.1 The sclerosing bone dysplasias with hearing loss.

Condition	Inheritance	Reference
Osteopetrosis with delayed manifestations	AD	Beighton et al., 1977
Craniometaphyseal dysplasia	AD/AR	Beighton et al., 1979
Craniodiaphyseal dysplasia	AR	MacPherson 1974
Frontometaphyseal dysplasia	XL/AD	Beighton and Hamersma, 1980
Endosteal hyperostosis AD type (Worth)	AD	Worth and Wollin, 1966
Endosteal hyperostosis AR type (van Buchem)	AR	van Buchem et al., 1962
Sclerosteosis	AR	Beighton, 1988
Diaphyseal dysplasia (Camurati-Engelmann)	AD	Sparkes and Graham, 1972
Osteopathia striata with cranial sclerosis	AD	Horan and Beighton, 1978
Oculodento-osseous dysplasia	AD/AR	Gorlin et al., 1963; Beighton et al., 1979

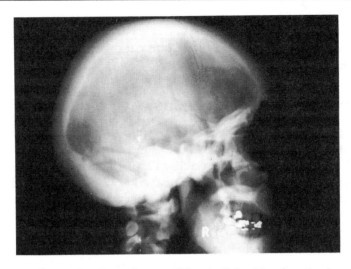

Figure 13.1 Sclerosteosis. Lateral X-ray of the skull. In this sclerosing bone dysplasia the bones of the calvarium and of the skull are hyperostotic and dense. Hearing loss and facial palsy are common complications, due to entrapment of the seventh and eighth cranial nerves in their foramina. Reproduced from Beighton P., Inherited Disorders of the Skeleton, 2nd ed, Churchill Livingstone, Edinburgh, 1988, with permission.

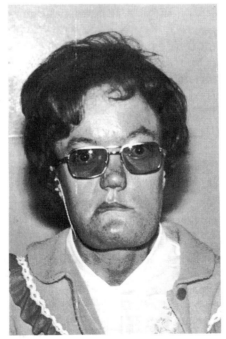

Figure 13.2 Sclerosteosis. The face of a woman with sclerosteosis. The mandible is asymmetrical and massive, the teeth are malpositioned and the eyes are proptotic. Bone overgrowth has resulted in cranial nerve compression, which has led to hearing loss and facial paralysis. Reproduced from Beighton P. and Cremin B. Sclerosing Bone Dysplasias, Springer Verlag, 1980, with permission.

skeletal disorders, and conditions of this type in which the hearing mechanism is often involved are briefly reviewed in this section. The molecular genetics of these conditions is particularly interesting; different mutations in the same gene may be responsible for different conditions, while in some cases the same condition can result from mutations in more than one gene. Knowledge in this area has advanced extremely rapidly over the past few years.

Achondroplasia, which is by far the most common of the dwarfing skeletal dysplasias, is characterised by limb shortening, a normal trunk and a typical facies, with a bulky forehead and a depressed nasal bridge. The root cause is a mutation in the fibroblast growth factor receptor 3 (*FGFR3*) gene at 4p16 that replaces glycine 380 by arginine (Shiang et al., 1994); remarkably, this particular aminoacid substitution is found in almost every case, even though most cases represent independent mutational events. Other mutations in the same gene can cause *thanatophoric dysplasia* (Tavormina et al., 1995) and *hypochondroplasia* (Bellus et al., 1995). Airway obstruction due to choanal stenosis predisposes to recurrent upper respiratory tract infection. These infections occur in the majority of affected children and may lead to chronic otitis media. This complication is exacerbated by malformation of the auditory ossicle which is sometimes present. Prompt and thorough treatment of middle ear infection is indicated, and removal of the adenoids and the insertion of grommets may be necessary. In the long term, with effective treatment, hearing loss is rarely severe in this disorder. Otosclerosis may be an additional cause of hearing loss in adult achondroplasts.

Progressive hearing loss has been documented in *spondylo-epiphyseal dysplasia congenita* (Spranger and Maroteaux, 1983) and *Kniest dysplasia* (Dobin and Daniel, 1988). The auditory dysfunction is very variable in these uncommon forms of dwarfism but it is usually conductive in type; it is likely that this complication is the consequence of bony malformation of the middle ear structures, perhaps with concomitant chronic otitis media. These two conditions form part of the spectrum of type II collagenopathies, a category that includes severe achondrogenesis II, hypochondrogenesis and spondyloepimetaphyseal dysplasias, all of which are usually caused by mutations in type II collagen (Mortier et al., 1995).

Diastrophic dysplasia is characterised by severe dwarfism in association with a rigid club foot and a stiff 'hitch-hiker' thumb. A notable otological feature is repeated episodes of spontaneous inflammation of the pinna of the ear during infancy, which lead to a 'cauliflower' or 'pugilistic' configuration. Hearing loss is infrequent in diastrophic dysplasia. Diastrophic dysplasia is especially common in Finland and following molecular investigations involving 84 affected individuals in 13 families, the faulty gene has been mapped to chromosome 5q31-34 (Hastbacka et al., 1991), and recently cloned (Hastbacka et al., 1994). The gene encodes a sulphate transporter, and other mutations in the same gene can cause achondrogenesis type IB and atelogenesis type II.

Osteogenesis imperfecta

Osteogenesis imperfecta (OI) is a well-known disorder in which bone fragility leads to frequent fractures. Other variable syndromic components include blue sclerae, dentinogenesis imperfecta and hearing loss. The condition is clinically and genetically heterogeneous; some affected individuals have severe disturbance of growth, while others have normal stature. Equally, the fracturing tendency may be severe, with residual limb and spinal malalignment, or comparatively trivial, with few fractures and little disability. The radiological appearances of the skeleton vary from normality to chaos, and the presence of Wormian bones in the cranial sutures is the only consistent feature (Figure 13.3).

Osteogenesis imperfecta is conventionally divided into four main categories, on a basis of the phenotypical appearances and mode of inheritance. In molecular terms, however, all forms can be caused by defects in one or other of the collagen I chains. The autosomal dominant type I OI, which is by far the most common form, is characterised by the classical stigmata in mild to moderate degree. Hearing loss develops in early adulthood in about 40% of persons with this form of OI. This auditory dysfunction does not usually progress to total deafness, but neverthe-

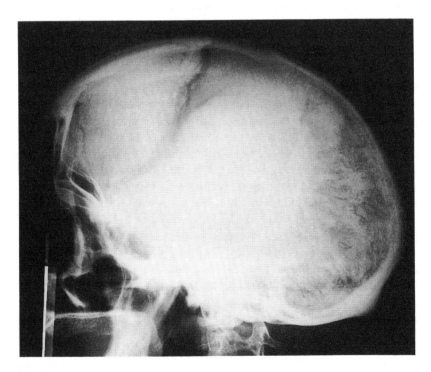

Figure 13.3 Osteogenesis imperfecta. Lateral X-ray of the skull showing marked Wormian bones in the occipital region.

less, it represents an important complication. The pathogenesis is an otosclerotic-like process in the middle ear in which the auditory ossicles are fixed by overgrowth of soft, chalky bone. The inner ear is sometimes involved and the hearing loss may be sensorineural or mixed in type (Riedner et al., 1980). There has been considerable controversy concerning the inter-relationship of OI and classical otosclerosis, but it is now generally accepted that these conditions are separate entities.

The auditory deficit in OI is managed along conventional lines. Hearing aids are often helpful, and if there is a significant conductive component, surgical exploration of the middle ear may be warranted. Excision of overgrown bone, stapedectomy or mobilisation of the stapes footplate may all be indicated, and some improvement of hearing is frequently obtained (Pedersen, 1985).

Mucopolysaccharidoses

The mucopolysaccharidoses (MPS) are a group of metabolic disorders which bear numerical and eponymous designations. Types I–VII are well established and several sub-types have been defined. All forms involve heteroglycan metabolism, and each has a specific enzymatic deficiency and a unique pattern of glycosaminoglycan excretion in the urine. The MPS group of conditions share the general manifestations of dwarfism, intellectual impairment, hepato-splenomegaly, a coarse facies, corneal clouding and generalised radiological changes in the skeleton (dysostosis multiplex). They are all inherited as autosomal recessive traits, with the exception of type II (Hunter syndrome) which is X-linked. The MPS disorders have been extensively reviewed by Whiteley (1992).

MPS type I (Hurler syndrome) and *MPS type II (Hunter syndrome)* are by far the most common forms, and it is significant that the hearing mechanism is involved in both these entities. The majority of children with Hurler syndrome have some degree of mixed hearing loss; this problem results from middle ear inflammation due to repeated upper respiratory tract infections which, in turn, are the consequence of malformation of the cranio-facial skeleton and distortion of the airways. The accumulation of glycosaminoglycans in the middle and inner ears contributes to the hearing loss, as does limitation of movement of the auditory ossicles (Schachern, 1984). Assessment of the hearing loss is difficult because of the mental retardation in this form of the disorder, and management is strongly influenced by the fact that the condition is progressive, with life expectancy not usually exceeding 10 years. Prompt treatment of the upper respiratory tract infections and the insertion of tympanic grommets are the conventional management modalities.

In MPS type II (Hunter syndrome) some degree of hearing loss eventually develops in the majority of affected persons. Although clinical features are comparatively severe, intellectual impairment is mild and survival into adulthood is frequent. The hearing loss, which is usually 'mixed' in type, results from a combination of chronic middle ear infection and glycosaminoglycan infiltration of the otic ganglion (Shapiro et al., 1985; Zechner and Moser, 1987). An otosclerotic process may also develop in the labyrinthine capsule. Management of the hearing loss revolves around prompt treatment of infections, adenoidectomy, insertion of grommets when necessary and, in appropriate circumstances, the provision of a hearing aid (Peck, 1984).

Hearing is usually normal in the *MPS type III* (*San Filippo syndrome*). In *MPS type IV* (*Morquio syndrome*), which is rare, progressive sensorineural or mixed hearing loss often develops in late childhood (Sataloff et al., 1987). In *MPS type VI* (*Maroteaux-Lamy syndrome*), which is also rare, conductive hearing loss consequent upon middle ear infection is common. The status of the hearing mechanism in *MPS type VII* (*Sly syndrome*) has not been documented.

Craniofacial malformation syndromes

A number of well established genetic entities are the consequence of craniostenosis and/or disturbance of growth of the facial bones and branchial arch structures (Cohen, 1975). The hearing mechanism is involved, to a greater or lesser extent, in the majority of these disorders. The more important of these conditions are briefly reviewed below.

Apert syndrome or acrocephalosyndactyly is characterised by a high forehead (turricephaly), proptosis, hypertelorism, a hooked nose and gross syndactyly of the fingers and toes ('mitten' hands and feet) (Figures 13.4 a,b). Variable mental retardation is an additional feature. Inheritance is autosomal dominant; the majority of affected persons represent new gene mutations and a paternal age effect has been demonstrated. The cause is certain specific mutations in the fibroblast growth factor receptor 2 (*FGFR2*) gene at 10q25 (Wilkie et al., 1995). Malformation of the bony components of the upper airways, sometimes with cleft palate, predisposes to recurrent otitis media, and hearing deficit may result (Bergstrom et al., 1972; Cohen and Kreiborg, 1992). Fixation of the stapedial footplate may also be present. Mental retardation and the unsightly cosmetic appearance overshadow the hearing loss, which may pass unnoticed.

Crouzon syndrome resembles Apert syndrome in craniofacial appearance, but the hands and feet are not involved and mentality is usually normal (Figure 13.5). Inheritance is autosomal dominant, with very variable phenotypic expression. The same gene, *FGFR2*, is involved as in Apert syndrome, but different aminoacids are mutated (Reardon et al., 1994). Some degree of hearing loss is present in about 55% of affect-

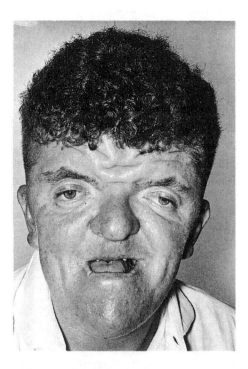

Figure 13.4a Apert syndrome. An adult male with turricephaly and hypertelorism. Mild mixed hearing loss and marked mental retardation were additional syndromic features. Reproduced from Beighton P. Inherited Disorders of the Skeleton, 2nd ed, Churchill Livingstone, Edinburgh, 1988, with permission.

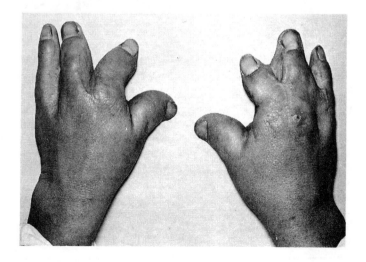

Figure 13.4b Apert syndrome. The hands of the patient showing the characteristic 'mitten' syndactyly.

ed persons (Kreiborg, 1981). This auditory deficit is conductive in type, and results from a combination of constriction of the external auditory meatus, calcification of the stylohyoid ligaments and chronic middle ear infection.

Treacher Collins syndrome or mandibulo-facial dysostosis is a well recognised disorder with a frequency of about 1 in 50,000 live births. The clinical features and genetics are described in detail in Chapter 20. The majority of affected persons have structural abnormalities of the external ears together with narrowing of the auditory meati (Lloyd and Phelps, 1979). The middle ear, auditory ossicles, cochlea and vestibules are frequently malformed and significant conductive hearing loss is present in about 30% of affected persons (Lloyd and Phelps, 1979). The inner ear is usually normal. The auditory deficit is often severe, and in several surveys of special educational facilities for persons with hearing impairment, the Treacher Collins syndrome has been recognised in

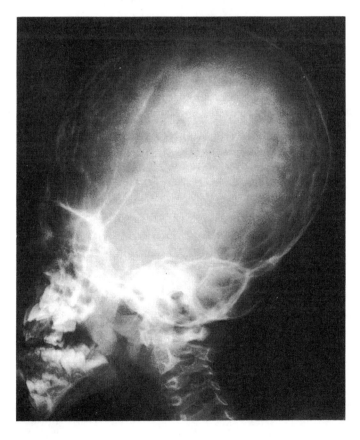

Figure 13.5 Crouzon syndrome. Lateral X-ray of the skull of an affected woman showing gross turricephaly.

about 1 – 2% of the deaf scholars (Sellars and Beighton, 1983). The accurate diagnosis of this condition is crucial, as the middle ear abnormalities may be amenable to surgical intervention, with prospects of significant improvement or restoration of hearing.

Miscellaneous skeletal or articular syndromes

Hearing loss is a variable component of a number of uncommon genetic skeletal disorders which are outside the scope of this chapter. For completeness, however, the most important of these conditions are listed in Table 13.2.

Table 13.2 Miscellaneous skeletal or articular syndromes with hearing loss.

Condition	Inheritance	Reference
Stickler syndrome (hereditary arthro-ophthalmopathy)	AD	Popkin and Polomeno, 1974
Trichorhinophalangeal dysplasia	AD	Weaver et al., 1974
Digital arthrogryposis-perceptive hearing loss syndrome	AD	Akbarnia et al., 1979
Otopalatodigital syndrome	XL	Gorlin et al., 1973
Orofacialdigital syndrome Type II (Mohr syndrome)	AR	Rimoin and Edgerton, 1967
Multiple synostosis-conductive hearing loss	AD	Herrmann, 1974
Dominant symphalangism-conductive hearing loss	AD	Spoendlin, 1974
Ectrodactyly, ectodermal dysplasia, clefting mixed hearing loss	AR/AD	Bixler et al., 1971; Bonafede and Beighton, 1979
Digital contractures, hypertelorism, perceptive hearing loss	AD	Bogard and Lieber, 1977
Radial ray hypoplasia, external ophthalmoplegia, thrombocytopenia and mixed hearing loss (IVIC syndrome)	AD	Arias et al., 1980
Fibrodysplasia ossificans progressiva	AD	Connor and Evans, 1982

This list is reproduced in modified form from the chapter on hereditary deafness in Principles and Practice of Medical Genetics, Eds Emery AEH and Rimoin DI, 1990 (Beighton, 1990).

Comment

Although they are individually rare, collectively the genetic disorders of the skeleton are not uncommon. The hearing mechanism is primarily or secondarily involved in many of them and taken together, they make a significant contribution to the overall burden of hearing dysfunction. Management of the hearing loss is dependent upon the nature of the underlying defect, which varies from disorder to disorder. In some of these conditions, hearing can be improved by surgical intervention, while in others the additional syndromic components and natural history greatly influence management directions. For all these reasons, diagnostic precision is crucial. Recent advances in molecular understanding have in some cases made diagnosis more secure.

Chapter 14
Usher syndrome

WILLIAM J KIMBERLING and RICHARD JH SMITH

Background

Usher syndrome (US) is an autosomal recessive disorder characterised by hearing loss and retinitis pigmentosa (RP). Von Graefe (1858) first noted the simultaneous occurrence of hearing loss with retinitis pigmentosa, and the heritable nature of US was recognised by Liebreich (1861). Usher (1914) described the recessive pattern of inheritance and is the clinical scientist for whom the disorder has been named. The phenotypic heterogeneity of Usher syndrome was remarked on by several early researchers (e.g. see Bell, 1933) but it was Hallgren (1959) who clearly pointed out that at least two distinct type of Usher syndrome existed in a study of a large series of Swedish Usher patients. Although most medical geneticists were suspicious that two or more different genes were involved (Merin et al., 1974; Davenport and Omenn, et al., 1977; Fishman, 1979; Fishman et al., 1983) the issue remained unresolved until the underlying genetic heterogeneity was revealed by a linkage analysis study (Kimberling et al., 1990). Over the next years, further linkage and positional cloning research established that the genetic heterogeneity of Usher syndrome was far more extensive than first thought and that at least five genetically distinct types exist.

Characteristic findings

Hallgren (1959) brought attention to the fact that two different US types appeared to exist. The first, Usher type I, is characterised by a profound hearing loss, vestibulocerebellar ataxia, and retinitis pigmentosa. Patients with Usher type II have a milder hearing loss, normal vestibular reflexes, and retinitis pigmentosa. The two phenotypes rarely occur together in the same family.

The severity of hearing impairment is highly correlated with the genetic type. Patients with type I have a profound hearing loss. They

141

seldom have any residual hearing, rarely use hearing aids, and always have poor speech. Type II patients show a sloping loss which is milder in the low frequencies and more severe in the higher frequencies; most type II patients benefit from hearing aids and can effectively use oral communication. The audiometric profile within subtypes is consistent and the extent of the variability for both types is quite limited. Hearing loss in both types I and II is stable over age and does not usually progress any more than expected by way of the normal ageing process. An exception to this rule occurs with Usher type III. These patients show a progressive hearing loss (Karjalainen et al., 1989). Type III patients may be erroneously diagnosed as either type I or II since in the younger patient the hearing impairment is milder and mimics type II, and in the older patient the hearing is more impaired and the phenotype mimics that of type I. Families with sibs who appear to have both type I and II may actually have Usher type III. For all types, the hearing loss is symmetrical and, for any single patient, of the same approximate degree in both ears (Möller et al., 1989, Smith et al., 1994).

The second important distinguishing sign between types I and II Usher syndrome is the presence or absence of vestibular responses. The vestibular system in type I Usher patients is non-functional while it appears to be normal in all type II patients. It is the vestibular areflexia, not a cerebellar defect, that gives rise to the apparent 'ataxia' seen in Usher type I patients. The issue of vestibular involvement in type III remains unresolved.

The diagnosis of retinitis pigmentosa is the *sine qua non* of Usher syndrome. Although fundus changes vary between patients, there is no recognised pattern of fundus involvement that is correlated with any specific type or subtype. The RP is responsible for the night blindness and restricted visual fields characteristic of this disorder.

Table 14.1 shows a summary of the characteristics of the Usher syndromes.

Prevalence

The frequency of US has been estimated at between 3 to 5 per 100,000 (Grondahl, 1986; Hallgren, 1959; Boughman, Vernon, and Shaver, 1983). Higher frequencies have been observed in certain regions such as Northern Sweden and Louisiana. The prevalence of US in the deaf population ranges from 0.6 to 28%, but most researchers accept the estimate that about 5% of all children in schools for the deaf have US. The frequency of hearing impairment in the RP population is estimated to range between 8.0 and 33.3% (Bell, 1933; Schleuren, 1935). Overall, there are about 16,000 deaf and blind people in the United States, of which more than half are believed to have Usher syndrome.

Table 14.1 Classification of Usher syndrome.

Type	Gene	Localisation	Hearing	Vestibular	Visual
I	*USHIA* uncommon *USHIB* (common) *USHIC* (Acadian)	14q31-ter 11q13-14 (Myosin VIIa) 11p13-14	Severe to profound hearing loss involving all frequencies (deaf). Congenital.	Absent vestibular responses.	Retinitis pigmentosa with diagnosis usually in the preteenage years.
II	*USHIIA* (common) *USHIIA* (rare)	1q32-41 Unknown	Sloping moderate to profound hearing loss (hard of hearing). Congenital.	Normal vestibular responses.	Diagnosis often made later, after puberty.
III	*USHIII* (rare)	3q	Progressive hearing loss. May have normal hearing at birth.	Hypoactive to normal vestibular reflexes.	Not well differentiated from types I and II.

The more severe type I appears to comprise about 90% of Usher syndrome in the United States, with type II accounting for nearly 10%, and other types accounting for only about 1%. The linkage subtypes have only recently been elucidated and so their relative proportions can only be roughly approximated. Type IB is the most prevalent severe subtype and type IIA the is the more prevalent milder form. Type III appears to have a higher frequency in the Finnish population and type IC is found in the Louisiana Acadian population. Type IA comprises 20 – 30% of US in the USA and may occur in a higher frequency in certain regions of France. Little is known about the ethnic distribution of the various Usher syndrome genes, and population studies are needed to appreciate whether any of the rarer types could be more frequent in some of the as yet unstudied populations.

Gene localisation and identification

Usher type I

The Usher syndrome type I gene was first localised to chromosome 14q by linkage with a DNA polymorphism (D14S13) in fifteen French families (Kaplan, et al., 1992). The test for genetic heterogeneity was significant, suggesting the possibility that two or more different genes were involved. Further work revealed that two other type I loci existed, one on 11q and another on 11p (Kimberling, 1992; Smith et al., 1992). The linkage to 11q occurred in families of mixed European ancestry while that to 11p occurred only in families from the French Acadian population in Louisiana. These loci have been given the designations of *USH1A* (14q), *USH1B* (11q), and *USH1C* (11p). Mutations at the *USH1B* locus appear to cause about 75% of all Usher type I cases while those at the *USH1A* locus are responsible for most of the remaining cases. *USH1C* is rare outside of the Acadian population.

The *USH1B* locus lies close to the region where the mouse mutation known as *shaker-1* (*sh1*) is found (Brown et al., 1992). *Sh1* causes hearing loss with vestibular disturbances. No retinitis pigmentosa has been observed. A mutation in the myosin VIIa gene was found to be responsible for the *sh1* phenotype (Gibson, et al., 1995). When Usher patients were screened for mutations in the human myosin VII gene, several mutations were observed, thus establishing the myosin VIIa gene to be responsible for Usher type IB (Weil et al., 1995). The exact role of this unconventional myosin in the inner ear and retina is not yet fully understood. However, myosin-like proteins are present in both tissues and it has been postulated that it may play a role as part of the transduction motor, or in some other not yet defined cytoskeletal function.

Usher type II

Usher syndrome type II was localised to chromosome 1q32 (Kimberling et al., 1990; Lewis, 1990). The gene has subsequently been shown to be flanked by the markers D1S237 and D1S229 and has been mapped to approximately 1 megabase of DNA. An autosomal homologue of the X-linked choroideraemia gene, known as *hCHML*, had been localised to 1q. This gene shows homology with a bovine protein which regulates the GDP/GTP exchange of GTP binding protein smg 25A. It is expressed in the choroid/retinal pigment epithelium and several other tissues. It is not known if it is expressed in the cochlea. This has been localised to 1q31-41 and hence must be considered a logical candidate for Usher syndrome.

A potential mouse model for Usher syndrome type II has recently been discovered by Chang et al. (1993). The RBF/DnJ albino mouse carries a recessive mutation, *rd3*, which causes a retinal degeneration similar to retinitis pigmentosa, but which does not produce any hearing impairment. Electroretinograms and retinal appearance are both suggestive of human type RP. The *rd3* gene maps to 10 cM distal to the alkaline phosphatase gene on mouse chromosome 1. This region shows considerable homology with human chromosome 1. The region where the *rd3* mouse gene would lie is theoretically close to the position where the mouse homologue for the Usher type II gene should lie.

Originally, only one family with Usher type II was observed not to be linked to markers in the 1q41 region (Pieke Dahl, et al., 1993). This family also failed to show linkage to markers on 11q, 11p, or 14q and was given the designation *USH2B*, leaving *USH2A* to refer to the original 1q locus. Subsequently, analysis of a larger series of USA and European

Usher type II families revealed that about 12% were not linked to 1q41 markers (Kimberling et al., 1995). Sankila et al. (1994) showed that a set of Usher families from Finland linked to markers on chromosome 3q. These families showed a characteristic progressive hearing loss with variable vestibular involvement. Of the 7 USA and European families unlinked to 1q41, 5 were found to be linked to the 3q region and re-evaluation of the phenotype revealed that they had a progressive hearing loss. We have observed two families with Usher type II symptoms that fail to link with any of the known Usher loci.

Conclusions

Usher syndrome was first described as hearing impairment with retinitis pigmentosa. Investigators have realised that at least two clinical types exist and that they can be consistently and reliably distinguished from each other. However, linkage analysis has shown that a minimum of five different genes are involved, 3 for type I and two for type II with possibly two additional genes. Unfortunately, no clear clinical differences between the different subtypes within each type has become evident.

The next stage of Usher research should be focused on identifying and cloning the responsible genes. The discovery that myosin VIIa is responsible for Usher IB is an important step forward in understanding the biological basis of these disorders. It certainly suggests that the other Usher genes may be coding for different unconventional myosins or genes which interact with myosin VIIa. It will also be of value to begin correlating the phenotype with the locus involved, in the hope of determining whether different mutations produce different phenotypes.

One important use of this genetic information is for genetic counselling. Given tight linkage and an informative family with one previously affected child, early diagnosis is possible for subsequent children. The markers showing tight linkage could also be used to determine which of the unaffected relatives are carriers. Effective screening of spouses who marry into a family will become more feasible as the Usher genes are identified and mutations are characterised.

The goal of genetic research is to develop a treatment for Usher syndrome. More information about the role of the unconventional myosins in the inner ear is needed. Furthermore, an understanding of the underlying pathological process occurring from mutant myosin VII gene to phenotype, and the elucidation of the roles of the other Usher genes will be important steps towards finding an effective method of remediation and/or prevention. Considering the tremendous burden imposed by the loss of both major senses and the fact that Usher syndrome is now the major cause of hearing loss/blindness, it is important to pursue research into the causes of Usher syndrome in the hope that an effective remediation may become possible.

Chapter 15
Pendred syndrome

WILLIAM REARDON and RICHARD C TREMBATH

Introduction

The natural history of the syndrome first described by Vaughan Pendred in 1896 has not followed a streamlined course, largely due to the variable clinical presentation and the absence of a specific diagnostic test. Pendred reported an Irish family, resident in the North of England, in which 2 adult females were deaf and had large goitres, the first evidence of which was dated from the age of 13 (Pendred, 1896). Over thirty years later and without reference to Pendred's report, Brain presented details of 4 families with 2 or more children affected (Brain, 1927). This report is noteworthy for the significant variability as to the extent of thyroid involvement and age of onset of goitre in the individuals described. Phenotypic variability and, occasionally, difficulty in classifying families/individuals as Pendred syndrome or otherwise, are central themes emerging from Fraser's study of 207 families, comprising 334 cases of Pendred syndrome (Fraser, 1965). Not only does this rigorous and carefully documented report represent the benchmark against which all other studies of Pendred syndrome have to be compared, but it clearly established the condition as an important and relatively common cause of inherited hearing loss, estimating a prevalence of 75 cases per million population.

That hearing loss and thyroid dysfunction are aetiologically related is beyond dispute. Trotter summarised the situation in 1960, distinguishing clearly between hearing loss in relation to endemic cretinism/goitre, and sporadic goitre with hearing loss (Pendred syndrome) (Trotter, 1960). He drew attention to the several reports identifying unusually high rates of hearing loss in geographically distinct areas noted to be regions of endemic goitre. Frequently the hearing loss and goitre were observed in the same individuals and a likely causative link was further substantiated by the observation in Switzerland of a positive correlation between the falling incidence of hearing loss over time and the extent of salt iodization. Citing the reports of Pendred and Brain as well as several other sibships documented in the intervening years, Trotter emphasised the intrinsically different condition represented by the association of sporadic goitre and congenital hearing loss, frequently seen in several members of the same family, in areas where the prevalence of goitre was low. He endorsed Brain's conclusion that a single gene defect was responsible for both the hearing loss and goitre. Trotter made several clinical observations which remain pertinent today. Vigilance is the key to the identification of cases – it is clear that once Trotter and colleagues, including Fraser, started to look for patients with the disorder, they were surprised at the high prevalence of a condition which was only beginning to be recognised as a distinct entity. They defined the syndrome as 'the association of some degree of congenital hearing loss with a demonstrable thyroid abnormality'. The variability of thyroid involvement was again demonstrated from Fraser's initial report of 13 families (Fraser et al., 1960). Finally, the limitations of surgical treatment were recorded, almost all cases of goitre recurring after partial thyroidectomy.

The proportion of genetic hearing loss attributable to Pendred syndrome is uncertain, Fraser's estimate of 7.5% of all childhood hearing loss considerably exceeding more recent estimates (Coakley et al., 1992). The 7.5% estimate was derived from an adult deaf population, the argument being that the lower figures, varying from 4.3 to 6.4% obtained in large scale studies of paediatric deaf populations masked those cases of Pendred syndrome in whom the goitre was not detectable in childhood (Fraser, 1965). That this high prevalence figure has not been corroborated in later studies may, at least in part, reflect difficulties in ascertainment, there being no single definitive diagnostic test for the condition. Fraser's criteria for the diagnosis were congenital hearing loss, goitre and a positive perchlorate discharge test (Figure 15.1). Latterly some authors have advocated that a Mondini malformation of the cochlea be included as an essential prerequisite to the diagnosis (Johnsen et al., 1989a) and have recognised a degree of plasticity in the matter of goitre.

Audiovestibular studies in Pendred syndrome.

Although minimal disturbance of hearing has been recorded, typically the disturbance is of moderate to severe degree sensorineural loss, being more pronounced in the higher frequencies. The hearing loss is thought to be congenital and is certainly prelingual in most cases (Fraser 1965). One report of seventeen unrelated cases found evidence of progression of the hearing impairment in three patients and also identified one case in which the hearing dysfunction escaped detection until the age of 16 years (Johnsen et al., 1987).

The data concerning vestibular disturbance are less uniform. While several authors refer to variable degrees of dysfunction

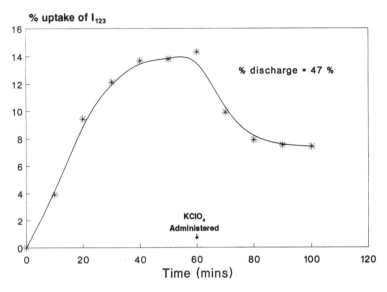

Figure 15.1 Perchlorate discharge test. Note the avid uptake of radiolabelled iodide by the thyroid gland and the sharp fall in radioactivity within the gland as the radiolabelled iodide is discharged immediately following perchlorate administration. In this patient the discharge was calculated at 47%.

(Arnvig, 1955; Fraser 1965; Johnsen et al., 1987), others have reported to the contrary (Illum et al., 1972; Das, 1987). Indeed McKusick referred to vestibular disturbance as a particular feature of one group of patients in his personal experience (McKusick et al., 1994). However, many of these references are dated, the diagnostic criteria being predominantly clinical. In addition, the only series of cases published (Johnsen et al., 1987) could hardly be considered definitive. For the record, ten of the fourteen cases investigated showed normal responses bilaterally.

Thyroid dysfunction in Pendred syndrome

Goitre was an essential element of the diagnosis in the initial report from Pendred (1896) and also in Brain's important paper (Brain, 1927). Indeed, the presence of goitre was critical to securing the diagnosis in all cases until supplanted by the application of the perchlorate discharge test, the diagnostic value of which was initially identified in a classically affected sibship who came to attention as a result of goitre (Morgans and Trotter, 1958). As the value of perchlorate discharge testing in securing the diagnosis was authenticated in thirteen families ascertained for hearing loss and goitre and the variable nature and extent of the goitrous involvement in Pendred syndrome became appreciated, the perchlorate discharge test replaced goitre as an essential element of the diagnosis (Fraser et al., 1960).

Exploiting the perchlorate test, Fraser was able to chart the natural history of the thyroid dysfunction in many of the families in his study (Fraser, 1965). Classically the goitre appears in mid-childhood, but is often postpubertal, especially in males. There are rare instances of congenital goitre. The goitre tends to be diffuse initially but may become nodular. There is distinct intrafamilial variability in the presence and extent of goitre between affected individuals. While Johnsen et al. suggested that up to 50% of cases are hypothyroid (Johnsen et al. 1987), Fraser's experience, in a far larger study, was that most cases are euthyroid (Fraser 1965). Many cases do come to surgery for tracheal decompression, this hazard being more common among females. Most cases undergoing subtotal thyroidectomy suffer recurrence of the goitre.

Histological examination of the excised thyroid tissue typically reveals a somewhat pleiomorphic histological appearance with a fairly marked degree of mitotic activity (Batsakis et al., 1963). These features also characterised the pathological descriptions of other forms of dyshormonogenic goitres (Vickery, 1981). As emphasised by Fraser (1965), this appearance, coupled with the general tendency to recurrence of the goitre, have led to suspicions of malignant involvement of the thyroid in Pendred syndrome (Thieme, 1957; Elman, 1958; Demeester-Mirkine et al., 1975; Abs et al., 1991). Whether a true association between Pendred syndrome, and indeed other forms of thyroid dyshormonogenesis, and thyroid carcinoma exists remains unclear. However, on those rare occasions when the pathological evidence of carcinoma has been accepted, the histological type is of a follicular thyroid carcinoma, supporting a possible role for chronic low level TSH stimulation in tumourigenesis (Williams 1979).

The perchlorate discharge test

We have already referred to the replacement, in diagnostic criteria, of goitre by a positive perchlorate discharge test, following the initial observations by Morgans and Trotter (1958). In a normally functioning thyroid gland, inorganic iodide, having been trapped, is immediately organified by binding to thyroglobulin. Iodination of thyroglobulin requires the generation of H_2O_2 and the oxidation of iodide and tyrosyl residues by the enzyme, thyroid peroxidase. The subsequent coupling of iodotyrosyls into iodothyronines T_4 and T_3 within the matrix of thyroglobulin is also governed by thyroid peroxidase (Vassart et al., 1995). Perchlorate and thiocyanate unmask defects of organification by provoking the discharge of inorganic iodide from the gland. As a result, administration of potassium perchlorate in the presence of an organification defect, having primed the thyroid with radio-iodide, results in a dramatic fall in the counting rate from sequestered radio-iodide over the thyroid, exactly as observed by Morgans and Trotter (1958). In the case of complete block of organification, thyroidal radioactivity declines in parallel with the plasma radio-iodide. This radioactivity is totally discharged from the gland within minutes of administration of perchlorate. The discharge in normal patients is small as sequestered iodine is usually organified. Consequently, a discharge in response to perchlorate of 10% or greater is considered abnormal.

Fraser studied the application of the perchlorate discharge test to 13 families with Pendred syndrome (Fraser, 1960). Whereas the unaffected individuals did not manifest an appreciable change in thyroid count rate after perchlorate, the affected group had significantly lower thyroid counts. Discharge rates in affected individuals varied from 15% to 80%. Intermediate discharge levels of this nature were taken to signify a partial defect in the thyroid peroxidase enzyme system. Comparison was made between the results obtained from the unaffected relatives and perchlorate discharge data from several control groups. No significant differences could be demonstrated, suggesting that perchlorate discharge characteristics might have a role in identifying homozygotes but not in heterozygote recognition. Fraser rightly recognised the poor discriminating value of perchlorate discharge response at the lower end of the range (10 – 15% levels) due to the high standard errors of the residual thyroid count rates in subjects with a low uptake.

Intermediate levels of discharge following perchlorate exposure have now become a hallmark of the disease (Vassart et al., 1995) (Figure 15.1). However this response is not specific to Pendred syndrome and has also been recorded in autoimmune thyroid disease (Morgans and Trotter, 1957) and thyrotoxic patients treated with radioactive iodine (Suzuki and Mashimo, 1972). Although several authors, in writing about Pendred syndrome, have tended to assume that the perchlorate discharge test is confirmatory (Johnsen et al., 1987, Das, 1987) a recent salutary report underlines the need to consider alternative diagnoses, the importance of interpreting the perchlorate discharge data in the context of thyroid autoantibody results and once again reiterates the non-specificity of the investigations for Pendred syndrome (O Mahoney et al., 1996). Although alterations to the standard perchlorate discharge test have been advocated as a means of improving the sensitivity of the investigation in identifying organification defects (Friis, 1987) and may clarify issues in a minority of cases, the perchlorate discharge data should always be viewed in the light of clinical and other available data and not as a sole diagnostic criterion. Fraser relates one instance of an initially negative perchlorate discharge test becoming positive when repeated after a goitre had developed (Fraser, 1965). The present authors have observed two instances of affected siblings, one of whom had unequivocally positive perchlorate discharge responses and the other of whom had a borderline response in the overlap between normal and pathological (Reardon and Trembath, 1995).

Several issues arising from the perchlorate discharge test remain to be addressed. Unaffected relatives of affected individuals in Fraser's study showed responses within the normal range (Fraser et al., 1960). Baschieri performed perchlorate discharge tests on 281 subjects, comprising normal individuals and patients with various types of thyroid disease and/or hearing loss (Baschieri et al., 1963). While family members of probands with normal perchlorate responses universally showed a normal response, a significant perchlorate discharge result was found in 9 of 42 relatives of 13 probands with a positive perchlorate discharge test. Three pedigrees were recorded in which the perchlorate test was positive in each of two generations, always associated with hearing loss in one generation only. These observations were taken to be suggestive of autosomal dominant transmission of positive perchlorate response. Similar findings have been reported in pedigrees with Pendred syndrome segregating, and the positive perchlorate response in some normally hearing individuals in these pedigrees has been proposed as evidence for autosomal dominant transmission of Pendred syndrome (Johnsen et al., 1989a).

The theory of metabolic flux suggests an explanation for why most inborn errors of metabolism are recessive (Kacser and Burns, 1981). The wide variability in perchlorate discharge response among definite Pendred syndrome cases is compatible with this framework. Likewise the intrafamilial variability in perchlorate response and, indeed, the apparently unusual examples in the literature which we have cited of positive perchlorate responses in successive generations, can be rationalised within this hypothesis. It is less easy though to explain the observation in Fraser's data (Fraser et al., 1965) that iodide uptake in affected subjects far exceeded that in the normal control group, but that this significant difference disappeared after the administration of perchlorate. The similarity of the means in the two groups after perchlorate was taken to indicate that the proportion of iodide 'converted to organic compounds by the thyroid is much the same in the two patient groups' (Pendred cases and normal controls). This would appear to suggest that organification is normal.

Radiological studies in Pendred syndrome

The association between Mondini malformation of the cochlea and Pendred syndrome can be traced to the histological study of the inner ear of a patient with Pendred syndrome (Hvidberg-Hansen et al., 1968), later confirmed in a further study of temporal bone studies from another 4 cases (Johnsen et al., 1986). Meanwhile the first radiological report appears to be that of Illum, who observed Mondini abnormalities in 8 of 13 cases examined by temporal bone tomography (Illum et al., 1972). Four of these patients were from the same pedigree and three siblings also investigated had normal cochlear morphology. Within a different sibship, the two affected cases were discordant radiologically. CT demonstration of the Mondini abnormality (Figure 15.2) was reported by Johnsen and colleagues in a cohort of cases already known to have the malformation from tomograms (Johnsen et al., 1989b). It is still unclear whether, as some authors suggest (Johnsen et al., 1986), the Mondini appearance is always present in Pendred syndrome, and a large scale sibship study of rigorously investigated cases is required to address this question. While the presence of a Mondini malformation is clearly supportive of the diagnosis in a patient with hearing loss and positive perchlorate discharge test with or without goitre, it needs to be borne in mind that Mondini malformation (Figure 15.2) is also non-specific and has been recorded in several other situations, both genetic and non-genetic (Phelps and Lloyd, 1990; Gorlin et al., 1995).

The inherited basis of Pendred syndrome

Brain considered a single recessive trait of pleiotropic effect, segregating in Mendelian manner affecting 'several children of normal parents in the absence of a family history of the complaint .... manifested by both males and females equally', as the likely basis of Pendred syndrome (Brain, 1927). Fraser concurred, the evidence for autosomal recessive inheritance in his study – the largest on record – being supported not only by segregation analysis but also by the observation of parental consanguinity in 22 of 186 fully documented pedigrees with Pendred syndrome (Fraser, 1965). More recently Gausden et al. (1996) have drawn attention to several examples of definitely affected, unrelated individuals marrying and producing only affected offspring. These observations are in themselves strongly supportive of autosomal recessivity. McKusick, while accepting that most cases are likely to represent an autosomal recessive condition, does cite a single example of 'pseudodominance' (McKusick et al., 1994). It seems clear that while Pendred syndrome does comply with the criteria for autosomal recessive inheritance in most families, some rare exceptions may exist.

The example of pseudodominance cited by McKusick relates to the family reported by Illum and colleagues, and indeed Pendred syndrome is observed in three successive generations of the same family (Illum et al., 1972). However, it is important to note that the partners marrying into generations I and II themselves came from families with incontrovertible evidence of Pendred syndrome. Indeed, of the two such Pendred-

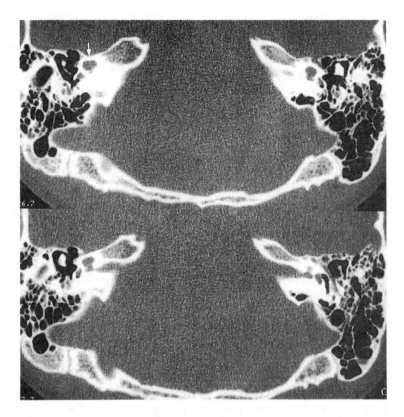

Figure 15.2 Axial CT section showing probable slight deficiency of the interscalar septum in the distal coils of the cochlea to give a bilateral Mondini cochlear malformation (arrow).

Pendred matings resulting, it is far more difficult to understand why three of the offspring are reported as unaffected, with five of the eight offspring clearly affected. It is noteworthy that no clinical details of these three cases are presented other than the figure of the pedigree and it is quite plausible that these cases would also have been found to be affected had the opportunity to study them been available. Another example of unusual inheritance was documented by Fraser in the case of the 'Northamptonshire Family'. Hearing loss was present in each of six successive generations and goitre, sometimes, though not exclusively, cosegregating with the hearing loss was seen in 5 of these generations. However the perchlorate discharge test was positive only in a single branch of the family and most individuals tested were within the normal range. Fraser was forced to the somewhat unsatisfactory conclusion that Pendred syndrome was present in a single branch of the pedigree and that the pathology in other family branches was different (Fraser, 1965). It is interesting to contrast Fraser's difficulties in this pedigree with the diagnostic problems posed by the Brazilian pedigree detailed by

Almeida et al., (1974) and subsequently re-studied by Billerbeck et al. (1994). There is a fundamental distinction in that this pedigree emanates from an area of endemic goitre. However, two individuals have goitre, hearing loss and a positive perchlorate discharge response, while several others have goitre and a positive perchlorate test but without hearing loss, while yet other individuals have goitre and/or hearing loss only. The pedigree is complicated by several consanguineous loops, but, as with the Northamptonshire family, the fact that certain individuals satisfy diagnostic criteria for Pendred syndrome serves only to emphasise the limitations of such criteria rather than offering a satisfactory explanation for the pedigree as a whole.

Bax (1966) identified a two generation family in which three of five sons were deaf and had goitre, but were euthyroid. The perchlorate discharge test was positive in two of the affected sons but was negative in the third. Their father, who had a demonstrable high tone hearing loss, also showed a positive perchlorate discharge response. Although not a satisfactory explanation for the discordant perchlorate discharge responses in the affected sons, it seems most likely that the family represents an example of a homozygote-heterozygote mating with resulting pseudodominance. A negative perchlorate discharge response was also reported by Cave and Dunn (1975), who reported a sibship of eight, three being affected by hearing loss, goitre and mental retardation of borderline degree. Perchlorate discharge was negative in the two patients available for study.

Johnsen et al. have presented six pedigrees in which Pendred syndrome has been diagnosed in at least two generations. They have advocated the use of the perchlorate discharge test for carrier detection (Johnsen et al., 1989a). The investigative evidence is patchy as the relevant individuals have not been uniformly studied. As a result, interpretation is fraught with difficulty. However, it is important to note the occurrence of positive perchlorate discharge tests in successive generations of three families in this report, as also seen by Baschieri et al. (1963).

It is worth considering these several possible deviations from straightforward recessivity in some detail. While each report is interesting in itself, cumulatively their importance is twofold – firstly to highlight occasional difficulty in securing a diagnosis of Pendred syndrome due to the nonspecificity of currently defined criteria and secondly, to draw attention to a range of clinical presentations closely resembling Pendred syndrome, which may or may not represent allelic variants. Indeed, they serve to highlight the importance of recognising that, even in its classical form, Pendred syndrome encompasses a wide range of presentations. As a consequence, linkage studies must focus initially only on multiple affected sibships of classical Pendred syndrome. Only when the locus for this has been identified will it be possible to tease out the relationship, if any, between Pendred syndrome and these deviant examples.

Genetic studies in Pendred syndrome

In light of the perchlorate discharge data, several authors have suggested that Pendred syndrome is likely to represent a defect of thyroid peroxidase. However *in vitro* studies cast doubt upon this suggestion, demonstrating a normal level of peroxidase activity (Burrow et al., 1973). The gene for thyroid peroxidase has been identified on the short arm of chromosome 2 (Kimura et al., 1989). The validity of interpreting the perchlorate test as a failure of organification has been shown in total iodide organification defect (TIOD), an autosomal recessive condition characterised by hypothyroidism and a greater than 90% iodide discharge following perchlorate administration, by the demonstration of a range of mutations in the coding sequence of the thyroid peroxidase gene in seven cases of TIOD (Abramowicz et al., 1992; Bikker et al., 1994; Bikker et al., 1995). However, the thyroid peroxidase locus has now been excluded as a major locus in Pendred syndrome (Gausden et al., 1996).

A cytogenetic clue to the location of the Pendred syndrome gene is given by the report of van Woude et al. (1986). The proband, a severely retarded girl, inherited this unbalanced karyogram from her father, who had a *de novo* balanced translocation t(8;10)(q24;p11). The unbalanced proband had a 10p duplication and an 8q deletion. Clinical studies were consistent with a diagnosis of Pendred syndrome in that hearing loss, hypothyroidism and a positive perchlorate discharge test were documented. However, recent linkage data by the present authors exclude 8q as the site of the Pendred syndrome locus.

Conclusions

The clinical, genetic and radiological evidence in support of a distinct autosomal recessive entity conforming to the condition described by Pendred is overwhelming. No single test is diagnostic but, taken in combination, the audiovestibular, radiological and perchlorate studies appear robust enough to identify most cases. This is especially so in sibships where single generations only are affected. Clarification at the molecular level will be required before some of the unusual pedigrees mimicking Pendred syndrome clinically and in perchlorate discharge characteristics can be interpreted correctly.

Note added in proof

Using the autosomal recessive model of inheritance, two separate groups have recently localised the gene for Pendred Syndrome to the long arm of chromosome 7 (Coyle et al., 1996; Sheffield et al., 1996)

Additionally, new data confirm the defect as a result of iodide organification.

Chapter 16
Waardenburg syndrome

ANDREW P READ and VALERIE E NEWTON

Introduction

The combination of hearing loss with pigmentary abnormalities has been known for many years in a variety of mammals. The underlying cause is absence of melanocytes in the skin, hair, eyes and stria vascularis. Usually the absence is patchy, giving spotting of the skin or fur, and a variable degree of hearing impairment. Melanocytes arise from the neural crest of the early embryo, and auditory-pigmentary syndromes reflect a failure of differentiation, migration and/or survival of melanocytes. Thus the primary action of the genes underlying these disorders is in the neural crest or in melanocytes, rather than in the inner ear.

In man, although auditory-pigmentary syndromes were described many years earlier (see Fraser (1976) for references), the first comprehensive description was by Waardenburg (1951). Waardenburg's interest had been aroused by a patient shown to him by David Klein, and Waardenburg syndrome (WS) is sometimes called Waardenburg-Klein syndrome.

Subtypes of Waardenburg syndrome: type I, type II, type III and type IV

Waardenburg (1951) described hearing loss with varying combinations of white forelock, heterochromia irides (different coloured eyes) and leukoderma (white skin patches), inherited as an autosomal dominant syndrome. He described the characteristic eye abnormality, dystopia canthorum, in some but not all of his cases. Later Arias (1971) pointed out that dystopia was seen in all affected people in some families, but in none in others, and suggested WS should be divided into type I WS (WS1), with dystopia, and type II (WS2), without dystopia. It turns out that the two types have different genetic causes.

Klein's original patient had severe hypoplasia of the arm and shoulder muscles, with contractures of the wrists and hand joints (Klein, 1983). The combination of WS1 with limb abnormalities has been called Klein-Waardenburg syndrome or WS type III (WS3). Very few cases have been reported, and most are much less severely affected than Klein's original patient. WS3, at least in the milder presentations, is not genetically distinct from WS1. The cause of the problems in Klein's original patient is not known.

Shah (Shah et al., 1981) described a series of Indian infants with Hirschsprung disease and white forelocks, and this combination, apparently inherited as an autosomal recessive character, has been called Shah-Waardenburg syndrome or WS type IV (WS4). Shah's patients had pale brown eyes and died before their hearing could be tested, thus the relationship to classic WS is not clear. Recently a recessively inherited combination of typical WS2 with Hirschsprung disease has been described in one or two families with mutations in the gene for the endothelin receptor B (see below).

Phenotypic features of Waardenburg syndrome

Liu et al. (1995) compared 60 WS1 patients with 81 WS2 patients (plus a further 210 WS1 and 43 WS2 patients collected from the literature). The frequency of various features is shown in Table 16.1. All features of the syndromes are variable both within and between families. The minimal set of auditory-pigmentary features needed to make a diagnosis is greater in WS2 than in WS1, because in WS1 dystopia canthorum gives a very reliable diagnostic handle.

Table 16.1 Phenotypic features in Waardenburg syndrome type I and type II.

	SNHL	HetI	HypE	WF	EG	Skin	HNR	Eyb
Type I								
Examined (n = 60)	52*	14*	10*	46*	40*	37	100	63
Literature (n = 210)	57	31	18	43	23	30	52	70
Type II								
Examined (n = 81)	78*	42*	3*	23*	30*	5*	0	7*
Literature (n = 43)	77	54	23	16	14	12	14	7

Percentage of patients with each feature (*calculated omitting proband from each family). SNHL: sensorineural hearing loss; HetI: heterochromia irides; HypE: hypoplastic blue eyes; WF: white forelock; EG: early greying; Skin: white skin patches; HNR: high nasal root; Eyb: bushy confluent eyebrows. Data of Liu, Newton and Read (1995).

Hearing impairment

The hearing loss is sensorineural, congenital and usually non-progressive. Hearing loss was noted in 58% of families with type I and 74% of families with type II investigated by Liu et al. (1995). It may be unilateral or bilateral and may vary in degree from slight to profound. The commonest degree of hearing loss, particularly in type I, is a profound bilateral loss. Audiogram shapes vary both between and within families. Unusual shapes include low frequency and U-shaped losses, bilateral or unilateral, and sometimes a combination of a low frequency sensorineural loss in one ear with a profound loss in the other. Asymmetrical loss is more common in type II. Subjects with normal hearing on pure tone audiometry may have dips on DP-grams. Wide notches were found between 1 kHz and 3 kHz in some type I and type II patients. In each case Audioscan testing showed no abnormality (Liu and Newton, in press).

The vestibular system has not received as much attention as auditory function, but vestibular hypofunction has been described in individuals with WS1 using caloric stimulation and rotational tests (Marcus, 1968; Hageman and Oosterveld, 1977). 17 out of 18 affected persons investigated by Marcus had abnormal vestibular function, but not all of these had a hearing loss. Radiological investigation of the auditory system has indicated a normal temporal bone or dysplasia of the lateral semicircular canal associated with a normal bony cochlea (Nemansky and Hageman, 1975). The histological appearance of one temporal bone studied by Fisch (1959) was consistent with the auditory features of WS1 being caused by a cochleosaccular degeneration.

Pigmentary anomalies

Iris heterochromia may be complete or partial. In complete heterochromia irides each iris is a different colour. In partial heterochromia the differently coloured area of the iris is sharply demarcated and is usually but not invariably a radial segment. Partial heterochromia may be unilateral or bilateral, and if bilateral may be symmetrical or asymmetrical. Hypoplastic blue irides are found where there is deficient iris stroma, and mainly in association with a severe/profound hearing loss. The fundus is reported to show pigmentary changes that correspond to those found on the retina (Goldberg, 1966).

In the hair, a distinctive white forelock is usually described, but the forelock may be red or black, and sometimes it is at the side or the back of the head rather than in the front midline (Reed et al., 1967; Arias, 1971). The forelock may vary in size from a few hairs to a large clump, and if present at birth it may persist or disappear only to reappear later, usually in the teens (Di George et al., 1960). Greying of the hair before age 30 is common; complete depigmentation may occur in the teens, and the hair may be sparse and of poor quality (Fraser, 1976). Pigmentation defects can affect the eyebrows, eyelashes and body hair as well as scalp hair (Fraser,1976).

Hypopigmentation of the skin is congenital and may be found on the face, trunk or limbs. It may be associated with an adjacent white forelock. Hyperpigmentation has also been described (Fisch, 1959), and this may develop after birth in a previously hypopigmented area. Arias (1971) noted that hypopigmented areas frequently had hyperpigmented borders. Pigmentation abnormalities are more likely to be associated with severe or profound hearing loss than with normal hearing, and the likelihood of a severe sensorineural loss increases with the number of pigmentation defects present (Newton et al., 1994).

Dystopia canthorum

Dystopia canthorum is the most penetrant feature of WS1, being present in 99% of those affected (Arias and Mota, 1978). Usually it is readily diagnosed clinically with the appearance of blepharophimosis and with fusion of the inner eyelids medially leading to a reduction in the medial sclerae. The inferior lacrimal ducts are displaced laterally, with the punctae opposite the cornea. However, reliable diagnosis of dystopia depends on computation of a biometric index based on the inner canthal (a), interpupillary (b) and outer canthal (c) measurements. The index, being dependent upon the relationship between the measurements rather than absolute measures, is unaffected by age, race or sex. Newton (1989) compared several indices; the index of choice is the W index of Arias and Mota (Arias and Mota, 1978):

$$W = X + Y + a/b,$$
where $X = (2a - 0.2119c - 3.909)/c$ and $Y = (2a - 0.2479b - 3.909)/b$

Genetic linkage analysis (Farrer et al., 1994) suggests that in WS1 the W value, averaged over all affected family members, is 1.95 or above, whilst in WS2 the index is below 1.95. In dystopic individuals it is not only the inner canthal distance which is increased but interpupillary and outer canthal distances are also greater than normal, indicating a degree of hypertelorism. Hypoplasia of the alae nasae and a high, broad nasal root are features associated with dystopia canthorum in WS1. Medial hypertrichosis and synophrys are more common in dystopic than non-dystopic individuals.

Other features of the syndrome have been described and include a patent metopic suture and square jaw (Fisch, 1959) and cupid's bow mouth (Di George et al., 1960). Strabismus may be more common with type I than normally (Delleman and Hageman, 1978). Other associated conditions include Hirschsprung's disease (Omenn and McKusick, 1979), Sprengel's shoulder (Frazer, 1976), cleft lip/palate (Giacola and Klein, 1969) and spina bifida (Pantke and Cohen, 1971).

Homozygous WS

All the features described here so far are the features of heterozygotes, with one normal and one abnormal gene. Homozygotes, with two abnormal genes, would probably be much more severely affected. In view of the high frequency of deaf x deaf marriages, this is a consideration to be borne in mind in genetic counselling. For WS1, knowing that the *PAX3* gene is mutated (see below), we can use the mouse model (*Splotch*, see Chapter 5) to predict the homozygous phenotype. We would expect homozygotes to have lethal neural tube defects, together with very severe expression of the normal features of WS1. In fact, the only definite homozygote described to date (Zlotogora et al., 1995), although severely affected, did not have any neural tube defect. Nevertheless, it is likely in general that homozygous WS1 would be lethal. The outlook for WS2 homozygotes is less clear, but again it is likely they would be much more severely affected than heterozygotes. When the parents carry different genes for auditory-pigmentary syndromes (e.g. WS1 x WS2 marriages), the risk of severe problems is much lower, although still not negligible.

Diagnostic criteria

The diagnosis of WS has been clarified by the criteria set out by the Waardenburg Consortium (Farrer et al., 1992). Individuals are scored as affected if they show two major criteria or one major and two minor criteria.

Major criteria are:

- Sensorineural hearing loss (> 25 dB) without other evident cause.
- Iris pigmentary abnormality (heterochromia, iris bicolour or characteristic brilliant blue eyes with hypoplastic stroma).
- Hair hypopigmentation (white forelock).
- Dystopia canthorum (defined as W > 1.95, see above) (type I only).
- Affected first degree relative.

Minor criteria are:-

- Hypopigmented skin patches.
- Synophrys or medial eyebrow flare.
- Broad high nasal root.
- Hypoplasia of the alae nasi.
- Premature greying of the hair (mainly white by age 30).

Liu et al. (1995) similarly suggested that a diagnosis of WS2 should be based on the presence of two of the major criteria (excluding dystopia canthorum). Minor criteria for WS2 include white skin patches and early greying, but not synophrys, broad high nasal root or hypoplastic alae nasi.

Prevalence of Waardenburg syndrome

Waardenburg (1951) estimated prevalence of the syndrome (WS1 + WS2) to be 1/42,000 of the population and 1.43 per cent of the congenitally deaf. Fraser (1976) in his school study of 2,355 deaf children found prevalence to be 2.12 – 3.01/100,000 and estimated the prevalence in the general population as 1.44 – 2.05/100,000. Prevalence, especially of WS2, is likely to be underestimated if cases with mild to moderate hearing loss are not specifically sought by audiolometric testing. Probably 60 – 70% of cases are type II and 30 – 40% type I (although Arias and Mota (1978) considered that type II is much more common). Type III and type IV are excessively rare. The mutation rate has been estimated as 0.4/100,000 gametes by Waardenburg (1951) and Fraser (1976).

Genetic analysis of Waardenburg syndrome

Genetic mapping

Linkage analysis has shown that the abnormality in essentially all WS1 families, but no WS2 families, maps to the distal long arm of chromosome 2 (Foy et al., 1990; Farrer et al., 1994). An initial clue to the location was provided by the description of a child with *de novo* WS1 who had a chromosomal inversion inv(2)(q35;q37.3) (Ishikiriyama et al., 1989). There has been some confusion about the exact location, which has been variously quoted as 2q35, 2q36 and 2q37.3, but it is now generally agreed that the WS1 locus is at the distal end of band 2q35. In about 20% of WS2 families the disease maps to the proximal short arm of chromosome 3 (Hughes et al., 1994). The genes responsible for the remaining 80% of cases have not yet been mapped, although mutations in either the endothelin receptor B (*EDNRB*) gene at 13q22 or the endothelin 3 (*EDN3*) gene at 20q13 have been detected in a few families with WS2 features, almost always in association with Hirschsprung disease (see below). There is some evidence for involvement of a locus on chromosome 1 (Waardenburg Consortium, unpublished data), but this has not yet been clarified.

The *PAX3* gene and type I WS

The gene at 2q35 responsible for WS1 has been identified as *PAX3* (Tassabehji et al., 1992; Baldwin et al, 1992). *PAX3* is one of a family of nine genes that contain a paired box, a 384 base pair sequence encoding a DNA-binding paired domain. *PAX* genes are transcription factors that are active in the early embryo, and are found in organisms as diverse as *Drosophila* and man (Read and van Heyningen, 1994; Strachan and Read, 1994). *PAX3* (and also *PAX6* and *PAX7*) additionally contain a homeobox that encodes a second DNA-binding element, the homeodomain, in the gene product. Homeodomains are found in the genes that specify the basic body plan of all metazoan organisms, and so are central to all genetic investigations of embryonic development. Waardenburg syndrome was the first human inherited disorder shown to be caused by mutations in a homeodomain gene. Perhaps it was a little unexpected that the consequences should be so relatively modest – some *Drosophila* homeodomain mutations cause the fly to be built in the wrong order, for example with legs growing out of its head where antennae should be.

Over 40 different *PAX3* mutations have been characterised in different WS1 families. They range from complete deletion of the gene, through various changes predicted to wreck the gene product (splice-site mutations, frameshifts and nonsense mutations, see Chapter 2), to a series of aminoacid substitutions that should leave the overall protein structure intact. In general each family has its own private mutation, although certain ones have been seen more than once. Figure 16.1 shows those detected by our group (Tassabehji et al., 1995). Despite the great variety of mutations, there is no obvious correlation between any clinical feature of WS1 and any particular change at the DNA or protein level. This implies that the molecular pathology depends on loss of function mutations of the gene. WS1 is an example of haploinsufficiency, where a half dose of the gene product is insufficient for normal function in all cells. The great variability of clinical features probably reflects a delicate and shifting balance of effects within cells as a sub-optimal quantity of *PAX3* protein interacts with DNA sequences and probably with other proteins in the cell.

The *MITF* gene and type II WS

The microphthalmia (*mi*) mouse mutation has long been recognised as a potential homologue of WS2, but attempts to predict the chromosomal location of its human homologue were not successful. When eventually *mi* was cloned, it became possible to isolate and map the human homologue, called *MITF* (Tachibana et al., 1994). *MITF* turned out to map to proximal 3p, precisely the region to which WS2 had just been mapped in some families (Hughes et al., 1994). Not surprisingly, *MITF* mutations were soon found in a few WS2 families (Tassabehji, Newton and Read, 1994).

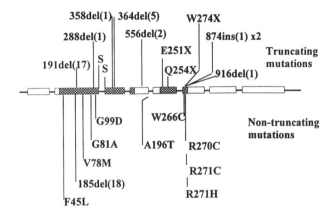

Figure 16.1 Mutations in the *PAX3* gene in type I Waardenburg syndrome. The gene has 8 exons. The paired box is in exons 2, 3 and 4, and the homeobox in exons 5 and 6 (see text). The mutations shown are those detected by the Manchester group (Tassabehji, Newton, Liu et al., 1995); other groups have described similar mutations. All these mutations inactivate the gene product, and the symptoms of WS1 are produced by reduced dosage of the *PAX3* protein at critical times during embryonic development.

MITF and the mouse *mi* gene encode a transcription factor of the basic-HLH-zip family (Hodgkinson et al., 1993; Steingrimsson et al., 1994). These proteins dimerise and the dimers bind DNA through a basic region. Dimerisation is determined by the HLH (helix-loop-helix) and zip (leucine zipper) domains. In the *mi* mouse, mutations that prevent dimerization produce recessive phenotypes – the mutant protein is inactive, but the cell can get by on a half dose of active protein. Dominant phenotypes are produced by mutations that leave dimerisation intact, but prevent the dimer functioning correctly as a transcription factor; the mutant protein sequesters the normal protein in inactive dimers. This is an example of a dominant negative effect. In humans, at the time of writing, the six known *MITF* mutations (Figure 16.2; Tassabehji et al., 1995) do not seem to fit this pattern very well. However, it is entirely likely that homozygotes for any of these mutations would be very severely affected, so that major parts of the phenotype may well be dominant.

The *EDNRB* and *EDN3* genes in type II WS

Endothelins are a family of three peptide hormones, endothelin-1, -2 and -3, long known to interact with two cell surface receptors, the A and B receptors, to regulate blood pressure. Evidently endothelins have some other actions as well, because mice lacking endothelin-1, endothelin-3 or the B receptor unexpectedly turned out to have problems

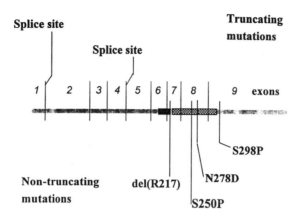

Figure 16.2 Mutations in the *MITF* gene in type II Waardenburg syndrome. The gene has 9 exons. The DNA-binding basic domain is encoded in exons 6 and 7, and the helix-loop-helix and leucine zipper dimerisation domains in exons 7-9 (see text).

indicative of malfunction of the embryonic neural crest. Following clues from the mouse work, mutations in *EDNRB* (the B receptor) or *EDN3* (endothelin 3) have been found in a small number of families with Hirschsprung disease and/or type II Waardenburg syndrome (Puffenberger et al., 1994 and unpublished data). Most patients, either with Hirschsprung disease or with WS2, show no signs of mutations in these genes. Only one WS2 family without Hirschsprung disease has so far been shown to carry a mutation in either of these two genes, but it is likely that a small proportion of WS2, especially in families where Hirschsprung disease occurs, will be found to be caused by *EDNRB* or *EDN3* mutations.

Chapter 17
Alport syndrome

HAN G BRUNNER

Introduction

Alport syndrome is characterised by a specific form of glomerulonephritis and progressive high frequency sensorineural hearing loss. There is a correlation between the severity of the renal disease, and the age at which hearing loss becomes manifest. In most instances, the hearing loss becomes clinically evident around the time that renal function starts to deteriorate. This may vary from approximately 10 years of age to well into adulthood, and some mildly affected cases never develop hearing loss. In cases with early onset disease, the hearing loss may progress to involve the lower frequencies as well. This causes clinically significant hearing impairment, and such cases may require the use of hearing aids.

The renal disease is characterised by microscopic haematuria from early childhood (which may become macroscopic during intercurrent infections) and by slowly deteriorating renal function in adolescence or adulthood. Renal failure occurs at different ages in different forms of Alport syndrome (Atkin et al., 1988). In some kindreds, end-stage renal disease occurs in late childhood and adolescence. In other kindreds affected individuals have normal or only mildly disturbed renal function in their thirties. Specific eye signs such as lenticonus anterior or perimacular flecs are found in patients with early onset renal disease. The macular flecks (if present) are asymptomatic. Anterior lenticonus causes myopia, and may rarely progress to rupture of the anterior lens capsule.

A diagnosis of Alport syndrome can be suspected if there is haematuria in combination with loss of renal function, high frequency sensorineural hearing loss, or a positive family history of these symptoms. The diagnostic procedure is a renal biopsy for electron microscopy which shows variable thinning and thickening of the glomerular basement membrane with a multilamellated aspect and granular inclusions.

Variants of Alport syndrome

Alport syndrome can be subdivided on the basis of:

* The age of end-stage renal disease.
* The pattern of inheritance.
* The presence or absence of hearing loss and/or other features.

Table 17.1 attempts to combine these data into a rational classification scheme.

By far the most common form of Alport syndrome is the X-linked variant, which is responsible for approximately 85% of cases. Autosomal recessive Alport syndrome may account for 10%, with autosomal dominant inheritance being rare. An unusual variant of X-linked Alport syndrome is caused by a combined partial deletion of the COL4A5 gene (which causes renal disease and hearing loss) and also a part of the COL4A6 gene. This combined genetic defect strongly predisposes to the development of multiple benign smooth muscle tumours of the oesophagus and/or the genitalia. It is assumed that the specific involvement of the COL4A6 gene is responsible for the development of the multiple leiomyomas in these cases. In a minority of cases Alport syndrome is inherited in an autosomal dominant or autosomal recessive manner. Mutations have been detected in the COL4A3 and COL4A4 genes on chromosome 2. For the variants of Alport syndrome with macrothrombocytopenia (Fechtner syndrome and Epstein syndrome, Table 17.1) the relationship to the other forms of Alport syndrome has not been established, and their primary defect is unknown.

Genetics of Alport syndrome

A diagnosis of Alport syndrome usually requires renal biopsy and a family study to determine the inheritance pattern. All major forms of inheritance (X-linked, autosomal dominant, autosomal recessive) can occur. In the X-linked forms, males are affected earlier and more severely than females. Often, the only detectable abnormality in a female carrier is microhaematuria, and some are entirely asymptomatic. Occasionally females are similarly affected to their male relatives and in these cases progressive renal failure may occur. The same is true for the hearing loss in X-linked Alport syndrome. For the autosomal dominant and autosomal recessive forms of Alport syndrome, males and females are clinically similarly affected.

Table 17.1 Alport syndrome variants.

Inheritence	Gene	Hearing Loss	Age At ESRD	Eye Signs	Other
XL	COL4A5	Yes	< 30 years	Perimacular flecks, lenticonus	
XL	COL4A5	Yes	> 30 years	No	
XL	COL4A5	No	> 30 years	No	
XL	COL4A5 + COL4A6	Yes	< 30 years	No	Oesophageal and/or genital leiomyomatosis, cataracts
AD	COL4A3	Yes	> 30 years	No	
AD	Unknown	Yes	> 30 years	Cataracts	Cataracts, macrothrombo-cytopenia 'Epstein syndrome'
AD	Unknown	Yes	> 30 years	Cataracts	Cataracts, macrothrombo-cytopenia and leucocyte inclusions 'Fechtner syndrome'
AR	COL4A3	Yes	< 30 years	Unknown	
AR	COL4A4	No?	< 30 years	Unknown	

ESRD = End-stage renal disease
COL4A5 = The gene encoding the fifth chain of type IV collagen
XL = X-linked inheritance
AD = Autosomal dominant inheritance
AR = Autosomal recessive inheritance

Pathogenesis of Alport syndrome

Alport syndrome has for many years been regarded as a disease of basement membranes, and type IV collagen has been considered as a candidate. This has now been confirmed for several different subtypes of
Alport syndrome (Table 17.1). Similar clinical features are observed in
patients with mutations of the X-chromosomal *COL4A5* gene, and in
those in whom *COL4A3* or *COL4A4* are mutated. A wide spectrum of
mutations has been described for the *COL4A5* gene in patients with X-
linked disease (Tryggvason et al., 1993). Both the *COL4A3* and *COL4A4*
genes are on chromosome 2, and mutations are found in autosomal
recessive Alport syndrome. The *COL4A6* gene on the X-chromosome
had not been reported to be mutated in cases with Alport syndrome
only, but it is involved in those cases where Alport syndrome is accompanied by leiomyomatosis of the oesophagus and/or genitalia (Zhou et
al., 1993, Antignac et al., 1992, Heidet et al., 1995). The genetic lack of
the third, fourth or fifth chain of type IV collagen has been confirmed on
tissue from renal biopsies by immunological studies (Kashtan et al.,
1986; Kleppel et al., 1987, 1992). The inherited lack of one of the component chains of type IV collagen may cause problems if patients are
transplanted with a renal allograft after their own kidneys have stopped
functioning. In some patients, the donor kidney has been rejected, and
this has been shown to be associated with the formation of antibodies
that are specific to the lacking collagen IV chain, or to other type IV collagen chains that are closely interacting with the missing chain (Hudson
et al., 1992; Kalluri et al., 1995).

X-linked Alport syndrome

Most cases of Alport syndrome are due to mutations in the X-chromosomal gene (*COL4A5*) that encodes the fifth chain of type IV collagen in
basement membranes (Tryggvason et al., 1993). Over 100 mutations in
this gene have been reported. Generally, mutations that completely
abolish gene function (such as deletions, frameshift mutations, or mutations introducing stop codons) are associated with early-onset Alport
syndrome, and prominent hearing loss.

More subtle (missense) mutations of the *COL4A5* gene change only a
single amino acid in the type IV collagen chain. Such mutations may be
associated with later onset of hearing loss and of end-stage renal disease. Some cases with single amino acid substitutions of the *COL4A5*
gene still have normal audiograms after the age of 30 years (Smeets et
al., 1992) As should be expected in an X-linked condition, the clinical
picture in females ranges from severe renal disease with prominent
hearing loss, to females who have neither detectable hearing loss, nor

haematuria. Using sensitive tests it has been found that carriers of X-linked Alport syndrome have either significant high frequency sensorineural hearing loss on pure tone audiometry or a mid-frequency notch on Audioscan testing (Sirimanna et al, 1995).

Nevertheless one should be cautious in interpreting such findings in an otherwise healthy family member. Although supportive, such findings are not by themselves sufficient to prove carrier status. The proportion of carriers of X-linked Alport syndrome who are undetectable by clinical tests approaches 15% (Tishler et al., 1979).

Alport syndrome and leiomyomatosis

This is a specific but rare combination that is associated with deletions of the X-chromosome that encompass part of both the *COL4A5* and *COL4A6* genes. Analysis of the X-chromosome breakpoints of the deletions suggest that leiomyomatosis occurs only if the break occurs within a specific part of the *COL4A6* gene (intron 2) (Heidet et al., 1995). Otherwise the clinical picture in males is typical of severe (early-onset) Alport syndrome with hearing loss. Females also develop leiomyomas, but have milder expression of renal and auditory symptoms. In several cases with both Alport syndrome and leiomyomatosis cataracts have developed at a relatively early age.

Autosomal recessive forms of Alport syndrome

Up to 10% of all Alport syndrome cases are due to autosomal recessive inheritance (Feingold et al., 1985). These cases are clinically similar to those with the X-linked form. Autosomal recessive inheritance is most likely if the parents are consanguineous and if males and females are equally severely affected. The molecular defect underlying autosomal recessive Alport syndrome can reside in either the third or the fourth component chain of the type IV collagen molecule. The genes encoding the third and fourth chain (*COL4A3* and *COL4A4*) are located on chromosome 2, and specific mutations have been described (Mochizuki et al., 1994). There are preliminary data to suggest that Alport syndrome patients due to a defect in the *COL4A4* gene have normal hearing. However, only small numbers of autosomal recessive patients have been studied at the molecular level.

Autosomal dominant Alport syndrome

This is probably the least common form of clinically diagnosed Alport syndrome (Feingold et al., 1985). Autosomal dominant inheritance must be assumed if there is father to son transmission of the disorder. However, X-linked inheritance needs to be excluded by urinalysis in the mother before autosomal dominant inheritance can be assumed. The autosomal dominant variety of Alport syndrome can have a relatively mild phenotype with late-onset hearing loss and slow progression of renal disease. It has been suggested that the mildest form of autosomal dominant Alport syndrome is familial benign haematuria or 'thin basement membrane syndrome' (Piel et al., 1982). On the other hand autosomal dominant inheritance of early-onset disease has also been reported (Atkin et al., 1988).

Males and females are equally affected, and the findings on renal biopsy are typical of Alport syndrome. The underlying genetic defect in autosomal dominant Alport syndrome may well involve the *COL4A3* and/or *COL4A4* genes. However, mutations in these genes have not yet been described in autosomal dominant families.

Epstein syndrome

This is a very rare condition of nephritis, cataracts, macrothrombocytopenia, and sensorineural hearing loss (Epstein et al., 1972). Inheritance is probably autosomal dominant, although X-linkage has not been excluded in all families. The renal disease and the high frequency hearing loss are very similar to the common forms of Alport syndrome.

Fechtner syndrome

Like Epstein syndrome, Fechtner syndrome is characterised by nephritis, macrothrombocytopenia and hearing loss. In addition specific leukocyte inclusions similar to May-Hegglin anomaly also occur as a specific feature (Peterson et al., 1985; Gershoni-Buruch et al., 1988). The inheritance pattern appears autosomal dominant.

Chapter 18
Neurofibromatosis type II

D GARETH R EVANS

Introduction

Type II neurofibromatosis (NF2) was probably first described by Wishart in 1820. However, following reports of patients with type I neurofibromatosis (NF1) by von Recklinghausen, various reports of NF2 cases around the turn of the century were assumed to be part of von Recklinghausen's disease. Although many reports emphasised the lack of skin tumours or café au lait patches in patients and families with bilateral vestibular Schwannomas (Gardner and Frazier, 1930; Young et al., 1971), the final separation of NF1 and NF2 came only in 1987. In that year the gene for NF1 was localised to chromosome 17, and NF2 to chromosome 22, by genetic linkage analysis (Rouleau et al., 1987). As a result of this and the increasing clinical evidence to implicate two distinct disorders (Kanter et al., 1980), the National Institutes of Health (NIH) Consensus statement published the following year (1988) formally separated them. The still widely held view that vestibular Schwannomas occur as part of NF1 has now been refuted (Huson et al., 1989). Previous reports of NF1 were clearly contaminated with NF2 cases (Crowe et al., 1956).

NF2 is a dominantly inherited disorder which predisposes affected individuals to the development of vestibular Schwannomas (usually bilateral), Schwannomas of the other cranial, spinal and peripheral nerves, meningiomas both intracranial (including on the optic nerve) and intraspinal, and some low grade CNS malignancies (ependymomas, gliomas). Two large studies have now confirmed the clinical phenotype (Kanter et al., 1980; Evans et al., 1992). The suggested diagnostic criteria for NF2 are shown in Table 18.1.

The original NIH criteria have been expanded to include patients with no family history who have multiple Schwannomas and/or meningiomas, but who have not yet developed bilateral eighth nerve

Table 18.1 Diagnostic criteria for NF2.

Basic Criteria	Additional Criteria
1. Bilateral vestibular Schwannomas OR 2. Family history of NF2 PLUS 2a Unilateral vestibular schwannoma OR 2b Any two of: meningioma, glioma, neurofibroma, Schwannoma, posterior subcapsular lenticular opacities.	a) Cerebral calcification should be added to the list in 2b. b) The diagnosis of NF2 can be made in an individual with unilateral vestibular Schwannoma PLUS 2b c) The diagnosis of NF2 can be made in an individual with multiple meningioma (2 or more) PLUS Unilateral vestibular Schwannoma OR Any 2 of: glioma, neurofibroma, Schwannoma, cataract, cerebral calcification.

tumours. Individuals may present with cranial meningiomas or a spinal tumour long before the appearance of a vestibular Schwannoma. As at least 50% of cases represent new dominant mutations (Evans et al., 1992b), the new criteria are more inclusive. The incidences of peripheral features and CNS tumours from the three major clinical studies (Kanter et al., 1980; Evans et al., 1992a; Parry et al., 1994) are shown in Table 18.2.

Table 18.2 Age at onset and frequency of tumour types in NF2.

	Kanter et al., 1980	Evans et al., 1992a	Parry et al., 1994
Number of cases	73	120	63
Number of families	17	75	32
Isolated cases	0	45	17
Age at onset (years)	20.4 (of 59)	22.2	20.3
Meningiomas	18%	45%	49%
Spinal tumours	Not known	25.8%	67%
Skin tumours	32% (73)	68% (of 100)	67%
> 10 skin tumours	Not known	10% (100)	Not known
Cafe au lait spots	42% (31)	43% (100)	47%
Cataracts	-	38% (90)	81%
Astrocytoma	Not known	4.1%	1.6%
Ependymoma	Not known	2.5%	3.2%
Optic sheath meningioma	Not known	4.1%	4.8%

Epidemiology

NF2 has a birth incidence of 1 in 35 – 40,000, (Evans et al., 1992b). However, as many cases do not develop features of the condition until the third decade or later and many other cases die before this time, the actual diagnostic prevalence is only 1 in 200,000. The annual incidence rate is 1 per 2,355,000, representing about one new case per year for each Health Region in the UK (Evans et al., 1993).

Presentation

The majority of cases of NF2 present with symptoms attributable to vestibular Schwannoma, such as hearing loss, tinnitus and imbalance or vertigo. The symptoms are usually (75%) unilateral initially. However, at least 20% of cases first present with complications of a cranial meningioma or spinal tumour. Occasionally a skin tumour will have been removed in childhood and this may well have led to a mistaken diagnosis of NF1. Only about 1 – 2% of NF2 patients fulfil the diagnostic criteria for NF1 (National Institutes of Health, 1988) and even these can be excluded after careful consideration. There is no convincing evidence of any patients having a mixed form of neurofibromatosis. Childhood cataracts are also common, and can probably be found in over 20% of NF2 cases before the presence of any tumour. This on its own is unlikely to alert a clinician to the diagnosis, but in the presence of a family history, or in a young patient presenting with bilateral hearing loss or a unilateral vestibular Schwannoma, should arouse a high degree of suspicion. After careful slit lamp examination a posterior lenticular opacity is found in up to 80% of NF2 cases (Kaiser-Kupfer et al., 1989). Patients may also develop a peripheral neuropathy which is not due to known spinal or other CNS tumours (Evans et al., 1992a).

Diagnosis

NF2 can be diagnosed if the criteria in Table 18.1 are fulfilled. There are several groups of individuals who should be considered at risk and investigated further. These include those with a family history of NF2, patients aged under 30 years presenting with a unilateral vestibular Schwannoma or meningioma, patients with multiple spinal tumours (Schwannomas or meningiomas) and individuals with minimal skin features of neurofibromatosis, but insufficient for a diagnosis of NF1. The gold standard in terms of diagnostic precision is the MRI scan with gadolinium enhancement (see Figure 18.1). This should include a complete spinal as well as a cranial scan. However, a careful skin and eye examination is also of great diagnostic importance. It is now also possible to make a presymptomatic DNA diagnosis (see 'Genetics' below).

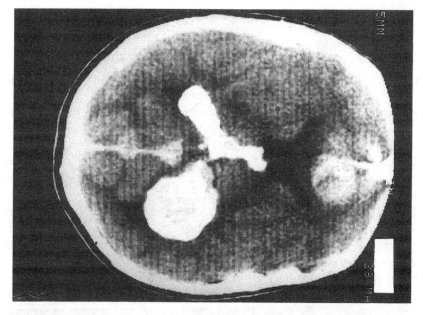

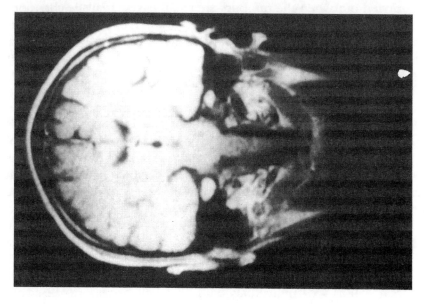

Figure 18.1 Gadolinium enhanced MRI image showing bilateral vestibular schwannomas.

Treatment

Until such a time as gene therapy becomes a realistic proposition, surgical intervention will be the mainstay of management for patients with NF2. Total removal of both eighth nerve tumours with preservation of hearing in one or both ears is rarely achievable, and in many instances may not necessarily be the correct management. Patients who present early with multiple rapidly growing tumours need careful evaluation and may well need spinal or other cranial tumours to be removed as the first priority. Other patients from families with a milder disease course, tend to present with bilateral eighth nerve tumours in the third and fourth decades and with few if any other intracranial or spinal tumours. The disease course is relatively benign with slow growth, and hearing may be preserved until late in life. The distinction between these two subgroups may not always be quite as well defined as this description may suggest, but nevertheless it is useful to recognise the heterogenous nature of the condition.

The failure to preserve hearing in the majority of cases has led many to suggest that the tumour should be observed until one of two situations obtains: either the hearing is lost 'naturally', in which case there is little point in not removing the tumour, or the tumour reaches such a size that there is neurological necessity to remove it regardless of the effect upon hearing (Baldwin et al., 1991). In the latter instance, subtotal removal may allow some hearing to be retained. However, operations carried out when the tumours are small have a realistic chance of long term preservation of hearing (Samii et al., 1985). Although other methods of hearing preservation such as stereotactic radiosurgery are also used, the long term consequences of this treatment have not yet been fully assessed.

Often the eighth nerve lesions are of less immediate importance than spinal tumours, which may threaten to cause paraplegia or bladder problems. Furthermore if surgery to the vestibular Schwannomas is planned, there is a very good case for compromising on the principle of total tumour removal in order to ensure that no facial nerve damage is caused. The importance of multidisciplinary regional or supraregional centres with experience in dealing with all aspects of NF2 cannot be over stated (Evans et al., 1993).

Hearing

The great majority of individuals with NF2 will become totally deaf. Patients who have both vestibular Schwannomas and both auditory nerves resected will of course be incapable of gaining any help from a conventional cochlear implant. Work from the House Ear Clinic in Los

Angeles (Nelson, 1992) indicates that the auditory brainstem implant (ABI) will have a very useful role in the rehabilitation of these individuals. The ABI stimulates the cochlear nucleus directly, and early results indicate an ability to hear environmental noise, to discriminate pitch differences, and an enhancement of lip reading skills. Patients should also be encouraged to investigate other means of communicating (lip reading, sign language), preferably before hearing loss ensues.

Genetics

Many studies have confirmed the autosomal dominant inheritance of NF2. The gene has a high degree of penetrance and is nearly always expressed by the late fifties (Evans et al., 1992c). The initial clue to the whereabouts of the gene came with the discovery of chromosome 22 abnormalities in meningiomas (Zang, 1982). This was confirmed at the molecular level in several different tumours from an NF2 patient, by showing loss of constitutional heterozygosity for chromosome 22q markers (Seizinger et al., 1986). This was a major indicator that the NF2 gene is a tumour suppressor, with both copies needing to be inactivated before tumorigenesis ensued.

Linkage to markers on chromosome 22 was then confirmed in one large family (Rouleau et al., 1987), and further studies showed that the NF2 phenotype is almost certainly caused by a single gene on 22q (Narod et al., 1992). The gene was further localised by the discovery of germ line deletions in NF2 families, one of which involved the neurofilament heavy chain gene (Watson et al., 1993). The NF2 gene itself was eventually identified as encoding a cell membrane related protein termed merlin (Troffater et al., 1993) or Schwannomin (Rouleau et al., 1993). Several studies have now confirmed the presence of constitutional and tumour deletions of this gene in NF2 patients.

Standard mutation detection techniques such as SSCP (single strand conformation polymorphism) or DGGE (denaturing gradient gel electrophoresis) detect between 35 and 60% of causative mutations (MacCollin et al., 1994; Bourn et al., 1994; Merel et al., 1995). The majority of these mutations are truncating mutations. This means that more rapid screening techniques such as the protein truncation test could be employed. There are early indications of a genotype/phenotype correlation (MacCollin et al., 1993; Watson et al., 1993; Evans et al., 1995a); a mild phenotype is seen with most missense mutations (which will give rise to a complete protein product) or deletions (which give no protein product). Truncating mutations (that may produce a partial gene product) tend to give a more severe phenotype. This may be due to a dominant negative effect, with mutant protein dimerising with the normal product and leaving less wild-type protein for tumour suppression.

Predictive diagnosis is now possible in the vast majority of families containing two or more living affected individuals by linkage analysis using flanking markers (Narod et al., 1992; Ruttledge et al., 1993; Evans et al., 1995a). Once a mutation has been identified in an affected individual, a 100% specific test is available for that family. However, mutation detection is time consuming and expensive and may not reveal the causative mutation. In most families with more than one affected individual, linkage analysis will still remain the test of choice, as this will give > 99% certainty by using intragenic or flanking markers. By combining this with a life curve, the risk to an unaffected 30 year old with a normal scan and favourable DNA result would be infinitesimally small. 100% confidence can still only be attained with the identification of family-specific mutations.

Recent evidence suggests that patients with what has previously been called Schwannomatosis have a variant form of NF2. In this condition the tumours are largely confined to the skin and spine, with sparing of the eighth nerve. Mutations in the NF2 gene are now being found in patients with this variant form of the disease. Therefore a vestibular Schwannoma should not be considered as an inevitable consequence of every disease causing mutation in the NF2 gene.

Modifying factors

There has been evidence to suggest that the condition may be worse if the disease is inherited from the mother (Kanter et al., 1980; Evans et al., 1992b). However, this could also be due to decreased genetic fitness in males, with only the less severely affected men having offspring. There is no evidence for genetic imprinting (selective expression of a gene depending on whether it is inherited from the mother or the father) of genes on chromosome 22q, therefore these reports of a maternal gene effect may be spurious. Some data (Gardner and Frazier, 1930; Evans et al., 1992b) suggest anticipation (a general worsening of the disease with successive generations), but true anticipation, as seen for example in myotonic dystrophy, seems unlikely. There has previously been a suggestion of a worse disease course in affected females (Parry et al., 1994). However, a more complete analysis would suggest that the effect is mainly on meningioma rather than Schwannoma growth and development (Evans et al., 1995b).

On the whole, NF2 disease course does breed true in families. Some families have a mild disease course with late onset and few if any CNS tumours other than vestibular Schwannomas, while other families have a more virulent course with early onset and death due to multi-tumour disease. The early evidence of a genotype correlation is encouraging and may well lend an insight into the disease process. None the less, even in monozygotic twins the disease course is not identical (Baser et al., 1995), and much will depend on stochastic events such as loss of the second NF2 allele.

Future possibilities

Localisation and cloning of the NF2 gene was a major step forward. This achieved, precise diagnosis is possible if a specific mutation can be found, and there is the possibility of predicting the disease course through genotype/phenotype studies. This will not be important in families where other affected members reveal the extent of the disease, but an insight into the likely speed of tumour progression and risk of other tumours would be very helpful in patients with new mutations. Although DNA predictive testing is now available with flanking markers, there is currently little demand for prenatal diagnosis. A less controversial option would be preimplantation diagnosis, and this is being evaluated in a limited sense for other diseases such as familial adenomatous polyposis and cystic fibrosis.

The real hope is that the discovery of the gene and its protein product merlin/schwannomin will lead to the development of somatic gene therapy. Intuitively, the prospects for NF2 appear promising. This is because of the lack of variation between individuals with the same mutation and the paucity of involvement of other genes in the tumours themselves. Replacement of the tumour suppressor product in the tumours through viral vectors or direct recombination of the NF2 gene, requires great advances in our knowledge but could be very rewarding.

Chapter 19
Branchio-oto-renal syndrome

RICHARD JH SMITH and WILLIAM J KIMBERLING

Introduction

Branchio-oto-renal (BOR) syndrome is an autosomal dominant disorder with branchial, otological and renal manifestations. The branchial manifestations usually are inconsequential, however the hearing impairment and renal malformations can be significant. The disease gene has been localized to chromosome 8q.

Background

Early reports of possible examples of BOR syndrome can be traced to the nineteenth century. Aucherson first recognized the familial occurrence of branchial anomalies in 1832, and the combination of preauricular pits, branchial fistulae and hearing impairment was reported by Heusinger in 1864 and by Paget in 1877 and 1878. Under the Nazi regime, this constellation of features was referred to as *Innenohrschwerhörigkeit*, or 'hereditary hardness of hearing' and provoked a great deal of discussion by several German authors, notably Albrecht (1933), Schneider (1937), Loebell (1938), Steinberg (1938) and Langenbeck (1938), because of the eugenic problems it raised (Fourman and Fourman, 1955).

The association of preauricular pits, bilateral branchial fistulae and progressive sensorineural hearing loss was diagnosed more frequently following the report of a large affected family by Fourman and Fourman in 1955. Twenty years later, Melnick et al. (1975) recognized the possibility of concomitant renal anomalies and suggested the term branchio-oto-renal syndrome to underscore the phenotypic anomalies of the branchial arches, otocysts and renal primordia. Nomenclature has varied, with terms applied to the disease often reflecting observation and author bias. Examples include: ear pits-deafness syndrome; preauricular pits, cervical fistulae, hearing loss syndrome; branchio-oto-dysplasia syndrome; branchio-oto-ureteral syndrome; branchio-oto-renal dysplasia; and Melnick-Fraser syndrome (Cremers and Fikkers-van Noord, 1980; Fraser et al., 1983).

Prevalence

Congenital hearing loss affects 1:1,000 children, and in approximately one half of these children, the hearing impairment is inherited (Fraser, 1976). BOR syndrome is a type of autosomal dominant syndromic hearing impairment. Although the precise prevalence of BOR syndrome is unknown, estimates have been made by George Fraser. In 1976, he surveyed 3,460 children with profound hearing impairment and found only 5 children (0.15%) with a family history of branchial fistulae and preauricular pits (1:700,000) (Fraser, 1976). Four years later, however, FC Fraser presented evidence to suggest that the prevalence of BOR syndrome is much higher (Fraser et al., 1980). In a study of 421 white children in the Montreal Schools for the Deaf, they diagnosed BOR syndrome in 2% of the profoundly deaf students. Using this information, they estimated disease prevalence at 1:40,000. The true value is probably somewhere between these extremes.

Characteristic findings

Numerous studies describing the BOR syndrome phenotype are available (Fraser et al., 1978; Cremers and Fikkers-van Noord, 1980; Chen et al., 1995a). In persons carrying the gene mutation, disease penetrance appears to be nearly 100%, although expressivity is highly variable. The most common manifestations of the syndrome occur in > 20% of affected persons and include hearing loss, preauricular pits, pinnae abnormalities, branchial fistulae and renal malformations (Table 19.1). Of these anomalies, hearing loss and renal malformations carry the greatest morbidity. Hearing loss also is the most common disease manifestation and can be detected in 85 – 90% of affected persons. Although the loss can be stable or progressive; and conductive, sensorineural or mixed, most studies report that mixed losses are most common (Cremers et al., 1981; Gimsing and Dymrose, 1986; Melnick et al., 1976; Ostri et al., 1991; Smith et al., 1984) (Table 19.2). Characteristic morphogenetic abnormalities of the temporal bone also have been described and include hypoplastic and displaced ossicles, cochlear hypoplasia, bulbous internal auditory canals, deep posterior fossa and acutely angled promontories (Chen et al., 1995).

Table 19.1 Phenotypic features of BOR syndrome (N=45).

Major Anomalies	Percentage
Hearing loss	93
Preauricular pits	82
Renal anomalies	67 (N=21)
Branchial fistulae	49
Pinnae deformities	36
External auditory canal stenosis	29

Minor Anomalies	Percentage
Preauricular tag	13
Lacrimal duct aplasia	11
Short palate	7
Retrognathia	4
Benign intracranial tumour	2
Cleft palate	2
Congenital hip dysplasia	2
Euthyroid goitre	2
Facial nerve paresis	2
Gustatory lacrimation	2
Non-rotation of the gastrointestinal tract	2
Pancreatic duplication cyst	2
Temporoparietal linear naevus	2

A complete spectrum of renal malformations occurs, running the gamut from complete agenesis, hypoplasia and dysplasia to ureteral-pelvic junction obstruction, caliceal cysts, diverticuli, caliectasis, hydronephrosis, pelviectasis, prominence of the collecting system and vesicular uretal reflux (Chen et al., 1995). This variability has suggested to several investigators that BOR syndrome is heterogeneous, and in support of this hypothesis, in 1978 Melnick et al. described three families, one with the regular features of BOR syndrome and two with only cup-shaped pinnae and branchial fistulae. The renal abnormalities and hearing impairment expected with BOR syndrome were not present in the latter families and their type of malformation was labelled branchio-oto (BO) syndrome (Fraser et al., 1980). However, when Fraser et al. (1983) re-evaluated intravenous pyelograms previously read as normal in persons with BO syndrome, anomalies were found in three of four individuals suggesting that BO and BOR syndromes may be the same entity. To further complicate the issue, a third disorder, branchio-oto-ureteral (BOU) syndrome has been described in two families with branchial and otological findings of BOR syndrome and renal abnormalities limited to duplication of the collecting system and bifid renal pelvises (Fraser et al., 1983).

Because the sensitivities of ultrasonography and intravenous pyelography differ, this apparent confusion in syndrome nosology may reflect test specificity. For example, by performing excretory urography, van Widdershoven et al. (1983) were able to demonstrate renal malformations in 16 of 16 patients with BOR syndrome. Both Heimer and Leibner (1986), and Chen et al. (1995) also have described multigenerational families in which individuals with manifestations of BO, BOU and BOR syndromes could be identified. In the latter case, linkage analysis with this family localised the defective gene to chromosome 8q, consistent with prior localisation of the gene for BOR syndrome to this same region (Kumar et al., 1992; Smith et al., 1992).

Phenotypic observations in several families have suggested the possibility of increased disease severity in successive generations, and recently seven three-generational families were assessed for anticipation with respect to severity of hearing loss and renal involvement. In four of these families, the degree of hearing loss showed anticipation, but in the remaining three, the degree of loss did not vary by generation. With respect to renal disease, generational progression was noted in three families, but in one family the reverse trend was found. These data are more consistent with statistical as opposed to biological anticipation and may reflect the variable expression and decreased fitness that occur in BOR syndrome. For example, persons with renal agenesis are unlikely to have descendants (Chen et al., 1995).

A review of recurrent renal agenesis in BOR syndrome also suggests that transmission does not implicate a parent-of-origin effect. Marked renal defects have been reported in six live-born offspring (including bilateral renal agenesis in three individuals) who had affected fathers (Carmi et al., 1983; Cremers and Fikkers-van Noord, 1980; Greenberg et al., 1988; van Widdershoven et al., 1983) and in four live-born offspring of affected mothers (Chitayat et al., 1992; Cremers and Fikkers-van Noord, 1980; Fitch and Srolovitz, 1976; van Widdershoven et al., 1983). An excess of unexplained foetal deaths, presumably a consequence of bilateral renal agenesis, occurred in all of these families, suggesting a higher recurrence risk for parents with a previously affected child.

Anomalies which have been reported in less than 20% of individuals with BOR syndrome are considered uncommon. Examples include lachrymal duct aplasia, short palate, retrognathia, cleft palate, congenital hip dysplasia, facial nerve paralysis, non-rotation of the gastrointestinal tract, pancreatic duplication cysts and temporal parietal linear naevus (Chen et al., 1995) (Table 19.1).

Gene localization

In 1992, the BOR gene was localized to chromosome 8q12-22 (Kumar et al., 1992; Smith et al., 1992). This localization was in accordance with an earlier report by Haan et al. (1989) of a family with an inherited rearrangement of chromosome 8q, dir ins(8)(q24.11 q13.3 q21.13). Individuals with this chromosomal abnormality have manifestations of both trichorhinophalangeal (TRP) and BOR syndromes. TRP syndrome has been linked to deletions involving 8q24.11-q24.13, however no person with a deletion of this part of chromosome 8q had been previously described with features of BOR syndrome (Bowen et al., 1985; Buhler and Malik, 1984; Buhler et al., 1987; Fryns and van den Berghe, 1986), suggesting that the BOR syndrome gene maps to 8q13-q21. Hearing losses associated with BOR are shown in Table 19.2.

Table 19.2 Hearing loss associated with BOR syndrome (N=64).

Type of Hearing Loss		Degree of Hearing Loss	
Mixed	45%	Mild	27%
Conductive	29%	Moderate	22%
Sensorineural	26%	Severe	33%
		Profound	16%

Although the disease gene has not yet been cloned, its location has been refined to the interval between markers D8S553 and D8S286 (Ni et al., 1994; Wang et al., 1994). To identify candidate genes within this interval, yeast artificial chromosomes (YACs) that span the region (Vincent et al., 1994) are being studied for expressed sequences common to both the ear and the kidney. Preliminary studies suggest that BOR syndrome is part of a contiguous gene deletion syndrome that includes Duane syndrome, a dominant form of hydrocephalus and trapezius aplasia (Vincent et al., 1994). The BOR syndrome gene is probably expressed during the fourth to tenth weeks of embryogenesis when the otic placode and renal anlage are developing, and may encode a protein important in extracellular matrix adhesion.

Chapter 20
Treacher Collins syndrome

MICHAEL J DIXON

Introduction

Treacher Collins syndrome was first reported in 1846 by Thompson, however it was E Treacher Collins, who reported the essential character- istics of the disorder in 1900, who is credited with its discovery. The first extensive review of the condition was detailed by Franceschetti and Klein in 1949, who used the term mandibulofacial dysostosis to describe the clinical features. Nevertheless, there is historical evidence in pre- Columbian sculptures that both the syndrome and its hereditary nature, were recognised as early as the seventh century (Poswillo, 1989).

Clinical features

Treacher Collins syndrome is a rare autosomal dominant disorder of craniofacial development, which has been estimated to occur with an incidence of 1/50,000 live births, although no formal population studies have been performed. However, up to 60% of cases do not appear to have a previous family history and are thought to arise as the result of a *de novo* mutation. The condition is characterised by:

- Abnormalities of the pinnae which are frequently associated with atresia of the external auditory canals and anomalies of the middle ear ossicles. As a result bilateral conductive hearing loss is common (Phelps et al., 1981) – see Figure 20.1.
- Hypoplasia of the facial bones, particularly the mandible and zygo- matic complex.
- Antimongoloid slanting of the palpebral fissures (see Figure 20.2) with colobomata of the lower eyelids and a paucity of lid lashes medial to the defect.
- Cleft palate.

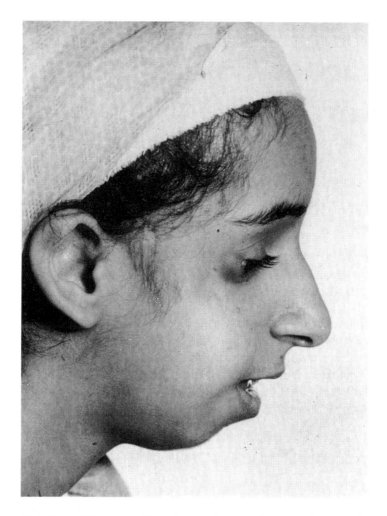

Figure 20.1 Typical features of Treacher Collins syndrome with anomalies of the pinnae and hypoplasia of the zygomatic complex and mandible.

Of these features, down-slanting palpebral fissures and zygomatic hypoplasia appear to be the most common, with anomalies of the ears also occurring in a high percentage of cases (Rogers, 1964). Audiological examination of patients with Treacher Collins syndrome is very important as 50%, or more, of patients have conductive hearing loss. Mixed or sensorineural hearing loss is rare (Hutchinson et al., 1977).

Whilst data from studies in the rat suggest that these features may occur asymmetrically (Wilkinson and Poswillo, 1991), clinical data suggest that, in humans, these features exhibit a striking degree of bilateral symmetry (Kay and Kay, 1989). The penetrance of the disorder is very high, indeed, there is only a single case in the literature where non-penetrance has been established (Dixon et al., 1994). There is, howev-

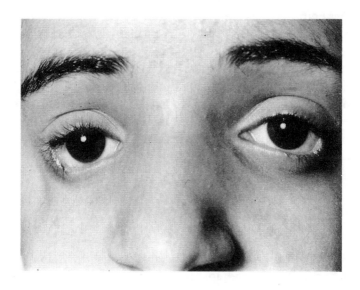

Figure 20.2 The same child as Figure 20.1 displaying down-slanting palpebral fissures with colobomata of the lower eyelids and a paucity of eyelid lashes medial to the defect. Note the bilateral symmetry of the clinical features.

er, extreme variation in the clinical features. At one end of the spectrum severe cases may result in perinatal death due to a compromised airway, whereas, at the other end of the spectrum, mild cases may be difficult to diagnose and a number of individuals are only diagnosed after the birth of a more severely affected child. A number of attempts have been made to classify the condition based on the severity of the clinical features; however these classifications are arbitrary and of little use as they can in no way be used to make predictions about future pregnancies. Nevertheless, the extreme variability in the degree to which individuals can be affected, together with the high rate of *de novo* mutations, can complicate the provision of genetic counselling, particularly where the diagnosis of either of an affected child's parents is equivocal. As Treacher Collins syndrome is inherited in an autosomal dominant fashion the risk to future pregnancies if either parent is affected is 50%; however genuinely unaffected parents who produce an affected child have a negligible recurrence risk, even though their affected child will itself possess a 50% chance of producing an affected child. In the case of mildly affected individuals, or where non-penetrance is suspected, it is very important to ensure that minimal features of Treacher Collins syndrome are not present. In this regard, the use of craniofacial radiographs, particularly the occipito-mental view, which enables visualisation of the zygomatic complex, may be useful in detecting zygomatic hypoplasia (Dixon et al., 1991a; Marres et al., 1995).

Anticipation, in which the severity of the disease increases with successive generations, has been suggested to be a feature of Treacher Collins syndrome. This observation is probably the result of ascertainment bias as it has not been borne out by studies of multigenerational families with large numbers of affected individuals (Dixon et al., 1994; Marres et al., 1995). Whilst concordance of severity in affected siblings has been reported (Nicolaides et al., 1984), it is not possible to predict how severely affected an individual might be, in view of the marked intrafamilial variability in severity seen in multiplex Treacher Collins syndrome families (Dixon et al., 1994).

Differential diagnosis

A number of conditions have a facial gestalt which may resemble Treacher Collins syndrome, including Nager and Miller syndromes, in which there are limb defects, and also the oculoauriculovertebral (OAV) spectrum. In Nager syndrome the limb defects are preaxial and most commonly include hypoplastic or absent thumbs, radial hypoplasia or aplasia, and radioulnar synostosis. In Miller syndrome the limb anomalies are postaxial, most commonly with absence or incomplete development of the 5th digital ray of all four limbs. Whilst most cases of Nager and Miller syndrome are sporadic, both autosomal dominant and autosomal recessive transmission have been reported.

OAV spectrum is a complex and heterogeneous set of conditions which includes hemifacial microsomia and Goldenhar syndrome, which primarily affect development of the ear, mouth and mandible. These conditions vary from mild to severe and usually affect only one side of the face. Bilateral involvement has occasionally been documented, but in such cases expression is usually more severe on one side of the face (Kay and Kay, 1989). Goldenhar syndrome has vertebral anomalies and epibulbar dermoids in addition to the facial involvement. In most instances, OAV spectrum occurs sporadically, although 1 – 2% of cases have a previous family history. Overall, the spectrum is characterised by a low empirical recurrence risk, although counselling should be provided on an individual family basis. While it is usually straightforward to exclude OAV from the differential diagnosis of Treacher Collins syndrome on the basis of the facial gestalt, caution should be exercised where individuals are only mildly affected so that the minimal diagnostic criteria that constitute Treacher Collins syndrome are not overlooked.

Treatment

Severely affected patients may need a tracheotomy to be performed to enable them to maintain their airway in the perinatal period. Generally, the tracheotomy will be maintained until reconstructive surgery can be performed. Facial surgery is generally delayed so that facial growth may proceed, thereby reducing the inhibitory effect that scarring may have on facial growth. Nevertheless, it is extremely difficult to achieve an ideal cosmetic result in patients with severe Treacher Collins syndrome. In a number of children affected by Treacher Collins syndrome, particularly those with mandibular hypoplasia, intubation may prove to be difficult, such that specialised anaesthetic care may be necessitated.

In terms of the audiological problems, in the vast majority of cases the hearing loss may be alleviated by the use of bone conduction hearing aids. The provision of percutaneous titanium implants allows prosthetic ears to be fitted for those patients with severe anomalies of the external ears and, in general, the aesthetic result achieved in this way is superior to that which can be achieved by surgery. Moreover, the implants can be used to attach bone anchored hearing aids behind the ear. The success of these procedures is such that in most cases of Treacher Collins syndrome, particularly those with the more severe forms of ear anomaly, there is seldom a good indication for reconstructive ear surgery.

Aetiology

On the basis that the tissues affected in Treacher Collins syndrome arise during early embryonic development from the first and second branchial arches, clefts and pouches, two main theories have been advanced to explain the pathogenesis of the disorder; both of which result from teratological experiments in animals. The mechanisms proposed are interference with neural crest cell migration, and excessive cell death in the ectodermal placodes. Poswillo (1975) produced a phenocopy of Treacher Collins syndrome in the rat by the administration of teratogenic doses of vitamin A palmitate early in development. This appeared to cause focal death of neural crest cells prior to, or during, their migration from the neural folds. Examination of affected embryos indicated that the pre-otic neural crest had disappeared. It was therefore proposed that selective destruction of those crest cells destined for migration into the first and second branchial arches had occurred. As morphogenesis appeared to continue normally, it was proposed that the anomalies resulted from a lack of available tissue.

A later study by Sulik et al. (1987) suggested that Treacher Collins syndrome resulted from excessive cell death in the ectodermal placodes. In this case, phenocopies of Treacher Collins syndrome and Nager or Miller syndrome were produced in mice via acute maternal exposure to 13-cis-retinoic acid (a vitamin A analogue, which is not stored in the maternal liver) at 9.0 – 9.5 days post-fertilisation. These studies demonstrated that the craniofacial and limb anomalies resulted from excessive cell death in the proximal aspect of the maxillary and mandibular processes of the first branchial arch and the apical ectodermal ridge of the limb bud. Nevertheless, despite these theories, the underlying genetic defect remained unknown until recently. For this reason, positional cloning strategies were used in an attempt to identify the gene mutated in Treacher Collins syndrome.

Positional cloning strategies

The gene mutated in Treacher Collins syndrome was initially mapped to chromosome 5q31-34 using genetic linkage analysis (Dixon et al., 1991a; Jabs et al., 1991b). Due to the low informativity of the majority of restriction fragment length polymorphisms, and the relative shortage of large families, subsequent linkage studies have concentrated on the use of highly informative short tandem repeat polymorphisms (STRPs). A large number of these STRPs have been isolated and a dense marker framework around the Treacher Collins syndrome locus (TCOF1) created. These studies have permitted the refinement of the localisation of TCOF1 to 5q32-33.1 and have allowed polymorphic markers flanking the disease locus to be identified. All the families that have been analysed to date (approximately 50) support linkage of the disease locus to markers in the same region of the genome with none showing unequivocal evidence of nonlinkage (Loftus et al., 1993; Jabs et al., 1993; Edery et al., 1994). Nevertheless, Treacher Collins syndrome has been associated with a number of different chromosomal anomalies involving other regions of the genome (Dixon et al., 1991b; Balestrazzi et al., 1983; Jabs et al., 1991a; Arn et al., 1993) which raise the possibility of genetic heterogeneity. However, in each of these cases, linkage analysis with a series of familial cases of well documented Treacher Collins syndrome families failed to show co-segregation with markers for the relevant region. Moreover, one of the translocations did not ultimately completely co-segregate with the disease phenotype (Dixon et al., 1991b), whilst in the remaining cases the facial gestalt of the patients did not entirely conform to the Treacher Collins syndrome clinical criteria. These data strongly suggest that Treacher Collins syndrome is genetically homogeneous.

The creation of a dense marker framework of highly informative polymorphisms around the TCOF1 locus has enabled post-natal diagnostic predictions to be undertaken in mildly affected, and apparently unaffected, individuals (Dixon et al., 1994). This has proven particularly helpful where the clinical diagnosis is equivocal. In this regard, a large Treacher Collins syndrome family with multiple affected individuals has been studied where linkage analysis had demonstrated that *TCOF1* was linked to markers in the 5q31-34 region. The family was analysed for linkage to eight STRP markers, and the genotyping results were used to make diagnostic predictions in certain mildly affected and apparently unaffected individuals. The linkage results supported the 'affected' diagnosis made in two individuals who exhibited only very minor stigmata of *TCOF1*, neither of whom had produced clinically affected offspring. The results further suggested that one child, who appeared to be clinically and radiographically normal, despite being at risk of having inherited the mutated gene, had, in fact, inherited the haplotype associated with the disease in the family and was therefore highly likely to be affected. This being the case, this was the first time that genetic linkage analysis has been used to demonstrate non-penetrance in *TCOF1* (Dixon et al., 1994). In a previous study, radiological investigation had revealed hypoplasia of the zygomatic arch in an apparently clinically normal individual (Dixon et al., 1991a). In this family, the pedigree structure did not permit diagnostic evaluation using linked DNA markers. Both of these studies emphasise the importance of performing a thorough clinical, radiological and, where the pedigree structure permits, genetic investigation of families in which there is a history of Treacher Collins syndrome.

First trimester prenatal diagnosis has also been performed (Edwards et al., 1996). Until recently, prenatal diagnosis had only been undertaken in affected families using either fetoscopy (Nicolaides et al., 1984) or ultrasound imaging (Meizner et al., 1991; Milligan et al., 1994). Although the quality of ultrasound imaging has improved markedly in recent years, allowing non-invasive prenatal diagnosis to be made, it can still be difficult to make a positive diagnosis where the foetus is mildly affected. Prenatal diagnosis using either fetoscopy or ultrasound imaging is not possible until the second trimester of pregnancy (approximately 18 weeks). At this time termination of pregnancy is a particularly traumatic procedure psychologically as it involves the induction of labour. Prenatal diagnosis using linked DNA markers allows first trimester diagnosis to be undertaken using DNA extracted from chorionic villus samples taken at 10 – 11 weeks of gestation, but does not allow severity to be predicted. Nevertheless, diagnostic predictions of the type noted above should be undertaken with caution, and only in families showing significant evidence of linkage to 5q32-33.2. Moreover, such diagnostic predictions can only be undertaken in a subset of families where there is a positive family history of Treacher Collins syndrome. The recent isolation of *TCDF1* (Treacher Collins Collaborative Group, 1996) makes DNA diagnosis for the vast majority of families a much stronger possibility.

In addition to providing the basis for diagnostic predictions, the creation of a high resolution genetic map around the Treacher Collins syndrome locus, and the identification of markers flanking the disease locus, has provided important anchor points for the cloning of the disease gene. Until recently, the creation of long range continuity over large physical (megabase) distances was extremely difficult due to the limitations of existing cloning vectors. The advent of cloning in yeast artificial chromosomes (YACs, see Chapter 2) has overcome some of these shortcomings. For instance, the amount of DNA that can be cloned in a single YAC is an order of magnitude greater than the size of a cosmid insert. This considerably reduces the number of clones required for the creation of a contig across the critical region encompassing a disease gene, thereby reducing the amount of work required to link up existing markers. Moreover, YACs have been shown to contain regions of the genome which are not recoverable in other cloning vectors. Nevertheless, whilst the increased length of YAC inserts enables more rapid map generation, they require a more complex protocol for the analysis of the inserts. Moreover, a significant proportion of YAC clones result from the co-ligation of non-contiguous DNA fragments (chimaeras). In addition, the clones themselves are frequently more difficult to use e.g. for the isolation of coding sequences. We have therefore used the joint advantages of YACs and cosmids in the creation of the contig map across the Treacher Collins syndrome critical region. Restriction mapping of the clones encompassing this region, with a panel of restriction enzymes, has permitted the identification of a large number of clustered restriction sites for rare-cutting enzymes, suggesting that the region contains a large number of different genes.

The calcium-binding protein, annexin 6, was found to lie within this region and was considered to be a candidate for the disease locus. However, genotyping of affected families with a short tandem repeat polymorphism isolated at this locus, resulted in the identification of two recombination events in affected individuals, effectively excluding mutations in this gene from a causative role in the pathogenesis of Treacher Collins syndrome. This observation simultaneously resulted in a reduction of the size of the critical region to less than 500 kb (Loftus et al. 1996). Cosmids encompassing the majority of this region have been assembled and the gene encoding the heparan sulphate N-deacetylase/N-sulphotransferase has been isolated from this region. This enzyme is required in the series of reactions that result in N-sulphation of the oligosaccharide backbone of heparan sulphate, N-sulphation being of required in the binding of the fibroblast growth factors to their receptors. Nevertheless, this gene has been excluded from a role in Treacher Collins syndrome as it has not been possible to demonstrate a mutation within the coding sequence of this gene in any affected individual.

The creation of a comprehensive transcription (gene) map of the Treacher Collins syndrome region has resulted in the identification of a number of additional genes, which have been searched for mutations in families with a history of Treacher Collins syndrome (Loftus et al., 1996; Treacher Collins syndrome Collaborative Group, 1996). The identification of five different mutations within one of these genes indicated that the Treacher Collins syndrome gene has finally been identified (Treacher Collins Syndrome Collaborative Group, 1996). Although the function of this gene, which has been named *Treacle*, is currently unknown, the investigation of its role during development will improve our understanding of facial development and provide important information regarding the development of the outer and middle ear. Moreover, this finding will increase the accuracy of diagnostic testing in the condition, as well as allowing the extension of such testing to a wider range of affected families.

Part IV
Non-Syndromal Hearing Loss

Chapter 21
Autosomal recessive non-syndromal hearing loss

CHRISTINE PETIT

Although a large variety of syndromes exist in which hearing loss is associated with developmental abnormalities of different organs, or with endocrine or metabolic disorders (Konigsmark and Gorlin, 1976; Gorlin et al., 1995), in the majority of patients with hearing loss, hearing loss is the only symptom. These forms are referred to as isolated hearing loss and represent about 70% of all cases of childhood hearing loss (Morton, 1991).

Prevalence of the autosomal recessive forms

Historical aspects

The first interest in the origin of hearing loss arose from observations by Pierre Ménière in 1846 (Ménière, 1846). In a lecture entitled 'Upon marriage between relatives considered as the cause of congenital deaf-mutism' at the French Academy of Medicine on April 29, 1856, Ménière (professor at the Faculty and physician at the Institut Impérial des Sourds-muets) was questioning the causes of deaf-mutism (Ménière, 1856):

> 'Given a deaf-mute, is it possible to determine the causes which led to this so serious disability? ... From these documents emerges a general fact, namely that the number of deaf-mutes is largely variable in each country; sometimes it is estimated to be one affected individual in 3000, sometimes one in 2000 and some villages have as many as one in 200 individuals affected or even more ... If in restricted, isolated villages, one marries his first cousin or an uncle marries his niece, as the scarcity of matrimonial elements may render it necessary, ... it is within these populations that one observes ... inborn deaf-mutism ...'

It is in these terms that Ménière acknowledged for the first time the autosomal recessive origin of deaf-mutism. In such families both parents are usually phenotypically normal heterozygotes, while the risk of being affected for each child is 25% and the risk of normal hearing offspring being heterozygous carriers is 66%. The role of genetics in congenital hearing loss was also emphasized in 1853 by William Wilde, through the analysis he carried out on more than 3,000 cases identified during the course of an Irish census (Wilde, 1853).

During the period between Mendel's formulation of his laws in 1866 (Mendel, 1866) and the rediscovery and appreciation of his work in 1900 by de Vries, von Tschermak and Correns (Stern, 1950), Alexander Graham Bell (of telephone fame) addressed the possible causes of congenital hearing loss. Bell's work, rather than contributing to understanding, resulted in the promotion of eugenic theories (Bell, 1883). In 1898, EA Fay published a very well documented study on marriage between two deaf persons, or one deaf and one normal hearing person, in the United States (Fay, 1898). These data were reinterpreted in the light of Mendel's laws, by H Lundborg (Lundborg, 1912; Lundborg, 1920). His interpretations, based on the assumption that a single gene is the cause of non-syndromal profound hearing loss, led him to conclude erroneously that all cases of hearing loss are autosomal recessive.

Present views on the prevalence of autosomal recessive hearing loss

Among the various forms of hearing loss, the proportion of autosomal recessive forms is far from certain. This reflects the paucity of our knowledge of the contribution of genetics to hearing loss; in particular, we know very little of the causes of hearing loss with adult onset (after 18 years of age).

High prevalence of autosomal recessive forms in childhood hearing loss

Most information on childhood hearing impairment concerns prelingual hearing loss, that is, congenital or very early childhood onset of a hearing impairment exceeding 70 dB HL (decibels hearing level) in the better hearing ear. The greatest attention has been given to profound prelingual hearing impairments (loss greater than 90 dB HL), as they dramatically impede speech acquisition and thus result in major communication and educational handicaps. It is nevertheless difficult to compile epidemiological data because the various population surveys have been conducted using different criteria. In the United States, it has been estimated that 1/1,000 children are affected by hearing loss at birth or in early childhood (Morton, 1991). In England and Denmark, Davis and Parving (1993) report that 0.7/1,000 children have a hearing loss greater than 70 dB HL by 5 years of age, among whom about 0.4/1,000 have a loss greater than 95 dB HL; in 90% of these cases the hearing loss is congenital. In China, Liu et al. (1993) estimated that 1.1/1,000 children were affected by profound hearing loss by 5 years of age.

Direct evidence for a genetic origin of childhood hearing loss, which is provided by a family history, is obtained in only 13 to 30% of the cases (Davis and Parving, 1993; Marazita et al., 1993). At least in industrialized countries where the size of the sibships is usually small, most cases are sporadic, with both parents having normal hearing. Among these families, the percentage of hereditary forms is derived from an estimate of the percentage of non-hereditary forms, calculated using a maximum likelihood method (Morton, 1958; Chung et al., 1959; Morton and Chung, 1959). This last proportion is itself derived by studying families with normal hearing parents in which the distribution of simplex and multiplex cases is analysed with regard to the size of the sibships. Alternatively, it can be evaluated from a comparison of the inbreeding coefficients of these simplex and multiplex families (Chung et al., 1959). The most recent study performed in the US has concluded that in 62% of deaf school age children, a genetic defect is responsible (Marazita et al., 1993). Previous studies in the same country had estimated the percentage as only 50% (Fraser, 1964; Nance et al., 1977). The major reason for this change is the improvement in the state of public health, leading to a progressive decrease in the infectious causes of hearing loss, such as postnatal meningitis, rubella during pregnancy, cytomegalovirus infection and otitis media (Marazita et al., 1993).

Aside from these severe forms of prelingual hearing loss, there are also postlingual severe forms appearing later on in childhood. Morton (1991) reports that an additional 1/1,000 children become deaf before adulthood. Less severe forms which seem to appear during youth are also encountered. Thus, 0.59/1,000 children have a hearing impairment between 40 and 70 dB HL (hindering perception of normal speech) by 5 years of age (Davis and Parving, 1993); an additional 0.1% of children between 6 and 11 years of age and 0.2% of children between 12 and 17 years present with a hearing loss of 41 to 55 dB HL (Leske, 1981). The genetic contribution to these forms has not yet been evaluated.

The first estimate of the frequency of the different modes of inheritance for prelingual hearing loss was made by Chung et al. (1959). They demonstrated the high prevalence of autosomal recessive forms, followed by autosomal dominant forms and, finally, X-linked forms. The frequency of autosomal recessive forms of hearing loss is obtained by taking the frequency of deaf children whose parents have normal hearing, and subtracting the estimated frequencies of both non-genetic cases (see above) and those due to non-penetrant autosomal dominant causes, each value being calculated according to the Morton method (Morton, 1958; Morton and Chung, 1959).

Estimates of the frequency of the autosomal recessive forms among prelingual hearing loss vary from 72 to 92% (72% (Fraser, 1965), 75% (Newton, 1985), 85% (Nance et al., 1977), 92% (Liu et al., 1993)). This frequency increases with the inbreeding coefficient of the population (Majumder et al., 1989). Among these forms of prelingual hearing loss, the prevalence of an autosomal recessive mode of transmission seems to be even higher among profoundly deaf children (Newton, 1985). Interestingly, a recent study of the US population shows a secular change in the relative contributions of the various modes of transmission. A study from data collected in the US in 1969 (the 1969 – 70 Annual Survey) indicated that 85% of early onset hearing loss was autosomal recessive (Nance et al., 1977) whereas a similar study conducted in 1989 showed that recessive forms account for only 75% of cases (Marazita et al., 1993). This decrease seems to be due to the increasing number of deaf people who marry and have children, which results in an increase in the frequency of cases with a dominant mode of transmission.

As already mentioned, there exist only limited genetic data on progressive or late-onset forms of childhood hearing loss; however several pedigrees showing autosomal recessive transmission of such forms have been reported (de Kleyn, 1915; Johnsen, 1954; Mengel et al., 1967; Cremers, 1979; Guilford et al., 1994a; Veske et al., 1996).

Paucity of data on late-onset forms of hearing loss

Epidemiologic studies revealed that the percentages of the population having a hearing loss exceeding 45 dB HL and 65 dB HL are approximately 1.3% and 0.3% respectively between ages 30 and 50, and 7.4% and 2.3% between ages 60 and 70 (Davis, 1989). Most of these defects are thought to be conductive. It has been generally assumed that the development of these adult-onset forms is due to interaction of environmental and genetic factors, which has dampened enthusiasm for investigating their genetic origins. However, the role of heredity seems to be more important than initially thought since half of the affected individuals report a family history of hearing loss. The mode of transmission seems more complex than a simple dominant or recessive monogenic pattern (Sill et al., 1994).

In the rest of this chapter we will focus on childhood recessive hearing loss.

Autosomal recessive hearing loss in children

Clinical aspects

In most cases, diagnosis of a recessive form of hearing loss remains difficult. The question arises each time that a first deaf child is born to parents with normal hearing. Recessive inheritance is considered when no environmental origin such as infections or ototoxic drugs is plausible. It should be mentioned that about a quarter of young children affected by a hearing impairment have remained in a neonatal intensive care unit (Davis and Parving, 1993). The hypothesis of autosomal recessive inheritance of the hearing loss becomes highly probable when a child with a bilateral hearing impairment has parents known to be related (consanguineous), or suspected to be relatives because of their geographic origin (see below). However, even if there is evidence for parental consanguinity, the different branches of the family should be investigated in sufficient detail to eliminate the possibility of dominant transmission with variable penetrance or of X-linked transmission.

The majority of these autosomal recessive forms of hearing loss are sensorineural (Davis and Parving, 1993). The sensorineural impairment is demonstrated by comparison of air and bone conduction, analysed by pure-tone audiogram, which permits elimination of the possibility of conductive hearing loss. Then, if no residual auditory function persists, the sensorineural defect cannot be further explored and any associated conductive hearing impairment could not be detected. At present, these forms of hearing loss remain clinically undifferentiated. When enough residual auditive function persists, the auditory brainstem response (ABR) can be recorded, which allows the distinction between cochlear and retrocochlear defects. Almost all autosomal recessive forms of childhood hearing loss have a cochlear origin. However, a moderately severe hearing loss of retrocochlear origin can be cited (Blegvad and Hvidegaard, 1983). In these cases also, the respective damage to inner and outer hair cells can be tentatively assessed by recording otoacoustic emissions and distortion products.

One criterion which could be used to distinguish the various forms of isolated hearing loss is the existence of vestibular defects. Vestibular defects are likely to be frequently associated with cochlear defects in humans. Vestibular and cochlear neuroepithelia are very similar and a large number of deaf mouse mutants also present with balance problems (Steel, 1995). In humans, these vestibular defects are almost asymptomatic; probably they are compensated for early on by other senses, so that they lead to only one clinical manifestation, a delay in walking. Analysis of vestibular function (electronystagmography, oculomotility tests, rotational chair sigmoidal harmonic acceleration tests) may, however, allow detection of such defects even in the adult (see Chapter 11).

High genetic heterogeneity

Segregation analysis of hearing loss in consanguineous populations has shown a frequency of affected offspring which is not significantly different from 0.25, thus indicating that, in most cases, autosomal recessive hearing loss is a monogenic disease (Kimberling et al., 1989; Ben Arab et al., 1990). However, the high genetic heterogeneity of autosomal recessive hearing loss has long been recognized (Stevenson and Cheeseman, 1956). In most cases the children of deaf-deaf matings have normal hearing, even when both parents have autosomal recessive forms of hearing loss; if the same gene was defective in each parent, one would expect all the children to be affected.

The first estimate of the number of genes responsible for autosomal recessive hearing loss was produced by Chung et al. (1959), using a calculation based on the comparison of the mean inbreeding coefficient of the general population and of deaf children from normal hearing parents. This led to a minimum estimate of 36 'hearing loss' genes segregating in the congenital deaf-mute population of Ireland. In parallel, it was estimated that 16% of the general population carry a gene for hearing loss (Morton, 1960). Several other estimates have since been given for various populations, sometimes based on slightly different calculations (Chung and Brown, 1970). These data, which are concerned only with prelingual autosomal recessive hearing loss (Brownstein et al., 1991; Morton, 1991), lead to a mean estimate of 40 (range 28 – 60) autosomal recessive genes in large Western populations (Chung et al., 1959; Sank, 1963; Chung and Brown, 1970; Furusho and Yasuda, 1973; Costeff and Dar, 1980) and 8 (range 4 – 13) genes in isolated regions with frequent consanguineous marriages amongst the population (Hu et al., 1987; Majumder et al., 1989; Ben Arab et al., 1990; Brownstein et al., 1991). However, these statistical estimates rely on disparate collected epidemiological data. In addition, they were based on the working hypothesis that each hearing loss gene contributes equally to the population prevalence, an assumption which results in an underestimate of the number of genes involved.

Lastly, although a minority, other more complex modes of segregation of autosomal recessive hearing loss do exist besides the highly predominant monogenic defects. Such is the case of a maternally inherited recessive form of hearing loss which results from the association of an autosomal recessive mutation within the nuclear genome and a mutation in the mitochondrial genome (Prezant et al., 1993; Reid et al., 1994; see Chapter 26). Additionally, as shown for retinitis pigmentosa (Kajiwara et al., 1994), a digenic mode of inheritance is not unlikely for some forms of autosomal recessive hearing loss.

Mapping of the *DFNB* genes

Genes for autosomal recessive hearing loss were initially termed *NSRD* (non-syndromal recessive deafness), but they are now referred to as *DFNB* genes ('B' signifies the autosomal recessive mode of transmission).

Until 1994, mapping genes responsible for autosomal recessive hearing loss was considered too difficult because of the extreme genetic heterogeneity combined with the absence of clinical or paraclinical criteria that would allow differentiation of the inner ear defects caused by the various genes, and the high frequency of unions between deaf persons, at least in developed countries (90% in the United States) (Reardon, 1992). As a result, several defective genes responsible for hearing loss may coexist within the same family. This obstacle has recently been circumvented.

It is reasonable to assume that the probability that several different hearing loss genes segregate within the same family is greatly reduced in a family that has lived in an isolated region for several generations. Such conditions can be found in geographic regions cut off from any immigration by mountains, deserts or sea. Two factors may then increase the homozygosity of individuals and thus favour the emergence of autosomal recessive defects; the small size of the isolates (increasing genetic drift), and a high frequency of marriages between relatives. Consanguineous marriages are frequent for cultural and religious reasons in several countries, especially around the Mediterranean sea, in Pakistan and in India.

It was by analysing large families meeting these criteria that the first gene, *DFNB1*, was mapped to the pericentromeric region of the long arm of chromosome 13 (Guilford et al., 1994b). This localization was obtained in a large consanguineous family living in an isolated village in Northern Tunisia, by genetic linkage analysis using lod scores (see Chapters 2 and 3); the interval was then narrowed down to the region of homozygosity. The same locus has been shown to be involved in another family living in a village situated 10 km away. This approach, lod score analysis followed by homozygosity mapping, has been subsequently used to map several other *DFNB* genes (*DFNB2*, *DFNB4*, *DFNB8*, *DFNB9*, *DFNB12*) (see below). A pedigree of one such family is presented in Figure 21.1. Despite the efficiency of this strategy, one should be wary of thinking that the geographic isolation of a family totally guarantees the segregation of only one gene. In another branch of the first identified *DFNB1* family, another hearing loss gene was found to be segregating (C. Petit, unpublished data). A similar situation has been reported in a large family affected by *DFNB4* (Baldwin et al., 1995). These two examples illustrate the requirement to carry out an exhaustive search of all relationships between the individuals and their ancestors in such families in order to identify branches in which another *DFNB* gene might contribute to the phenotype. The second gene that was identified, *DFNB2*, was segregating in a large consanguineous family living in an isolated village in Southern Tunisia, and has been localized to the long arm of chromosome 11 (Guilford et al., 1994a). Three other genes, *DFNB4*, *DFNB9* and *DFNB12*, segregating in large

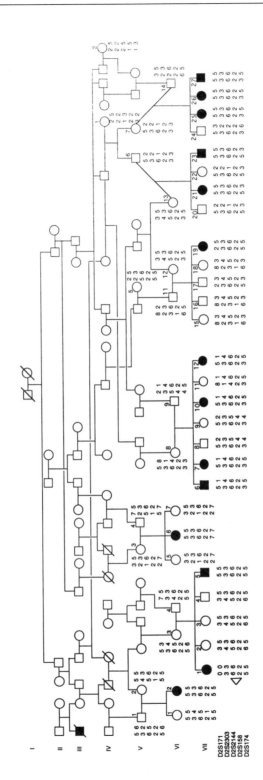

Figure 21.1 Segregation analysis of 5 polymorphic markers in a family affected by an autosomal recessive form of hearing loss. The gene responsible for deafness in this family, *DFNB9*, maps to chromosome 2p22-23 (Chaïb et al., 1996a). Haplotypes for the 5 markers are indicated, and the region of homozygosity is marked with a triangle (see generation VII).

consanguineous families of the Middle East, were mapped respectively to 7q31 (Baldwin et al., 1995), 2p22-23 (Chaïb et al., 1996b) and 10q21-22 (Chaïb et al., 1996b). The first gene was segregating in a Druze family living in Israel, the second and the third in Sunni families living respectively in Lebanon and in Syria; these families belong to two different Moslem communities which separated several centuries ago in the Mediterranean area. These communities are living as independent groups in scattered villages. Finally, the *DFNB8* gene, segregating in a large highly consanguineous family in Pakistan, has been assigned to chromosome 21q22 (Veske et al., 1996).

A different approach was used by Friedman et al. (1995) to map the *DFNB3* gene to the pericentromeric region of chromosome 17 (17p11.2-q12). In a small remote village of Bali, about 2.5% of the population are deaf; however within this geographic isolate no marriage between relatives has occurred. It was noted that all deaf couples with normal hearing parents had only deaf children, indicating that a single *DFNB* gene was segregating in this village. Moreover, a founder effect for an auditory deficiency was hypothezised based on historical documents. The mapping strategy developed consisted of searching in affected individuals for a homozygous chromosomal region containing specific alleles of polymorphic markers in significantly higher proportions than in normal hearing individuals from the same village.

Finally, three other *DFNB* genes were mapped using direct homozygosity mapping (Lander and Botstein, 1987). This efficient strategy is based on identifying homozygous regions shared by inbred affected children. It allows mapping of rare recessive genes in small consanguineous families (Lander and Botstein, 1987). A significant lod score can be obtained from a single family consisting of first cousin parents with normal hearing who have three affected children. *DFNB5* (initially referred to as *DFNB4*) (Fukushima et al., 1995a), *DFNB6* (Fukushima et al., 1995b) and *DFNB7* (Jain et al., 1995b) were mapped to chromosomes 14q12, 3p14-21 and 9q13-21, respectively, in small or middle-sized consanguineous families from Western and Southern India.

Thus, a significant breakthrough has been recently accomplished in this field. From the estimates quoted above, a number of other *DFNB* genes remain to be mapped. What strategies are most likely to identify them? Although the simplest strategy is to study large consanguineous families living in geographically isolated regions, this approach may encounter a limit due to the rarity of such families. The elegant mapping strategy used for *DFNB3*, based on population analysis combining homozygosity mapping and linkage disequilibrium, requires such particular characteristics of the population that it may find only a few applications. If the founder mutation was introduced too long ago, the chromosomal region of homozygosity surrounding the disease gene may be so small as to be exceedingly hard to detect. Homozygosity mapping is by far the least demanding strategy in terms of the size of the family. However, to be efficient, this strategy requires genome screening with a high density of markers. Rather than embarking on such an analysis of the complete genome, the screening may initially be focused on candidate regions (see below) which can be covered with a sufficiently high density of polymorphic markers.

Whatever the approach chosen, attention must be given to clinical examination of family members, in order to identify any individual whose hearing loss may have an environmental origin, most often infectious.

Preliminary clinical characterization of auditory defects involving the *DFNB* genes

The simple localization of a *DFNB* gene individualizes a form of hearing loss. Characterization of the new nosological entity should include a detailed description of both auditory and vestibular functions. Intra-familial variability of the clinical symptoms and of the progression of the defect (suggesting the existence of modifier genes) should be appreciated. Inter-familial variability should also be estimated through the clinical examination of affected individuals belonging to separate families for which a significant linkage with the same *DFNB* locus has been obtained. Rigorously speaking, considering the predicted high number of *DFNB* genes and therefore the not inconsiderable probability of having two *DFNB* genes tightly linked, it would be desirable to demonstrate mutations within the gene. Finally, estimates of the prevalence of a gene defect would rely upon large family surveys conducted in different regions of the world.

At present, only some scattered information is available. Compilation of the data reported so far can provide only the rudiments of such a medical textbook. All the *DFNB* genes presently mapped are responsible for sensorineural hearing loss; in all but two, *DFNB2* and *DFNB8*, the hearing loss is prelingual. Because all the *DFNB* genes have so far been mapped through analysis of families living in non-industrialized countries, the inner ear investigations have been almost entirely restricted to a pure-tone audiogram (or ABR recording for young children). Table 21.1 summarizes some clinical characteristics of the *DFNB* associated auditory deficiencies. Additional information related to the first mapped *DFNB* genes, i.e. *DFNB1*, *DFNB2* and *DFNB3*, subsequently obtained through the analysis of other families is detailed below.

Table 21.1 Characteristics of the *DFNB* associated hearing loss.

Locus	Localization	Onset	References
DFNB1	13q11.5	Prelingual	(Guilford et al., 1994b; Guilford et al., 1995; Maw et al., 1995; Scott et al., 1995) (Brown and Mueller, personal communication)
DFNB2	11q13.5	Prelingual to second decade	(Guilford et al., 1994a; Fukushima et al., 1995a) (Brown and Mueller, personal communication) (Chaïb et al., unpublished)
DFNB3	17p11.2-q12	Prelingual	(Friedman et al., 1995) (Brown and Mueller, personal communication)
DFNB4	7q31	Prelingual	(Baldwin et al., 1995)
DFNB5	14q12	Prelingual	(Fukushima et al., 1995a)
DFNB6	3p14-p21	Prelingual	(Fukushima et al., 1995b)
DFNB7	9q13-q21	Prelingual	(Jain et al., 1995a)
DFNB8	21q22	First-second decade	(Veske et al., 1996); (Bonné – Tamiv et al., 1996)
DFNB9	2p22-p23	Prelingual	(Chaïb et al., 1996a)
DFNB10	10q21-22	Prelingual	(Chaïb et al., 1996b)

DFNB1

Most individuals affected by *DFNB1* belonging to the two Tunisian families initially analysed, presented with prelingual profound bilateral sensorineural hearing loss affecting all frequencies; a few individuals presented with severe hearing loss. More recently, profound hearing loss segregating in a very large consanguineous Bedouin family from Israel (Scott et al., 1995), was shown to be linked to the *DFNB1* locus. In addition, moderate to profound hearing loss has been reported to co-segregate with the *DFNB1* region in 9 out of 19 non-consanguineous nuclear New Zealand families of western European Caucasian origin, suggesting that this gene might be an important contributor to hearing loss in this population (Maw et al., 1995). However, linkage to *DFNB1* was found in only one of 27 consanguineous families from Pakistan being studied by Brown and Mueller (personal communication) and in none of 26 consanguineous families from Southern India (Fukushima et al., 1995a). Interestingly, in two French families, a gene responsible for an autosomal dominant form of hearing loss, *DFNA3*, has been mapped to the same chromosomal region as *DFNB1* (Chaïb et al., 1994; and unpublished). Refined mapping of *DFNB1* (Scott et al., 1995) supports the hypothesis that the same gene could be responsible for both the recessive *DFNB1* and the dominant *DFNA3* forms of hearing loss (Chaïb et al., 1994). That the same gene can be responsible for a dominant and a recessive disease has already been shown in other genetic disorders, in particular certain forms of myotonia (Koch et al., 1992), osteogenesis imperfecta (Byers et al., 1991), epidermolysis bullosa (Hovnanian et al., 1992) and retinitis pigmentosa (Rosenfeld et al., 1992).

DFNB2

Individuals from the Tunisian family affected by *DFNB2* presented with a sensorineural bilateral hearing loss, with loss greater than 70 dB HL for all frequencies, accompanied by vestibular problems for some of them (Guilford et al., 1994a). However, the age of onset of the hearing loss was variable. For half of the cases it was postlingual. One person who was homozygous for the defective haplotype was still unaffected at 20 years of age. In one of the 26 Southern Indian families (Fukushima et al., 1995a), this same gene seemed to be involved. Finally, in a very large non-consanguineous Druze family from Lebanon, a lod score greater than 3 for this chromosomal region has been observed (Chaïb et al., unpublished). Interestingly enough, the eight affected individuals of this family, as well as those from the Southern Indian and Pakistani families, suffer from profound congenital sensory hearing loss. Assuming that the same gene is involved in all these families, this defective gene would be responsible for features ranging from undetectable auditory impairment up to profound hearing loss.

DFNB3

In Bali, the individuals from a *DFNB3* affected family suffered from congenital profound hearing loss (Friedman et al., 1995). In 2 out of 27 Pakistani families suffering from congenital profound hearing loss, linkage to the *DFNB3* locus was found (Brown and Mueller, personal communication), whereas this locus did not seem to be involved in any of the 26 Southern Indian families (Fukushima et al., 1995a).

Candidate *DFNB* genes

So far no *DFNB* gene has been isolated. However, *DFNB2* has been mapped to the same chromosomal region as the gene responsible for Usher syndrome type IB (Guilford et al., 1994a). Usher type I (USH1) associates profound congenital sensorineural hearing loss, vestibular dysfunction and retinitis pigmentosa. The *USH1B* phenotype results from a mutation in the gene encoding a cytoskeletal motor protein, myosin VIIa (Weil et al., 1995). The sequence of the myosin VIIa cDNA, as well as the gene structure, have been determined (Weil et al., 1996). The gene consists of 48 coding exons. Since mutations of the murine orthologous gene in *shaker-1* mice (Gibson et al., 1995) solely manifest by hearing loss and vestibular dysfunction without any evidence for an impairment of retinal functions, and thus present a phenotype similar to that of *DFNB2* patients, the human myosin VIIa gene has been proposed to be responsible also for *DFNB2* (Guilford et al., 1994a; Weil et al., 1995). The search for mutations of the myosin VIIa gene in *DFNB2* affected patients is currently underway (G. Lévy, submitted). If the *DFNB2* gene turns out to be the myosin VIIa gene, comparison of the mutations in DFNB2 and in USH1B patients could contribute to understanding the role of this protein with respect to retinal and cochlear functions. It would also lead to consideration of the other *USH* loci as candidates for isolated forms of hearing loss.

The cloning of a *DFNB* gene can at first be attempted by a candidate gene approach and, if unsuccessful, by a positional cloning strategy (see Chapter 3). Both approaches are, however, impeded by the genetic heterogeneity that constrains linkage analysis of *DFNB* genes. Only families exhibiting a significant lod score can be used for defining the chromosomal location of *DFNB* genes.

The candidate gene approach at present encounters another limit. Among the *DFNB* genes, one can anticipate that some of them will be expressed in several tissues. Others will be exclusively expressed in the inner ear sensory organ, in the same way as some of the genes responsible for retinitis pigmentosa are exclusively expressed in the retina (Dryja et al., 1990; Farrar et al., 1991; Kajiwara et al., 1991; McLaughlin et al., 1993). For ubiquitously expressed genes the candidate gene approach will benefit greatly from the high density cDNA maps of the human genome that are now being generated. Conversely, the isolation of the second category of genes will be hindered by the almost complete lack of identified molecular components specific to the inner ear, with a few rare exceptions (Elgoyhen et al, 1994; Chen, H. et al., 1995), including those involved in the mechanotransduction process. This situation itself results from the very small number of sensory cells contained in this organ, about a thousandfold less than in the retina or in the olfactory epithelium. In this respect, the generation of subtracted cDNA libraries from the mammalian inner ear (Robertson et al., 1994), followed by the mapping of the relevant cDNA clones, is a promising approach (see Chapter 4).

Finally, cloning of *DFNB* genes can benefit greatly from the numerous (circa 90) deaf mouse mutants which have been identified (Steel, 1995; see Chapter 5). Some of them have already been shown to involve genes responsible for hearing impairment in man, the phenotypic expression often being different from one species to the other (Epstein et al., 1991; Baldwin et al., 1992; Tassabehji et al., 1993; Tassabehji et al., 1994; Tachibana et al., 1994; Gibson et al., 1995; Weil et al., 1995; Steel, 1995, for a review). In each case where the comparative human and murine maps lead to the hypothesis that the mouse homologue of a

DFNB gene may be mutated in a deaf mouse mutant, cloning the *DFNB* gene will be more efficiently accomplished by first isolating the murine homologue. Similarly, cloning of the genes responsible for hearing loss in mouse (Avraham et al., 1995) would focus the search for a *DFNB* locus within the homologous region in man. Table 21.2 presents for each *DFNB* gene the homologous murine region and potential corresponding mutants. In 5 out of 10 homologous regions (*DFNB2*, *DFNB3*, *DFNB6*, *DFNB7* and *DFNB12*), some deaf mouse mutants have been mapped which, according to their phenotypic features, are likely to represent animal models for the human *DFNB*-associated auditory defects.

Table 21.2 Homologous murine region and potential corresponding mutants for each *DFNB* gene.

DFNB locus	Corresponding Mouse Chromosomal Region*	Candidate Mouse Mutants	References
DFNB1	Not known		
DFNB2	7 (47 cM)	*shaker-1 (sh1)*	(Deol, 1956; Gibson et al., 1995)
DFNB3	11 (33 cM)	*shaker-2 (sh2)*	(Deol, 1954)
DFNB4	6 (1 cM)	*Sightless ** (Sig)*	(Deol, 1980)
DFNB5	Not known		
DFNB6	9 (59 cM)	*Spinner (sr)*	(Deol and Robbins, 1962; Fox et al., 1978)
DFNB7	19 (15 cM)	*Deafness (dn)*	(Bock and Steel, 1983; Deol and Kocher, 1958; Keats et al., 1995)
DFNB8	16 (69 cM)	(Inner ear defect associated with segmental trisomy)**	(Reeves and Citron, 1994)
DFNB9	12 (15 cM)	*Audiogenic seizure prone-1** (asp-1)*	(Collins, 1970; Collins and Fuller, 1968)
	17 (distal)	Not known	
DFNB12	10 (33 cM)	*Waltzer (v)*	(Deol, 1956)
	(34 cM)	*Jackson circler (jc)*	(Southard and Dickie, 1970)
	(48 cM)	*Ames waltzer (av)*	(Osako and Hilding, 1971)

* Distance from centromere (Jackson Laboratory DataBase)
** Relation with the human defect has to be considered with caution

Perspectives

Medical aspects

Characterization of DFNB nosological entities

The identification of a *DFNB* gene should lead to a clinical characterization of the corresponding form of hearing loss based on directed audiological and electrophysiological cochlear and vestibular investigations, as well as high resolution radiological examinations (NMR imaging, tomodensitometry). The detection of minimal defects in healthy carriers of the mutation could also contribute to defining the nosological entities. This process will hopefully allow the vast collection of hearing impairments at present categorized as 'undifferentiated sensorineural autosomal recessive hearing loss' to be split into subgroups.

Molecular diagnosis

Molecular diagnosis would be particularly efficient if it could establish the genetic origin of hearing loss for the first affected child in a kindred, which in turn would contribute to the genetic counselling. Molecular diagnosis will also be helpful for presymptomatic diagnosis of late onset forms of hearing loss. Such a diagnosis could guide a suitable choice of profession. However, as long as no efficient and economical method exists to detect mutations and deletions on a whole genome scale, the multiplicity of the *DFNB* genes will be a major obstacle for molecular diagnosis. In this regard, definition of clinical criteria for splitting undifferentiated autosomal recessive hearing loss will be particularly beneficial, since it will focus the search for mutations on to a subset of *DFNB* genes.

For each gene, development of a molecular diagnosis is dictated by a preliminary study, the purpose of which is to estimate:

- The frequency, penetrance and expressivity of the various mutations.
- Possible correlations between the nature of the mutations and the clinical signs.
- The reliability and performance of the detection test used.

Therapeutics

Today, the main therapeutical resource is prosthetics. The development of alternative therapeutic approaches for certain defects, will require a minimal understanding of the role of the defective proteins. In addition, for congenital sensorineural forms of hearing loss, a means to initiate regeneration of the damaged neuroepithelium has to be discovered.

Physiological aspects

One should not be surprised by the multiplicity of genes responsible for
hearing loss, considering the architectural complexity of the sensory
auditive organ. This frequency analyser comprises particular sensory
cells which all have a different fine structure, providing them with
unique mechanical properties which condition their activation by a specific frequency. Isolation of genes responsible for hearing loss, followed
by the characterization of the functions of the defective proteins, should
help clarify the molecular and cellular interactions that are involved in
the development and functioning of the inner ear. The molecular
approach to understanding cochlear and vestibular functions, to which
the contribution of mouse models would be essential, should also aid
the study of other auditory disorders, such as the sensitivity of the
ciliary cells to noise-induced hearing loss and sudden hearing loss.

Chapter 22
Autosomal dominant non-syndromal hearing loss

GUY VAN CAMP, PAUL COUCKE and PATRICK J WILLEMS

Introduction

Hearing loss is the most frequent condition affecting human communication. It has been known for a long time that genetic factors play an important role. Hearing loss is most probably due to a combination of genetic and environmental factors in many cases. However, many families with pure genetic hearing loss have been reported. On the basis of the age of onset, these families can be subdivided into prelingual and postlingual groups. Most studies on the aetiology of hearing loss have been carried out on the prelingual group (for a review see Cohen and Gorlin, 1995). The incidence of prelingual hearing loss is approximately 1/1,000 births, of which about 50% is thought to have a genetic origin (Fraser, 1976; Morton, 1991). These studies indicate that 75 to 80% of prelingual hearing loss has an autosomal recessive mode of inheritance, 20 to 25% shows autosomal dominant inheritance, and 1 to 4% X-linked inheritance (Fraser, 1976; Morton, 1991; Reardon, 1992).

Comparable data on postlingual hearing loss are not available. Most cases of hereditary postlingual hearing loss are non-syndromal, and a large number of families have been described in the literature (McKusick et al., 1994; Cohen and Gorlin, 1995). In all patients with postlingual hearing loss, hearing loss is progressive, which is not surprising as, by definition, sufficient hearing to develop normal speech is present at least in the first few years of life. Postlingual hearing loss has been classified into different types by several authors (Königsmark and Gorlin, 1976; McKusick et al., 1994; Gorlin, 1995). These classifications are based on phenotypic characteristics such as the affected frequencies (high, mid, low), type of hearing loss (conductive, sensorineural of mixed), uni- or bilateral loss, and the involvement of vestibular dysfunction. Classifications have also been based upon the mode of inheritance. It is striking that the inheritance pattern in nearly all published families with postlingual hearing loss is autosomal dominant. In an extensive recent survey (Gorlin, 1995), only 3 families with autosomal recessive postlingual progressive hearing loss were mentioned, while more than 50 papers about autosomal dominant progressive hearing loss are cited. This suggests that, in contrast to prelingual hearing loss, postlingual genetic hearing loss is for the most part inherited in an autosomal dominant manner.

Although many families with autosomal dominant progressive hereditary hearing loss have been reported in the literature, no systematic study to determine its frequency in the general population is known to us. This is probably the consequence of the problems that are inherently connected to this kind of study. In contrast to prelingual hearing loss, where large numbers of families can be collected relatively easily through institutions for the deaf, families with progressive hearing loss are more difficult to collect. In many of these families, the age of onset of the hearing loss is late, and affected family members often develop significant hearing loss only in late adulthood. Although the familial character of the hearing loss is frequently recognised by family members, many of them do not consult a geneticist as this type of hearing loss is mild compared to congenital deafness.

Adult onset progressive hearing loss can be caused by mutations in a single gene. It can also be caused by a number of environmental factors, including excessive noise exposure, infection, injury and ototoxic drugs. Even in the absence of obvious environmental or genetic causes, the sensitivity of hearing decreases with age. This decrease is more pronounced in the high tones, and the hearing loss is more pronounced in males than in females. According to international standards for thresholds of hearing by air conduction (ISO-standards), more than half of the otologically normal male population of 70 years of age have a hearing threshold at 8,000 Hz of 60 dB worse than the average hearing threshold for the otologically normal population aged 18. At 4,000 Hz, the difference between ages 70 and 18 is on average 43 dB, and at 2,000 Hz it is 19 dB. There is also a large variability in the degree of hearing loss between individuals. For example, at 4,000 Hz, the bottom 10 percent of the population aged 70 has a threshold 64 dB below the top 10 percent of the same age.

The mechanisms of this gradual hearing deterioration are poorly understood, and it is not known what causes the large differences between individuals. They cannot be accounted for by environmental causes only, and it is likely that this difference is caused by an interaction of genetic and environmental factors. Therefore, age-related hearing loss might be seen as a multifactorial condition in many cases. It is possible that mutations in some genes render the ear more susceptible to environmental factors causing hearing loss. In contrast to a number of environmental factors known to provoke hearing loss, no genes are known today that play a role in progressive hearing loss.

In many affected families hereditary postlingual progressive hearing loss of the high tones resembles age-related hearing loss. In a majority of families the hearing loss is sensorineural, and the high tones are more severely affected. It is therefore possible that the same genes are involved in purely genetic hearing loss as in multifactorial age-related loss. Such genes might therefore be involved in the pathogenesis of the very frequent hearing loss of the elderly. Families in which progressive hereditary hearing loss segregates as an autosomal dominant condition present a unique opportunity for identifying genes responsible for hearing loss. Further study of these genes will lead to a better insight into the mechanisms causing deterioration of hearing. These mechanisms might also be similar for pure genetic hearing loss and for multifactorial age-related hearing loss.

DFNA genes

In the McKusick catalogue the older phenotypic classification of families with hereditary hearing loss is gradually being replaced by a molecular classification on the basis of the underlying gene (McKusick et al., 1994). The loci for non-syndromal hereditary hearing loss have been numbered separately for dominant and recessive inheritance. Dominantly inherited hearing loss is given the prefix *DFNA*, and recessively inherited loss is named *DFNB*. For both categories, the loci are assigned a number in the order of discovery. At this moment (October 1995) 6 different loci for dominantly inherited hearing loss have been published, and 3 others have been reported at The Molecular Biology of Hearing and Deafness meeting in Bethesda, October 6-8, 1995. Unfortunately, the names that were given to loci have been subject to confusion, and reports with erroneous numbers have been published. A summary of the principal data for the correctly numbered loci, as approved by Dr P McAlpine, chair of the HUGO nomenclature committee, is given in Table 22.1. For each locus, a short description is given below.

DFNA1

In 1992, Léon et al. were the first to report the localisation of a gene for autosomal dominant non-syndromal hearing loss on the long arm of chromosome 5. Hearing loss in an extended pedigree from Costa Rica with autosomal dominant inheritance could be traced back to a single individual called Felix Monge, born in 1754. Therefore, *DFNA1* is sometimes referred to as Monge's deafness. The sensorineural hearing loss generally starts in the first decade of life in the low frequencies and progresses slowly to profound losses at all frequencies in affected adults (Léon et al., 1981). *DFNA1* was first localised in a region of approximately 7 cM between markers *IL9* and *GRL* (Leon et al., 1992), and later the localisation was refined to a 2 to 3 megabase region between markers *D5S89* and *FGFA* (Lynch et al., 1992).

Table 22.1 Published loci responsible for non-syndromal autosomal dominant hearing loss.

Locus	Localisation	Frequencies most affected	Onset (Decade)	Severe hearing loss over all frequencies	Families linked	References
DFNA1	5q31	Low	First	Fourth decade	1	Léon et al., 1992
DFNA2	1p32	High	First- third	Third-fifth decade	4	Coucke et al., 1994
DFNA3*	13q12	High	First	Moderate to severe hearing loss, slowly or non-progressive	1	Chaib et al., 1994
DFNA4	19q13	All	Second	Fourth decade	1	Chen et al., 1995
DFNA5	7p	High	First-second	Fourth-fifth decade	1	Van Camp et al., 1995b
DFNA6	4p16.3	Low	First-second	Variable, moderate to severe	1	Lesperance et al., 1995

*Several families with autosomal recessive prelingual profound hearing loss are linked to the same chromosomal region (Guilford et al., 1994; Scott et al., 1995; Guilford et al., 1995).

DFNA2

A second locus for autosomal dominant progressive hearing loss was reported in 1994 (Coucke et al., 1994). Linkage to the short arm of chromosome 1 was detected in a large Indonesian family and an American family with dominant hearing loss. Later, linkage with *DFNA2* was also found in two additional families originating from the Netherlands and from Belgium (Coucke et al., unpublished observation). In all four families, the hearing loss is most pronounced in the high tones, and with increasing age lower frequencies also become involved, leading to a profound hearing loss later in life. However, differences in age of onset, progression rate and audiometric curve shape can be seen between the four families. *DFNA2* is most probably an important locus for progressive hearing loss as the number of families linked to *DFNA2* is now 4, and these four families originate from three different continents.

By combining the information from key recombinants in the four families, the candidate region for *DFNA2* could be reduced to a region of 1 to 2 million base pairs between *D1S432* and the proto-oncogene *MYCL1* (van Camp et al., unpublished observation). This region has been cloned into overlapping yeast artificial chromosomes (YACs, see Chapter 2), which made it possible to exclude a number of candidate genes that are known to be located close to *MYCL1*. These candidate genes include collagen 8a2, collagen 9a2, collagen 16a1, connexin37 and syndecan-3 (van Camp et al., unpublished observation).

DFNA3

A gene localisation was reported for a French family with moderate to severe sensorineural hearing loss most pronounced in the high frequencies (Chaïb et al., 1994). The hearing loss has a prelingual onset and an autosomal dominant mode of inheritance. In some cases, the hearing loss is non-progressive, while in others it progresses moderately. Linkage was found close to the centromere of chromosome 13, in a region where a form of recessive congenital profound hearing loss (*DFNB1*) has been mapped in consanguineous families from ethnic isolates living in Tunisia and Israel (Guilford et al., 1994; Scott et al., 1995). The hearing loss in these families is characterised by prelingual profound hearing loss. It is likely, but not proven, that the recessive and dominant forms are caused by mutations in a single gene *DFNA3/DFNB1*. As the short arm of chromosome 13 mainly contains repetitive sequences and no polymorphic markers, the *DFNA3* candidate region could be defined only by informative crossovers with markers on the long arm of chromosome 13. It is also generally accepted that the short arm of chromosome 13 contains no genes except for ribosomal RNA genes, and therefore *DFNA3* is most likely to be located between the centromere of chromosome 13 and *D13S143*, a marker located on proximal 13q.

DFNA4

Linkage to chromosome 19q was reported in a US pedigree with autosomal dominant inheritance of sensorineural hearing loss across all frequencies (Chen AH et al., 1995). The hearing loss is progressive, starting in the second decade of life and leading to severe to profound loss by the age of 40. Obligate crossovers localise *DFNA4* in an interval of approximately 20 cM, flanked by markers *D19S414* and *D19S246*. The gene responsible for myotonic dystrophy (DM kinase) is a candidate gene for *DFNA4* as it is located in this region. In addition, it has been reported that a progressive sensorineural hearing loss can be found in some patients with myotonic dystrophy (Huygen et al., 1994).

DFNA5

Linkage to chromosome 7p was found in an extended Dutch family with autosomal dominant progressive hearing loss starting in the high tones (van Camp et al., 1995). This family has been the subject of several detailed audiological studies since 1966. It is one of the largest families ever reported, and has been a reference family for high frequency progressive hearing loss (McKusick et al., 1994). Hearing loss starts between the ages of 5 and 15 years in the high frequencies and increases to a severe hearing loss also affecting the mid and low frequencies by the age of 50. Key recombinations delineate a region of 15 cM between markers *D7S493* and *D7S632* containing *DFNA5*.

DFNA6

Linkage to a new locus for autosomal dominant low frequency hearing loss was reported in a large family from the US (Lesperance et al., 1995). This family was first described in 1968 (Vanderbilt University hereditary deafness study group, 1968). The majority of patients develop a progressive hearing loss below 1,000 Hz in the second decade of life. In some cases higher frequencies become involved with age and increasing hearing loss, but in others hearing loss remains confined to the low frequencies. Linkage was detected with markers located in 4p16.3, a gene-rich region containing the gene for Huntington's disease. *DFNA6* was mapped to a region of 1.7 million base pairs between markers *D4S412* and *D4S432*. This chromosomal region has been mapped in detail in the search for the Huntington gene, and over twenty genes are known to reside in this region. These genes include a regulatory myosin light chain gene (*MYL5*) (Collins et al., 1992). Several mouse mutations have been located in the region corresponding to human 4p16.3, including the *Bronx waltzer* phenotype, characterised by hearing loss and circling behaviour (Lyon, Rastan and Brown, 1995).

Unpublished loci

At the Molecular Biology of Hearing and Deafness meeting in Bethesda, October 6-8, 1995, three new loci for autosomal dominant hearing loss were reported. Close linkage to marker *D1S194*, located on chromosome 1q, was reported in a Norwegian family with progressive hearing loss, preferentially affecting the high tones (Tranebjaerg et al., 1995). Linkage to chromosome 15q15 was reported in an Austrian family with non-progressive moderate to severe sensorineural hearing loss, with a maximum lod score of 3.01 for marker *D15S132* (Kirschhofer et al., 1995). Linkage for a dominant form of hearing loss was reported in the proximal region of the long arm of chromosome 14 (Morton et al., 1995), in a region where a recessive form of hearing loss is also located (Fukushima et al., 1995a).

Progress in *DFNA* gene identification

One of the reasons for the initial slow progress in the localisation of non-syndromal hearing loss genes has been the considerable genetic heterogeneity. As different genes are responsible for hearing loss in different families, pooling of linkage data from several small families is impossible. Therefore, extended families are needed for gene localisation studies. Researchers have turned to ethnic isolates where families live close to each other, thereby facilitating the construction of a large pedigree, the clinical examination of many affected family members, and the collection of many blood samples. Not surprisingly, the first two genes for dominant hearing loss were localised using families from isolated populations in Costa Rica (*DFNA1*) and Java (*DFNA2*). However, large dominant families of this type have been described in countries all over the world, and in the past year, linkage has been reported for several families from the Western world (*DFNA3-6*).

At the present time, nine different loci have been reported in a limited number of families, and the majority of families remain unlinked. However, as gene localisation studies in hereditary hearing loss have accelerated from a slow start, it is to be expected that a large series of new gene loci will be reported in the next few years. The localisation of genes responsible for postlingual progressive hearing loss can provide a predictive test in the families that are linked. This is potentially important for young children with respect to school choice and career planning.

At the moment none of the genes for autosomal dominant hearing loss that have been localised, has actually been identified, and for only a few loci are candidate genes available. With the current technology, much time will have to be spent in narrowing the candidate region and isolating new genes from this region by molecular techniques. On the other hand, in the course of the Human Genome Project, a large percentage of all human genes will very probably be cloned and mapped within the next few years, allowing efficient gene identification through a positional candidate approach (see Chapter 3 and Collins, 1995). Thus, it can be expected that a significant number of hearing loss genes will be identified in the next few years. More time will then be available for actually studying these genes and their function. The function of these genes will hopefully teach us more about the molecular processes underlying hearing in the cochlea. At that moment, it will also become easier to evaluate the possibilities of therapeutic intervention or prevention of hearing loss in some cases.

The Hereditary Hearing Loss Homepage: on-line information on hereditary deafness research

Genes responsible for non-syndromal hereditary hearing loss are being localised at an increasing rate. In order to provide researchers in the field with easy accessible and up to date information, we have set up a world-wide-web site summerizing genetic information on non-syndromal hearing loss. The information is collected in collaboration with many researchers in the field and with Dr. Ph. McAlpine, chair of the HUGO nomenclature committee. The address for the Hereditary Hearing Loss Homepage is http://alt-www.uia.ac.be/u/dnalab/hhh.html. This site lists continuously updated information on the known loci for non-syndromal deafness, including the official name, the chromosomal localisation, the best microsatellite marker to perform linkage analysis, and references. Information about the families linked, the candidate region, and the type of hearing loss can also be found for most loci.

Chapter 23
Otosclerosis

FRANK DECLAU and PAUL VAN DE HEYNING

Introduction

Otosclerosis affects the bone homeostasis of the labyrinthine capsule resulting in abnormal resorption and redeposition of bone. This bone dysplasia, limited to the otic capsule, originates in the endochondral bone layer. Otosclerosis neither affects other endochondral bones in the human, nor is found in animals. We present here an analysis of the literature pertaining to the phenotypic expression, the mode of inheritance, prevalence, age of onset, and the occurrence of sporadic cases of otosclerosis.

Phenotypic expression

The foci of otosclerotic bone are symptomatically quiescent until the movement of the stapes is impaired by invasion of the stapedovestibular joint (Schuknecht, 1974). Fixation of the stapes as a cause of hearing loss was first recognized by Valsalva as early as 1704. In 1894, Politzer called this type of ankylosis 'otosclerosis'. In 1912, Siebenmann's microscopic examinations showed that the lesion apparently began as a spongification of the bone; hence, the term 'otospongiosis'. In commenting on otosclerosis, Guild (1944) emphasized the importance of distinguishing between clinical and histological otosclerosis. 'Histological otosclerosis' refers to a disease process without clinical symptoms or manifestations and it can be discovered only by routine sectioning of the temporal bone at autopsy. 'Clinical otosclerosis' refers to the presence of otosclerosis at a site where it causes a conductive hearing loss by interfering with the motion of the stapes or of the round window membrane (Shambaugh, 1949; Arnold et al., 1987). The primary symptom produced by the otosclerotic lesion is a conductive hearing loss, the magnitude of which is directly related to the degree of fixation of the stapes footplate.

221

Many otologists believe that otosclerosis also damages the inner ear to cause progressive sensorineural hearing loss (Schuknecht, 1974; Ramsay and Linthicum, 1994). In a histopathological survey of 248 temporal bones with otosclerosis, Kelemen and Alonso (1980) found that 40% of patients with clinical otosclerosis had an otosclerotic focus involving the cochlear endosteum. Any encroachment of the membranous labyrinth usually occurs in the lateral part of each cochlear turn (Schuknecht, 1974). In these areas, the inner periosteal layer is deformed, and subjacent atrophy of the spiral ligament may be seen (Friedman, 1974). However, severe alterations in the bony labyrinth and spiral ligament may occur with no observable histological alterations in the structures of the cochlear duct (Schuknecht, 1974); there does not appear to be a consistent spatial relationship between areas of atrophy of the spiral ligament and atrophy of the organ of Corti. Several reports correlate the size of the lesions, their activity and the degree of cochlear endosteal involvement with the magnitude of the sensorineural hearing loss (Lindsay and Beal, 1966; Linthicum, 1967; Linthicum et al., 1975; Hueb et al., 1991).

On the other hand, Guild (1944) has failed to establish a correlation between otosclerosis and sensorineural hearing loss. The concept of 'cochlear otosclerosis', that is, pure sensorineural hearing loss caused by otosclerosis of the bony labyrinth without stapes fixation, has been the subject of much debate (Shambaugh, 1965). Causse and Causse (1984) believe that a number of cases with low, mid and high frequency sensorineural hearing loss and a dominant mode of inheritance, described as separate syndrome entities by Konigsmark and Gorlin (1976), virtually represent cochlear otosclerosis. However, a temporal bone study of patients with pure sensorineural hearing loss of unknown cause has failed to show otoslerotic foci of significant incidence or size to explain the inner ear changes (Schuknecht and Kirschner, 1974). Also Hueb et al. (1991) found significant differences in sensorineural hearing loss in otosclerotic patients only if two or more otosclerotic sites of endosteal involvement were present.

Otosclerosis usually involves both ears. However, Morrison (1967) and Cawthorne (1955) found clinically unilateral otosclerosis in 13%, and Larsson (1960) in 15%. Guild (1944) reported histologically unilateral otosclerosis in 30% and Hueb et al. (1991) in 24.4%.

Low pitched tinnitus is usually present. Vertiginous spells or dizziness are uncommon. Virolainen (1972) found the objective disturbances in order of frequency to be caloric hypoexcitability and elevated thresholds of angular acceleration and deceleration, directional preponderance, and positional nystagmus. At the initial stages, paracusis Willisii, or the ability to hear better in a crowd, may be present.

Epidemiology

Clinical otosclerosis is a common hearing disorder, although its exact prevalence is unknown. Information on this is, however, important for health care planning. In Sweden, the clinical incidence has recently been estimated as 6.1/100,000 (Levin et al., 1988). This figure is lower than others reported previously: (12/100,000: Stahle et al., 1973; 13.7/100,000: Pearson et al., 1974). Levin's estimate was based on the number of patients admitted to hospital with otosclerosis for stapedectomy. The recent decline of operations for otosclerosis and hence the incidence calculations may be explained by the widespread publicity for stapedectomy and stapedotomy operations during the nineteen fifties, sixties and seventies. However, McKenna (1994) has argued that systematic vaccination for measles also accounts for the decreased incidence of otosclerosis.

Elucidation of the prevalence of otosclerosis is confused by the differentiation of clinical and histological otosclerosis. The prevalence of clinical otosclerosis in the Caucasian population has been studied by various authors (Table 23.1). In the early studies (Davenport, 1933; Shambaugh, 1949; Cawthorne, 1955), no attempt was made to relate the clinical condition to a known population at a given time. The mean prevalence can be estimated as 3/1,000 (0.3%) (Causse and Causse, 1984).

Table 23.1 Prevalence of Clinical Otosclerosis in the Caucasian population.

Author	Prevalence (Per cent)
Davenport et al. (1933)	0.1 – 0.25
Shambaugh (1949)	0.5 – 1
Cawthorne (1955)	0.5
Morrison (1967)	0.2
Hall (1974)	0.3
Pearson et al. (1974)	0.28
Gapany-Gapanavicius (1975)	0.044 – 0.1
Ben Arab et al. (1993)	0.6

The prevalence of histological otosclerosis has also been studied by various authors (Table 23.2). The mean prevalence in the Caucasian population can be estimated as 8.3% (Altmann et al., 1967). According to Guild's figures, 15% of the temporal bones with histological otosclerosis demonstrated an ankylosis of the stapedio-vestibular articulation; hence, 1.2% of all the temporal bones studied could be considered as having clinical otosclerosis. In Altmann's review on histological otosclerosis (1967), 0.99% of all temporal bones (with and without otosclerosis) had stapes fixation (12% of the temporal bones with histological otosclerosis). Calculating the prevalence of clinical otosclerosis, these extrapolations derived from temporal bone findings (0.99 and 1.2%) do not correlate well with the clinical data of otosclerotic families (0.3%). Morrison (1967) suggested that the diagnosis of histological otosclerosis may be biased by the overestimation of otosclerotic foci in the temporal bone sections. Having made some allowance for this possible error, there is no doubt that histological otosclerosis (genotype) occurs in the absence of clinical otosclerosis (phenotype). In the interpretation of the prevalence figures, two considerations have to be made: Firstly, Schuknecht and Kirchner (1974) counted all specimens with evidence of stapedial fixation as clinical otosclerosis – the other authors considered such cases to be in the category of histological otosclerosis and included them as such; secondly, the prevalence figures may refer either to the percentage of individuals, or to the percentage of temporal bones studied.

Table 23.2 Prevalence of Histological Otosclerosis in the Caucasian population.

Author	Number of Temporal Bones Studied	Number of Cadavers	Prevalence (Per cent)
Weber (1935)	Not known	200	11
Engström (1939)	145	100	12
Guild (1944)	Not known	518	8.3
Jorgensen and Kristensen (1967)	237	155	11.4
Schuknecht and Kirchner (1974)	734	Not known	4.4
Hueb et al. (1991)	1452	Not known	12.75

Otosclerosis is predominantly a Caucasian disease and follows their geographic distribution throughout the world. It is quite rare among Blacks, Orientals, and American Indians (Altmann et al., 1967).

Age of onset

The exact age of onset is difficult to determine, since a patient may not become aware of a hearing impairment for a number of years. Based on the similar findings of Davenport (1933), Larsson (1960) and Morrison (1967), the greatest period of risk appears to be between 11 and 45 years. Cawthorne (1955) reported that 70% of patients with clinical otosclerosis first noticed hearing losses between the ages of 11 and 30. Hearing loss interpreted as otosclerosis and beginning as early as age 5 years in some cases was described by Kabat (1943). The age of onset is similar in males and females. There is also a striking similarity within families and especially within sibships. On the other hand, Morrison (1967) found a tendency towards an earlier age of onset with succeeding generations.

Mode of inheritance

The first pedigrees in which the transmission of otosclerosis from generation to generation was demonstrated, were published by Hammerschlag (1905), Körner (1905), Albrecht (1922) and by Bauer and Stein (1925). Albrecht (1922) concluded that otosclerosis is due to a simple dominant factor, but Bauer and Stein (1925), with larger material and more advanced genetico-statistical standards, postulated a double autosomal recessive mode of inheritance. These early twentieth century studies show much bias due to inadequate otological diagnosis, especially in secondary cases, and inappropriate selection strategies.

The majority of the more recent studies on otosclerosis indicate an autosomal dominant mode of inheritance. Recent studies have been conducted by Larsson (1960), Morrison (1967), Gapany-Gapanavicius (1975) and Causse and Causse (1984). These studies have included all patients without regard to family history, age or prior therapy. A firm clinical diagnosis was made by otoscopic and audiometric analysis and also, to a large extent, by surgery. Exclusion of phenotypes has also been done. Bias of ascertainment has been eliminated by Weinberg's proband calculation (1925; also known as incomplete multiple ascertainment). This calculation calls for omission of the proband and for inclusion of the sibship each time it is ascertained.

The mode of inheritance was based on the following conclusions (Morrison, 1967):

- The expected frequencies of affected individuals for autosomal dominant traits were compared with the observed frequencies for relatives of otosclerotics.
- Many families had transmission of otosclerosis through three or more generations.
- Analysis of families with secondary cases outside the sibship of the proband revealed that they inherited the gene from only one side of the family.
- In the offspring of two affected parents, no accelerated or early onset cases were detected. There is no evidence for a phenotypical difference between the heterozygous and homozygous state.

The assumption of autosomal dominant inheritance is based on the existence of particular pedigrees and the exclusion of other modes by statistical analysis. However, it may be difficult to draw definite conclusions from isolated pedigrees for the following reasons (Gordon, 1989):

1. Individual families may demonstrate exceptions to the rule. Their attention may have been attracted by noteworthy accumulations of secondary cases or particularly serious cases (Larsson, 1960).
2. Individual pedigrees may mimic a mode of inheritance, especially if a carrier state, incomplete penetrance or variable expressivity exists.
3. More than one mode of inheritance may be responsible for a given disease (e.g. retinitis pigmentosa).
4. A give entity may actually represent a heterogeneous group of diseases.

Multifactorial inheritance is likely to play a role in the expression or penetrance of otosclerosis. Modifying genes and environmental factors may be responsible for the high degree of variability between families. This is in no way inconsistent with the accepted autosomal dominant mode of inheritance (Morrison, 1967). Also Ben Arab et al. (1993), postulated an autosomal dominant major gene with a high polygenic background.

Other modes of inheritance are highly unlikely as can be concluded from the detailed mathematical analyses of Larsson (1960) and Gapany-Gapanavicius (1975). Autosomal recessive inheritance is unlikely given the presumed degree of penetrance, but cannot absolutely be ruled out.

Polyhybrid inheritance has been claimed by Bauer and Stein (1925), Davenport et al. (1933) and by Hernandez-Orozco and Courtney (1964). These research groups postulated two genes. Bauer and Stein (1925) came to the conclusion that otosclerosis is determined by two autosomal recessive genes. The critical mating to test this hypothesis of double recessive genes is the mating of two otosclerotic parents. However, their own data are more conclusive against their own hypothesis (Davenport et al., 1933). Davenport et al. (1933) postulated two domininantly inherited genes – one autosomal and the other X-linked. Hernandez-Orozco and Courtney (1964) postulated two interacting genes – one autosomal recessive and the other X-linked dominant. These types of polyhybrid inheritance were suggested to explain the doubled incidence of otosclerosis in females compared with males. It is relatively easy to create a hypothesis to fit existing data with polyhybrids. Moreover, this type of inheritance is quite uncommon in humans. Morrison (1967) studied the results of back-cross matings where either the father or the mother was otosclerotic and came to the conclusion that the hypothesis of Davenport et al. (1933) could not be supported by his pedigree findings (Table 23.3).

Table 23.3 Expected frequencies for back-cross matings: autosomal dominant + X-linked dominant.

| | % Affected | | % Normal | |
	Males	Females	Males	Females
Father otosclerotic	0	25	50	25
Mother otosclerotic	12.5	12.5	37.5	37.5

By analogy, the same conclusion can be drawn for the hypothesis of Hernandez-Orozco and Courtney (1964; Table 23.4).

Table 23.4 Expected frequencies for back cross-matings: autosomal recessive + X-linked dominant: (unaffected parent heterozygous autosomal).

| | % Affected | | % Normal | |
	Males	Females	Males	Females
Father otosclerotic	0	25	50	25
Mother otosclerotic	12.5	12.5	37.5	37.5

Penetrance

Two methods for determining the degree of penetrance of otosclerosis have been reported in the literature. A first method was employed by Morrison (1967) and by Causse and Causse (1984). These authors calculated the difference between observed and expected ratios in relatives of otosclerotics. In both cases, the authors concluded that penetrance approximated 40%.

A second method was used by Larsson (1960). This author based his calculations on a formula devised by Weinberg (1925). The formula used was $P = D / A - B - (0.5 \times C)$ where P is the penetrance of otosclerosis, D is the number of patients who had clinical otosclerosis (phenotypic) during their lifetime, A is the number histologically (genetically) affected who died prior to the age period of risk, (B is the number of histogually (genotypically) affected who died prior to the age of risk) and C is the number histologically affected who died during the age period of risk. Larsson (1960) employed Guild's (1944) postmortem material to calculate the degree of penetrance as 25%. Larsson (1960) and Morrison and Bundey (1970) defined the degree of penetrance as the percentage of patients with histologic otosclerosis in whom the otosclerotic foci interfere with the hearing mechanism.

The use of Weinberg's formula and the application of Guild's figures has been criticized by Gordon (1989). According to this author, the following considerations should be made:

• The assumption that histological otosclerosis and the otosclerosis genotype are equivalent is not correct: a person who has inherited

the gene(s) for otosclerosis may not exhibit histologic otosclerosis at all. Environmental factors may influence the outcome.
- The presence of an otosclerotic focus does not imply the otosclerosis genotype: phenocopies may exist. The prevalence of histological otosclerosis exceeds that of clinical otosclerosis by more than can be accounted for by accepted penetrance figures alone.
- From the statistical point of view, the numbers in the above calculation are small and, subsequently, the standard error is large. Moreover, subtraction of half of the individuals histologically affected who died during the period at risk appears not to have any specific mathematical basis.

Sporadic cases

Anamnestic data on the occurrence of sporadic cases in otosclerosis are generally reported to be positive in about half of the cases. According to most studies (Table 23.5), the percentage of isolated cases ranges from 40 to 50%.

Table 23.5 Frequency of sporadic cases with clinical otosclerosis.

Author	% isolated cases
Nager (1939)	42
Cawthorne (1955)	46
Shambaugh (1949)	44.5
Larsson (1960)	49
Morrison (1967)	30
Gapany-Gapanavicius (1975)	48.4

According to Morrison and Bundey (1970), the presence of isolated cases can be explained as follows:

- Isolated cases of otosclerosis may be phenocopies of the disease. Without surgical exploration it may be difficult to exclude acquired or congenital ossicular fixations or defects.
- New mutations may account for a small fraction of these isolated cases (Morrison, 1967: 50×10^{-6}).
- Given the presence of a reduced penetrance between 25 and 40%, it would seem reasonable to suppose that sporadic cases are due to failure of manifestation in other family members (though they might be expected to have histological otosclerosis).

However, the prevalence of histologic otosclerosis exceeds that of clinical otosclerosis by far more than can be accounted for by accepted penetrance figures alone. Therefore, Morrison and Bundey (1970) proposed the concept of an alternative mode of inheritance for these isolated cases. According to these authors, clinical otosclerosis could be explained by more than one genetic mechanism. They calculated the theoretical prevalence of histological otosclerosis on the assumption that isolated cases follow a recessive inheritance, while the pedigree cases follow a dominant inheritance. According to their theory, the homozygous state would produce clinical otosclerosis, while the heterozygous 'carrier' state might result in areas of histological otosclerosis without stapedial ankylosis. The frequency of histological otosclerosis was the sum of the heterozygous recessive state, the dominant genotype (as seen in pedigrees) and the (less significant) mutation rates for each mode of inheritance. This was estimated as 6.14%, close to the frequency recorded by Guild (8.3%).

There is no evidence that the hearing loss in sporadic otosclerosis is of greater severity than the obvious hereditary cases (Morrison, 1967). However, in contrast to pedigree cases, there is a consistent tendency for later birth ranks to be associated with more cases of otosclerosis. Both maternal and paternal ages do not differ from those expected, so this tendency must be due to either parity or environmental factors. The sex ratio in sporadic cases is exactly equal. According to Larsson (1960), there is a lower morbidity risk for siblings of probands. He explains this finding as follows:

- There may exist a lower degree of penetrance, owing to modifying genes.
- It is also possible that they follow a different mode of inheritance.
- An admixture of environmental factors can also not be excluded.

Conclusions

The authors suggest that otosclerosis represents a heterogeneous group of inherited diseases in which different genes may be involved in regulating the bone homeostasis of the otic capsule. It is hypothesized that in response to various gene defects, the physiological inhibition of bone turnover in the otic capsule is overruled due to a greater susceptibility to environmental factors, resulting in a localized bone dysplasia known as otosclerosis.

Due to the heterogeneous character of the disease, linkage analysis cannot be performed by pooling different families. Search for huge otosclerotic families with at least 15 positively identified cases is warranted, so that a genome search within each family becomes possible. Smaller families may only be diagnostic if otosclerotic patients are present with associated chromosomal or additional abnormalities. Moreover, the diagnosis of otosclerosis is clouded by the differentiation of clinical and histological otosclerosis; clinically unaffected members cannot be considered as genetically unaffected due to the limited penetrance and the variable expression. Also, in family members with only cochlear hearing loss, we fail to discriminate these individuals with cochlear otosclerosis from those with other types of genetic hearing loss. Therefore, to find the aetiology of otosclerosis and to define candidate genes, more temporal bone research on bone metabolism is needed.

Chapter 24
X-linked hearing loss

HAN G BRUNNER

Introduction

X-linked inheritance accounts for approximately 1% of all congenital hearing loss, and for 5% of hearing loss in males that is genetically determined. Many X-linked syndromes have been reported which have hearing loss as one feature. These are listed in Table 24.1. For extensive discussion of various X-linked syndromal forms of hearing loss, the reader is referred elsewhere (McKusick, 1994; Gorlin et al., 1995; Brunner et al., 1990). In the following sections the different forms of X-linked non-syndromal hearing loss will be discussed. The current classification of X-linked hearing loss is based on audiometric characteristics which are usually relatively constant and reproducible between affected males in a given pedigree. It is clear, however, that within a clinically defined category such as congenital sensorineural hearing loss more than one gene may be involved. Also, mutations within a single gene may cause different types of hearing loss in different pedigrees.

The majority of X-linked hearing loss pedigrees are due to mutations in the *POU3F4* gene which cause either progressive mixed hearing loss or severe congenital sensorineural hearing loss (de Kok et al., 1995). In some pedigrees with maternally inherited hearing loss, mitochondrial rather than X-linked inheritance is responsible (Prezant et al., 1993; see Chapter 26) and this has to be considered, especially if other symptoms such as diabetes mellitus (Ballinger and Wallace, 1995), ataxia, or myoclonic epilepsy are also present in all or some of the cases.

X-linked congenital sensorineural hearing loss

This condition is characterised by severe to profound congenital hearing loss affecting all frequencies in males. Carrier females may have mild to moderate sensorineural hearing loss, or have normal audiograms. Vestibular function is consistently abnormal in some pedigrees, especially those in which it is associated with a structural abnormality of the

Table 24.1 X-Linked hearing loss.

Disorder	McKusick No.	Type of Hearing Loss	Genetic Localisation	Defective Gene
Congenital sensorineural hearing loss XR	304500	Severe congenital sensorineural	Heterogeneous	POU3F4 in ± 50 %
Moderate sensorineural hearing loss XR	304600/ 304700	Adolescent-onset sensorineural		
Progressive mixed hearing loss with gusher	304400	Severe progressive mixed	Xq13 - q21	POU3F4
Abruzzo-Erickson syndrome	302905	Mixed	Xq26.3 – q27	
Albinism-hearing loss	300700	Congenital subtotal sensorineural		
Alport syndrome	301050	High-tone sensorineural	Xq21 – q22	Collagen 4A5
Ataxia-hearing loss syndrome XR	301790	Early-onset sensorineural	Xp22.3	
Chondrodysplasia punctata + Xp22.3 deletion	302950	Mixed conductive		
CMTX and hearing loss	310490	Early-onset sensorineural	Xq24-26	
Hearing loss optic atrophy, dementia	311150	Profound early-onset sensorineural		
Fabry disease	301500	Mild sensorineural	Xq21.33 – q22	α-galactosidase A
FG syndrome	305450	Sensorineural		
Focal dermal hypoplasia	305600	Mixed in 5 – 10%		
Frontometaphyseal dysplasia	305620	Progressive mixed		
Hunter syndrome (mucopolysaccharidosis type II)	309900	Sensorineural/mixed	Xq27 – q28	Sulphoiduronate sulphatase
Hyperuricaemia, hearing loss and neurological involvement	311850	Sensorineural	Xq21 - q24	

Condition	OMIM / Reference	Hearing loss	Location	Gene
Hypogonadism and hearing loss	304350	Congenital mixed		POU3F4
Hypophosphataemia + hearing loss	307810	Sensorineural	Xp22	PEX
Mental retardation, hearing loss, short stature microgenitalism	309590	Mild/severe, type not specified	Xq12-q21	XNP
Mental retardation, microcephaly ophthalmoplegia hearing loss	312840 (Villard et al., 1996)	Severe sensorineural		
Mental retardation, ataxia, hearing loss, optic atrophy, hypotonia, death in childhood	301835	Unknown, severe, probably sensorineural	Xq 22.1 - q24	
Nephritis with mental retardation, sensorineural hearing loss, and macrocephaly	(Lane et al., 1994)	Sensorineural		
XR progressive hearing loss, blindness, spastic paraplegia and dystonia	304700	Childhood-onset progressive sensorineural	Xq21	
High frequency sensorineural hearing loss (XR)	(Lalwani et al., 1994)	High frequency sensorineural non-progressive	Xp21	
Norrie disease	310600	Progressive adult-onset sensorineural in 1/3	Xp11.3 – p11.4	NDP
Ocular albinism, hearing loss	300650	Late-onset sensorineural	Xp22.3	
Optic atrophy, neural hearing loss, polyneuropathy	311070	Progressive sensorineural	Xq26 – q27	
Oto-palato-digital syndrome type I	311300	Conductive		
Oto-palato-digital syndrome type II	304120	Conductive/mixed		
Spastic paraparesis and hearing loss	312910	Adolescent-onset sensorineural		
Toriello syndrome (maxillo-facial dysostosis XR)	301950	Mixed		

For references see the catalogue of Mendelian Inheritance in Man (McKusick, 1994) or Brunner et al., 1990. XR X-linked recessive inheritance. *PRPS* Phosphoribosyl Pyrophosphate Synthetase (Becker et al., 1995) CMTX X-linked Charcot Marie Tooth Disease (Priest et al., 1995). *NDP* Norrie disease protein gene (Berger et al., 1992). *PEX* Phosphate regulating gene with homologies to endopeptidases, X chromosome (HYP Consortium 1995).

inner ear (Reardon et al., 1993). This bony abnormality is identical to that found in patients with X-linked progressive mixed hearing loss with perilymphatic gusher. Mutations of the *POU3F4* gene have been detected in such families (de Kok et al., 1995). At least two (and probably more) genetic defects can cause a similar clinical picture of congenital severe X-linked sensorineural hearing loss (Table 24.2). Thus X-linked congenital sensorineural hearing loss is both clinically and genetically heterogeneous.

Table 24.2 Genetic subtypes of X-linked severe sensorineural congenital hearing loss.

Localisation	Gene	CT-scan	Vestibular function	Reference
Xq21	*POU3F4*	Abnormal	Abnormal	de Kok et al., 1995
Xq21	Unknown	Normal	Normal	Reardon et al., 1991
Xp21	Unknown	Normal	Unknown	Lalwani et al., 1994
Unknown, Xq21 excluded	Unknown	Normal	Normal	Reardon et al., 1994

X-linked progressive mixed hearing loss with perilymphatic gusher

This is the most common form of X-linked non-syndromal hearing loss. Mixed hearing loss becomes evident in the first years of life, and is progressive. In some instances progression of the sensorineural component may eventually mask the conductive element. Air conduction levels in males are typically 80 – 100 dB while bone conduction is around 60 – 80 dB involving all frequencies, although the lower frequencies may have slightly better thresholds (Nance et al., 1971).

Abnormal audiograms are found in approximately 50% of carrier females. Either sensorineural or mixed hearing loss may be present. Carrier females rarely require hearing aids, and in many, hearing loss is not noticed prior to audiometric examination. Vestibular function tests are abnormal in all affected males. Affected males, as well as some carrier females, have a characteristic abnormality of the inner ear which can be demonstrated on CT-scan (Phelps et al., 1991). There is a bulbous internal auditory meatus, dilated facial nerve canal, and incomplete separation of the basal coil of the cochlea from the internal auditory meatus. The inner ear abnormality allows communication of cerebrospinal fluid from the subarachnoid space in the internal auditory meatus to the perilymphatic space of the scala vestibuli (Reardon et al., 1993). This explains the occurrence of a perilymph 'gusher' if the stapedial footplate is opened during surgery. For this reason, operative correction of stapes fixation should always be preceded by CT-scan investigation of the inner ear. It has been suggested that a perilymphatic gusher can be provoked for a few seconds by lightly touching the stapedial footplate without opening the oval window (Cremers et al., 1985). This may provide an alternative intra-operative test.

Progressive mixed hearing loss with perilymphatic gusher is caused by mutations of the POU-domain gene *POU3F4*. The *POU3F4* gene resides in band q21 of the X chromosome, and encodes a transcription factor which presumably regulates multiple morphogenetic events during embryonal development of the inner ear (de Kok et al., 1995).

X-linked moderate sensorineural hearing loss

This condition has been described in 2 pedigrees from Italy and France, respectively (Livan, 1961; Pelletier and Tanguay, 1975). It is characterised by slowly progressive sensorineural hearing loss, beginning around adolescence, and affecting predominantly the high frequencies. Vestibular function tests were normal. The genetic defect for this condition is unknown and additional cases have not been reported over the past 20 years. There are similarities to X-linked high frequency sensorineural hearing loss, although hearing loss was reported to be non-progressive in that condition.

X-linked high frequency sensorineural hearing loss

A single Australian kindred has been reported in which affected males had a moderate hearing loss of approximately 60 dB affecting the higher frequencies (1.5 – 8 kHz). Hearing loss was non-progressive and vestibular tests were not reported (Wellesley and Goldblatt, 1994). There are similarities to X-linked moderate sensorineural hearing loss, although hearing loss was reported to be progressive in the latter condition. The defective gene is unknown.

Chapter 25
The X-linked recessive progressive mixed hearing loss syndrome with perilymphatic gusher during stapes surgery (*DFN3*)

COR WRJ CREMERS

Introduction

X-recessive inheritance is quite rare in genetic hearing loss (Brunner et al., 1991). Nance et al. (1971) were the first to describe the syndrome as 'X-linked mixed hearing loss with congenital fixation of the stapedial footplate and perilymphatic gusher', in a large Caucasian population of children (McKusick, 1992, 304400). The existence of this entity had been suggested earlier by Olsen and Lehman (1968) and has since been confirmed (Thorpe et al., 1974; Cremers et al., 1985; Cremers and Huygen, 1983; Wallis et al., 1988; Phelps et al., 1991; Reardon et al., 1991; Bach et al., 1992; Tang and Parnes, 1994).

The term perilymphatic gusher refers to a heavy flow of perilymph after the stapedial footplate has been opened in surgery. The gush of perilymph is actually cerebrospinal fluid (CSF). It is believed that these cases may have an abnormally wide cochlear aqueduct. Progressive sensorineural hearing loss in childhood is also associated with the large vestibular aqueduct syndrome (Arcand et al., 1991; Okumura et al., 1995). In view of the quantity of CSF which is expelled in association with the stapes gusher, it is probable that the fluid flows via the internal auditory canal and not via the cochlear aqueduct. This assumption was supported by observations during surgery (Glasscock, 1973) and dilatation of the internal auditory canal in these patients has been confirmed radiologically (Glasscock, 1973; Cremers et al., 1985; Phelps et al., 1991; Michel et al., 1991; Talbot and Wilson, 1994; Tang and Parnes, 1994).

The mode of inheritance and the audiological, radiological and genetic aspects of this syndrome are discussed below.

Hearing loss

Only a small number of families have been described with this syndrome. In two studies, fairly detailed audiometric findings in affected males were reported (Nance et al., 1971; Cremers et al., 1985; Cremers, 1985) and two reports presented the audiometric findings in female carriers of this syndrome (Nance et al., 1971; Cremers and Huygen, 1983). Table 25.1 shows the hearing loss found in eight affected males from the family shown in the pedigree (Figure 25.1). For two males, cases 13.16 and 13.01.04, the pure tone audiograms and speech threshold audiograms are shown in Figures 25.2 and 25.3, respectively. There were considerable discrepancies between the pure tone audiograms and speech recognition. Figure 25.4 shows the tympanogram and the stapedial reflexes elicited on the contralateral side for case 13.01.04. There was slight hearing loss at frequencies of 2,000 Hz and higher, while conductive loss was particularly noticeable at the lower frequencies (Cremers, 1985; Glasscock, 1973). Moreover, provided that the hearing loss was not too severe and despite the presence of conductive hearing loss, a stapedial reflex could still be elicited (Cremers, 1985).

This phenomenon was also observed in three isolated patients with a stapes gusher during stapedial surgery (Cremers et al., 1983). A stapedial reflex could be elicited even when the stapes was fixed, if the stapedial tendon was attached to the long process of the incus. Recently all three showed different mutations of the X-chromosome close to the locus of the gene locus for this syndrome.

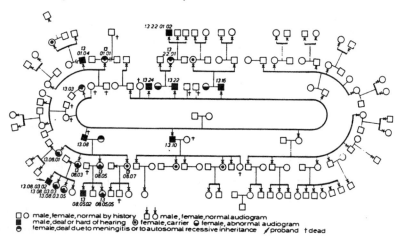

Figure 25.1 Pedigree of family with the X-linked mixed progressive, mixed hearing loss.

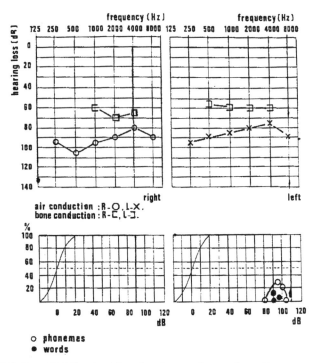

Figure 25.2 Case 13.16, mixed hearing loss and speech audiogram.

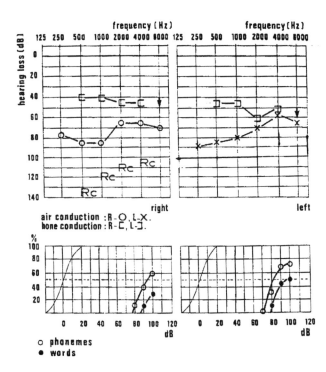

Figure 25.2 Case 13.01,04, mixed hearing loss and speech audiogram.

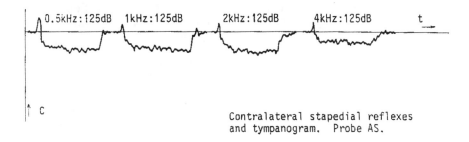

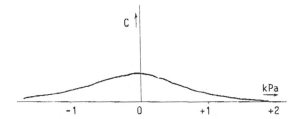

Figure 25.4 Case 13.01.04, stapedial reflexes.

Table 25.1 Sensorineural component in three younger and five older affected males.

Case	Age	Ear	250 Hz	500 Hz	1000 Hz	2000 Hz	4000 Hz	8000 Hz
13.10	74	R	>80	50+40	40+45	55+10	70+10	45+15
		L	>80	55+40	45+45	70+10	65+10	70
13.16	71	R	>90	100	60+35	70+20	65+15	90
		L	95	50+40	60+25	60+20	60+15	90
13 22	65	R	> 90	95	55+40	60+10	60+30	> 70
		L	>90	95	70+20	70+0	70+10	70
13.24	64	R	5+60	30+55	50+50	50+20	50+20	55+15
		L	10+60	25+55	30+55	40+30	55+10	55+10
13 01 04	55	R	80	40+35	40+35	45+20	45+20	70
		L	90	45+40	40+35	60+10	50+10	65
13.08.03.02	25	R	60	20+20	35+30	45+25	20+20	40+0
		L	75	25+60	40+50	50+15	45+05	30+0
13.08.05 02	21	R	70	40+35	50+25	55+15	50+20	55+15
		L	65	45+20	50+25	60+15	55+20	60+0
13.22.01.02	11	R	35	20+20	20+15	25+10	30+0	35+0
		L	75	35+50	30+50	45+25	55+30	40+25

Another explanation for the presence of the stapedial reflex, is that the components of the hearing loss are not localised in the middle ear, but that the total hearing loss originates on the medial side of the stapes in the enlarged vestibulum and the cochlea. If the cause of the hearing loss lies in the enlarged vestibulum it should be possible to detect a conductive loss using pure tone audiometry, whereas the findings of auditory brainstem response audiometry will suggest pure cochlear hearing loss. Our own recent measurements support this assumption (Snik et al., 1995). Hearing loss progression was clear from the medical history of each affected male and it has also been observed in the audiometric follow-up of some of the affected males over 20 to 30 years (Cremers et al., 1985; Glasscock, 1973). Family studies have shown that the younger affected males have better hearing but that it deteriorates as they grow older. Glasscock reported that the adult males in his kindred A were never offered the opportunity of early amplification and did not learn oral communication. Hearing loss in the younger proband was discovered at an early age so he was able to develop adequate speech and language skills (Glasscock, 1973).

It is assumed that progression of sensorineural hearing loss is caused by the conduction of pressure variation in the CSF in the perilymph to the cochlea, to the endolymph and the organ of Corti. Possibly the degree of hearing loss and its progression correlates with the size of the anomaly of the lateral end of the internal acoustic canal.

Radiological aspects

Glasscock (1973) was the first to describe abnormalities of the inner ear and internal auditory canal in this syndrome using conventional polytomography. The lateral part of the internal auditory canal was dilated and the vestibulum was also enlarged. Cremers et al. (1985) confirmed these findings with conventional polytomography. Phelps et al. (1991) described similar radiological findings using CT scanning. They studied seven pedigrees in which hearing loss was inherited as an X-linked trait. Dilatation of the lateral end of the internal auditory canal was a common finding, as was the deficiency or absence of bone between the lateral end of the internal acoustic canal and the basal turn of the cochlea. CT scanning of the petrous bones in a new affected male of the Dutch family (Cremers et al., 1985) show these anomalies (Figure 5). Some of the obligate female carriers had a mild form of the same anomaly which was associated with a slight hearing loss.

Otological aspects

Glasscock (1973) produced new evidence that the CSF gusher flows along the dilated internal auditory canal to the vestibule, enters the middle ear cavity via the opened stapes footplate and floods the auditory canal. The perilymphatic system is believed to be connected to the subarachnoid space in two ways, through the cochlear aqueduct and along the perineural sheaths of nerves supplying in the internal auditory canal. Another possibility is connection via the endolymphatic duct which passes through the vestibular aqueduct. In normal subjects, there must be a physiological mechanism which reduces the CSF pressure from 200 to 70 mm Hg and prevents the profuse flow of fluid from the oval window after the stapes footplate has been opened. It is assumed that this is the result of tight fitting connections along the nerve sheaths in the internal auditory canal, and the size of the cochlear aqueduct. In this way, the CSF pressure will be too low to pump a large quantity of CSF into the vestibule or cause a stapes gusher after the footplate has been opened.

Glasscock (1973) performed conventional polytomography on his patients and found that, in at least two cases with X-recessive mixed hearing loss syndrome who had undergone surgery, there was unusual dilation of the lateral end of the internal auditory canal and enlargement of the vestibule. These radiological findings have been confirmed (Cremers et al., 1985; Phelps et al., 1991; Michel et al., 1991; Talbot and Wilson, 1994; Tang and Parnes, 1994) and they also confirmed the surgical findings that the communication between the subarachnoid space and the vestibule is widened along the nerve sheaths in the internal auditory canal of patients with this syndrome.

The few reports which contain details of surgical findings nearly always mention stapes fixation, but the fact that it is possible to elicit stapedial reflexes in these patients contradicts the surgical findings. For the time being, it remains unclear whether there is any real histological fixation of the stapes. The question arose earlier as to whether conductive hearing loss forms part of this syndrome. Arguments can be put forward in favour of accepting the notion that the conductive component in the pure tone audiogram indicates an inner ear loss which is caused by enlargement of the vestibule and dilatation of the internal auditory canal.

Localisation and identification of the genetic defect

In a large Dutch kindred, Brunner et al. (1988) found close linkage (maximum lod score 3.07 at theta = 0.00) with *PGK*, which is located at Xq13 (McKusick, 1992). They drew attention to the fact that hearing loss is one of the predominant clinical features in males with deletions of Xq21. Wallis et al. (1988) showed close linkage to *DXYS1* (lod score 6.32 at theta = 0.00) which placed the gene defect at Xq13-q21. Bach et al.

(1992) studied thirteen unrelated male probands with X-linked hearing loss in an attempt to detect deletions. Microdeletions could be identified in two cases. The gene involved was called *DFN3* and it maps in close vicinity to *DXS26* locus. Some cases with X-linked hearing loss and stapes gusher also have other features, such as choroideraemia, and microdeletions in the same region on the X chromosome (Merry et al., 1989).

Brunner et al. (1988), Wallis et al. (1988), and Reardon et al. (1991, 1992) showed that X-linked hearing loss is invariably coinherited with DNA markers on the proximal long arm of the X chromosome. This region of the X chromosome is referred to as Xq13-q21. Brunner et al. (1988, 1991) and Merry et al. (1989) reported hearing loss, sometimes associated with a band on the X chromosome. These males also have choroideraemia, because the gene for this form of inherited retinal degeneration is also located in the Xq21 band (Frans Cremers, 1989). Further molecular studies on the thirteen male probands with various forms of X-linked hearing loss without choroideraemia, revealed two microdeletions at Xq21 which were invisible using normal chromosome analysis, but which could be detected using DNA analysis (Bach et al., 1992). The latter studies isolated the region where the X-linked hearing loss gene is located to only a tiny subsegment in the Xq21 band. This very precise localisation was helpful in allowing the identification of the POU gene as the gene responsible for this X-linked hearing loss (De Kok et al., 1993). In a number of the patients concerned, there is a mutation close to the locus for the POU gene. The mechanism causing this syndrome in those patients has not yet been clarified. Knowledge about the basic genetic defect will improve our insight into the pathogenesis of this disorder.

Discussion

The X-recessive mixed hearing loss syndrome with perilymphatic gusher during stapes surgery, has very striking audiological, radiological, otological and genetic aspects. The isolation of the *DFN3* gene can be used to confirm the clinical diagnosis. This is not only of importance for genetic counselling, but it will also help to prevent inappropriate and unsuccessful stapes surgery in these patients.

Some audiological characteristics can alert the audiologist to the fact that a particular anomaly may carry the risk of a stapes gusher – for example, mixed hearing loss with an extremely small air bone gap at 2,000 Hz, in combination with elicitable stapes reflexes. At present, such findings are an indication to perform CT scans of the petrous bone, even in isolated cases, to detect the presence of dilatation of the lateral part of the internal auditory canal and an enlarged vestibular labyrinth.

These radiological anomalies were first detected using polytomography and are much easier to see on CT scans. If surgery is being considered for suspected congenital conductive or mixed hearing loss, CT scanning of the petrous bone as a preoperative screening method is imperative so that the risk of a stapes gusher can be recognised well in advance. The application of these aspects to clinical practice has proved to be very worthwhile for making an accurate diagnosis and sparing patients from pointless surgery.

Further research is required to answer the question of whether the conductive component of the hearing loss can be explained by an enlarged vestibulum, and/or whether progression of the sensorineural component in the hearing loss can be explained by variation in CSF pressure in the cochlea. Now the POU gene has been identified as the *DFN3* gene, the future aim is to understand the reason why mutations close to the *DFN3* gene can also cause this syndrome. The possibility of being able in the future to identify potentially all affected persons and carriers will add extra impulse to this clinical research.

Chapter 26
Mitochondrially determined hearing impairment

NATHAN FISCHEL-GHODSIAN

Introduction

Over the last five years mutations in mitochondrial DNA have been found to be associated with a variety of hearing defects. This chapter will, after a short introduction to mitochondrial genetics, outline the spectrum of clinical presentations of mitochondrially determined hearing impairments, and the clinical and biological implications of these presentations.

Normal mitochondrial genetics

There are hundreds of mitochondria in each cell and they serve a variety of metabolic functions, the most important being the synthesis of ATP by oxidative phosphorylation. Each mitochondrion contains 2 – 10 mitochondrial chromosomes, so that each cell contains thousands of mitochondrial chromosomes. Each of these mitochondrial DNA molecules in humans is 16,569 base pairs long, double stranded, forms a closed circle, and replicates and is transcribed within the mitochondrion. The mitochondrial DNA molecule encodes 13 mRNA genes, as well as two rRNAs and 22 organelle-specific tRNAs which are required for assembling a functional mitochondrial protein synthesising system. The 13 mRNAs are translated on mitochondrion-specific ribosomes, using a mitochondrion-specific genetic code, into 13 proteins. These proteins interact with approximately sixty nuclear encoded proteins to form the five enzyme complexes required for oxidative phosphorylation. These complexes are bound to the mitochondrial inner membrane, and are involved in electron transport and ATP synthesis (reviewed in Attardi and Schatz, 1988).

Mitochondrial DNA is transmitted exclusively through mothers, as shown by restriction fragment length polymorphism analysis in pedigrees, with sperm apparently contributing no mitochondrial DNA to the zygote. This leads to the expectation that a defect in a mitochondrial gene should lead to disease equally in both sexes, but can only be transmitted through the maternal line. These basic rules of mitochondrial genetics are complicated by at least four factors:

1. Some mitochondrial mutations might lead to disease only in the presence of a specific nuclear genotype or environmental agent (Jaber et al., 1992; Prezant et al., 1993).
2. Some autosomal recessive and autosomal dominant inherited genetic disorders, as well as medications such as AZT, can lead to mitochondrial DNA pathology, such as acquired mutations/deletions or depletion (Arnaudo et al., 1991; Zeviani 1992; Suomalainen et al., 1994).
3. Although most healthy individuals appear to have only a single mitochondrial DNA genotype, i.e. are homoplasmic, in most mitochondrial disease states the mitochondrial DNA population is mixed (a condition called heteroplasmy). The amount of heteroplasmy varies from tissue to tissue, and for cells within a tissue, and the severity of the symptoms does not always correlate well with the proportion of mutant mitochondrial DNAs. While for most of the multisystemic mitochondrial syndromes the homoplasmic state would presumably be lethal, homoplasmy of the mutant mitochondrial DNA is observed for two tissue specific diseases, the ocular disorder Leber's hereditary optic neuroretinopathy (LHON) (Howell, 1994) and some hearing disorders as described in the sections on non-syndromal and ototoxic hearing loss below.
4. The identical mitochondrial mutation can lead to entirely different phenotypes, examples of which are given in the section on syndromal hearing loss.

Mitochondrial DNA mutations and hearing loss

Over the last few years hearing loss has been found to be associated with a multitude of different mitochondrial defects.

Syndromal hearing loss

Initially mitochondrial DNA defects were described in a number of systemic neuromuscular diseases, such as Kearns-Sayre syndrome, MERRF and MELAS (Moraes et al., 1989; Shoffner et al., 1990; Goto et al., 1990). In each of these diseases the pathogenic mutation is heteroplasmic and varies from large deletion/insertions to point mutations. It is not surprising that a patient with generalised neuromuscular dysfunction will also present with hearing deficits, and thus these diseases were of no particular interest to clinicians or researchers in the hearing field.

This changed with the surprising description of several families with mitochondrial mutations, in whom sensorineural hearing loss and diabetes mellitus occur with significant penetrance but not always together (Ballinger et al., 1992; van den Ouweland et al., 1992; Reardon et al., 1992). Even more surprisingly, in most of these families the pathogenic heteroplasmic mutation is the same A→G transition mutation at nucleotide 3243 in the mitochondrial gene for tRNA[Leu(UUR)] as in MELAS (van den Ouweland et al., 1992; Reardon et al., 1992), while in one family it was a heteroplasmic large deletion/insertion event (Ballinger et al., 1992). This association between diabetes mellitus, hearing loss, and mitochondrial mutations has been confirmed in population studies of diabetic patients (Oka et al., 1993; Kadowaki et al., 1994; Alcolado et al., 1994; Katagiri et al., 1994). Kadowaki et al., for example, found the heteroplasmic nucleotide 3243 mutation in 2 – 6% of diabetic patients in Japan, and in 3 out of 5 patients with diabetes and hearing loss. 27 of their 44 patients with diabetes and the nucleotide 3243 mutation had hearing loss. In none of these cases were other neurological symptoms present. The hearing loss is sensorineural, and usually develops only after the onset of diabetes. We are not aware of a study that has looked for the frequency of the nucleotide 3243 mutation in a population of patients with adult onset sensorineural hearing loss. In addition, diabetes mellitus, diabetes insipidus, optic atrophy and hearing loss have been well described as the Wolfram or DIDMOAD (an acronym for the major features) syndrome, usually an autosomal recessive condition, but which may also occur on the basis of mitochondrial deletions (Rotig et al., 1993; Bu and Rotter, 1993).

Non-syndromal hearing loss

The first hint that non-syndromal hearing loss can be caused by mitochondrial mutations came from an Arab-Israeli pedigree, in which the striking pattern of transmission only through mothers was first noted (Jaber et al., 1992). Formal segregation analysis of the inheritance pattern in this pedigree predicted a two locus disorder, in which the presence of both a homoplasmic mitochondrial mutation and an autosomal recessive mutation is required for phenotypic expression of the hearing loss phenotype (Jaber et al., 1992). Clinically the deaf family members predominately have the onset of severe to profound hearing loss during infancy, but a minority of family members had the onset during childhood or even adulthood, with the loss sometimes occurring over a relatively short time period and then remaining stable. Audiologically the hearing loss is sensorineural and of cochlear origin, and the vestibular system is unaffected. A homoplasmic mutation at nucleotide 1555 in the mitochondrial 12S rRNA gene was identified as the pathogenic mutation (Prezant et al., 1993), and the same mutation was also found to predispose to aminoglycoside induced hearing loss as described below.

A second family with a maternal inheritance pattern and non-syndromal hearing loss was then described in Scotland, and confirmed and established in a third unrelated pedigree from New Zealand (Reid et al., 1994; Fischel-Ghodsian et al., 1995; Figure 26.1). The mutation in these families was at nucleotide 7445, which is the last nucleotide of both the tRNA$^{Ser(UCN)}$ gene on one strand and the cytochrome oxidase I gene on the other strand. Since the sequence change in the cytochrome oxidase gene is a conservative change of the termination codon, it is most likely that the change of the 3' end of the tRNA molecule affects aminoacylation, and thus translational fidelity. The mutation is hetero-plasmic in lymphoblastoid cells, with the abnormal molecules corresponding to over 95% of the population of mitochondrial chromosomes. The clinical phenotype is sensorineural hearing loss with onset usually during childhood or adolescence. Interestingly, the penetrance of this mutation in the Scottish pedigree is quite low, while in the New Zealand pedigree every individual over the age of 20 has hearing loss. Thus, in similarity to the Arab-Israeli pedigree, the mitochondrial mutation by itself does not appear to be sufficient to cause hearing loss, but requires an additional genetic or environmental factor, which seems to be rare in the Scottish pedigree and ubiquitous in the New Zealand pedigree.

Recently a potential fourth extended population in a remote village in Zaire was described (Matthijs et al., 1994). Like the Arab-Israeli pedigree, they have the homoplasmic 1555 mutation. Both congenital hearing loss and acquired hearing loss later in life are common. However, because of the widespread use of streptomycin for tuberculosis, and the difficulties in obtaining reliable historical information from the village, the precise inheritance pattern remains elusive at the present time.

Interestingly, Shoffner et al. recently described an unrelated pedigree with maternally inherited Parkinson disease and hearing loss, which has the homoplasmic nucleotide 1555 mutation (Shoffner et al., 1994). However, since the group has not yet determined whether a hetero-plasmic mitochondrial mutation exists in a different mitochondrial gene, in addition to the homoplasmic 1555 mutation, it is too early to draw any conclusions from this finding.

Ototoxic hearing loss

Aminoglycoside ototoxicity is a common cause of acquired hearing loss. Although vestibulo-cochlear damage is nearly universal when high drug levels are present for prolonged periods, at lower drug levels there appears to be a significant genetic component influencing susceptibility to aminoglycoside ototoxicity. Numerous families have been described in which several individuals became deaf after exposure to aminoglycosides (Konigsmark et al., 1976; Higashi, 1989; Hu et al., 1991), and dramatic species differences in susceptibility to these drugs also suggest a genetic component (Stebbins et al., 1981).

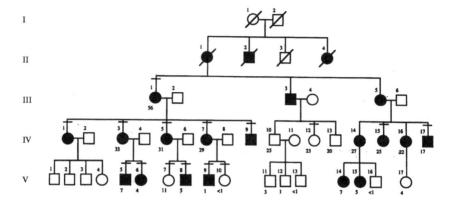

Figure 26.1 Pedigree of family with sensorineural hearing loss and the nucleotide 7445 mutation in the tRNA$^{Ser(UCN)}$ gene. Solid symbols indicate deaf individuals. Horizontal bars above the symbols indicate that audiological test results are available. Ages at time of study are indicated in years below the symbols. Individuals V1-V4 are in their early childhood. Hearing status of individuals in generation I is unknown.

We analysed three Chinese families in which several individuals developed hearing loss after the use of aminoglycosides (Prezant et al., 1993; Figure 26.2). The pattern of maternal inheritance in these pedigrees, the known effect of aminoglycosides on ribosomal translation ability, and the presence of resistance mutations in a range of prokaryotic and eukaryotic organisms, implicated the mitochondrial ribosomes, and in particular the mitochondrially encoded 12S rRNA gene, as the most likely locus of such predisposition to toxicity. In all three families a mutation was identified in the 12S mitochondrial rRNA gene that affected a site known to be important both in the binding to aminoglycosides and in resistance to the antibiotic (Prezant et al., 1993). Also, a small proportion of 'sporadic' patients, without a positive family history for aminoglycoside ototoxicity, exhibit this particular mutation (Fischel-Ghodsian et al., 1993). These findings were confirmed in two Japanese families and additional Chinese sporadic cases (Hutchin et al., 1993). Subsequently an additional heteroplasmic nucleotide deletion/insertion mutation around nucleotide 961 in the 12S rRNA gene, and two potential homoplasmic mutations in the same gene, which also appear to predispose to aminoglycoside ototoxicity, were described (Bacino et al., 1995). Most interestingly, in one streptomycin induced deaf individual with a strong familial history of aminoglycoside induced hearing loss and the mitochondrial 1555 mutation, detailed vestibular examination revealed severe hearing loss with completely normal vestibular function.

It appears at this time that, at least in China, Japan, and Mongolia, nearly every case of familial aminoglycoside induced ototoxcity, as well as a small proportion of the sporadic cases, has the 1555 mutation.

About a third of all aminoglycoside induced hearing loss cases in China appear to be due to the 1555 mutation (Hu et al., 1991). Since amino-glycosides are used much more extensively in those countries than they are in Western countries, and since the aminoglycoside induced ototox-icity associated with the 1555 mutation has been identified in all races, it is possible that a significant proportion of sporadic cases in countries with sparing use of aminoglycosides have the 1555 mutation. Most recently we have shown that 7/41 (17%) of unrelated American individ-uals with hearing loss after aminoglycoside exposure had the 1555 mutation (Fischel-Ghodsian et al., in press).

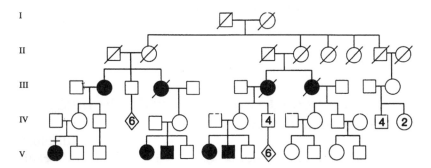

Figure 26.2 Pedigree of a Chinese family with maternally transmitted aminoglycoside induced hearing loss due to the nucleotide 1555 mutation in the 12S ribosomal RNA gene. Solid symbols indicate individuals treated with streptomycin before high frequency sensorineural hearing loss ensued. Horizontal bars indicate individuals whose DNA was sampled.

Presbyacusis

The relationship between mitochondrial DNA defects and presbyacusis is entirely speculative at this time, but has become not unlikely, given that acquired mitochondrial DNA mutations, and the resulting loss of oxidative phosphorylation activity, seem to play an important role in the ageing process (reviewed by Nagley et al., 1993). These mutations are thought to be associated with the insidious decline in physiological and biochemical performance of an organ and to contribute significantly to the ageing process and ultimately death. Because of the higher energy requirements of muscle and nervous tissue, and the fact that small num-bers of dysfunctional muscle and nerve cells can interrupt the function of many neighbouring normal cells, mitochondrial DNA mutations of those particular tissues are thought to be particularly harmful.

In man, accumulation of mitochondrial DNA defects has been docu-mented in the greatest detail in brain and heart. In general, investigators have concentrated on the detection of deletions, and in particular a 4977 nucleotide deletion, which is also called the 'common deletion'.

This deletion has been found in high concentration in many sporadic mitochondrial disorders, and is thought to arise by illegitimate recombination involving the 13-basepair repeats found at both deletion breakpoints. One particularly fascinating and perplexing finding in the human studies was the dramatic difference in the levels of acquired mitochondrial DNA deletions among different tissues in the same individual. For example, the 4977 nucleotide common deletion was found consistently at levels of hundreds to 2,000 times more commonly in the caudate, putamen, and substantia nigra than in the cerebellum, with the cortex having intermediate levels of deletion acquisition (Soong et al., 1992; Corral-Debrinski et al., 1992). No detailed investigation of mitochondrial DNA changes with age has been made of the auditory system, but such investigations in individuals with and without presbyacusis may reveal the role of mitochondrial DNA in the hearing loss associated with ageing.

Clinical relevance of mitochondrially induced hearing loss at this time

The clinical relevance of the findings on the role of the mitochondrial genome in hearing loss is so far mainly limited to the prevention of aminoglycoside induced hearing loss. Physicians need to inquire about a family history of aminoglycoside induced hearing loss prior to the administration of systemic aminoglycosides as antimicrobials, as well as prior to the local administration of aminoglycosides into the cochlea as treatment for Meniere's disease. In addition, every individual with aminoglycoside induced hearing loss should be screened at least for the presence of the mitochondrial 1555 mutation, since presence of the mutation will allow counselling to all maternally related relatives to avoid aminoglycosides. Insufficient data are currently available to know whether vestibular testing can consistently distinguish between aminoglycoside induced ototoxicity due to mitochondrial predisposition and other causes.

Hearing maternal relatives of deaf individuals with non-syndromal hearing loss and the 1555 mutation are also at risk for aminoglycoside induced hearing loss. However, since the 1555 mutation will only extremely rarely be responsible for non-syndromal hearing loss, clinical screening of such patients for the 1555 mutation is not warranted at the present time.

With the exception of aminoglycosides and mitochondrial mutations in the 12S rRNA gene, there are no proven preventive or therapeutic interventions for mitochondrially related hearing impairments. The diagnosis of such defects is, however, useful for genetic counselling and is indicated in all families with an inheritance pattern of hearing loss consistent with maternal transmission, and possibly in all patients who have both diabetes mellitus and adult onset hearing loss.

The remaining challenges

Elucidation of the interrelationship between defects in the mitochondrial DNA and hearing loss is in its infancy. In particular, the spectrum and relevance of mitochondrial mutations in syndromal, non-syndromal, ototoxic, and especially with age-associated hearing loss remain to be defined in more detail. Differentiation between homoplasmic mitochondrial disease mutations and benign rare polymorphisms remains a challenge in aiding this characterisation (Howell, 1994). In addition, the biological process leading from the mitochondrial DNA mutation to hearing loss can be understood at this time only for generalised neuromuscular mitochondrial diseases and aminoglycoside induced ototoxicity, and the finding that mitochondrial mutations can lead to non-syndromal or syndromal tissue-restricted hearing loss has been rather unexpected for the two following reasons:

1. If a mutation affects oxidative phosphorylation (the only known function of the human mitochondrial chromosome and an essential process in every nucleated cell of the human body), it is unclear how the clinical defect remains confined to the cochlea, rather than affecting every tissue in the body.
2. How can the same mutation in the mitochondrial genome lead to entirely different phenotypes? As described above, the nucleotide 3243 mutation can lead either to MELAS, a systemic neuromuscular disorder, or to a specific syndrome including only diabetes and hearing loss.

The factors that lead to the phenotypic expression of a mitochondrial mutation in a given tissue are thus unknown. For all heteroplasmic mitochondrial mutations it remains possible that some minor tissue differences in the quantity of the abnormal chromosomes account for the phenotypic differences, although this may be only a very partial answer. For example, the distribution of the abnormal mitochondrial chromosome has not been shown to be different in patients with MELAS and those with the diabetes/hearing loss syndrome. For the two homoplasmic mitochondrial diseases, Leber's hereditary optic neuroretinopathy (LHON) and our Arab-Israeli pedigree, the reasons for the tissue specificity remain entirely unknown. We have proposed two different mechanisms in which the tissue specificity in these, as well as in many heteroplasmic mitochondrial disorders, can be explained (Bernes et al.,

1993; Fischel-Ghodsian et al., 1995): Firstly, it is possible that tissue specific subunits of mitochondrial ribosomes or oxidative phosphorylation complexes interact specifically with the mitochondrial defect only in affected tissues. While there is no *a priori* reason that such tissue specific subunits should exist for a generalised cellular process, tissue specific subunits for general cellular processes, including oxidative phosphorylation, have been described (Arnaudo et al., 1992). We have therefore proposed that the molecular basis of non-syndromal hearing loss might in at least some of the cases be due to defects in general cellular processes (limited to the target organ because of tissue specific subunits), rather than due to unique structural or functional defects in hair cells or cochlear nerve fibres which are specific to the hearing mechanism. Secondly, it cannot be entirely excluded that human mitochondrial genes have functions in addition to their functions in oxidative phosphorylation. In this model the mitochondrial mutations would then not significantly interfere with oxidative phosphorylation, but with a tissue specific secondary function of the mitochondrial gene. Again, there is no *a priori* reason that such double functions should exist, but a precedent for precisely this hypothesis can be found in mice and *Drosophila* (Wang et al., 1991; Kobayashi et al., 1993). For example, the mitochondrial large ribosomal RNA gene in *Drosophila melanogaster*, in addition to being involved in mitochondrial translation, has also been identified in the cytoplasm where it induces pole cell formation in embryos, a key event in the determination of the germ line and entirely unrelated to oxidative phosphorylation (Kobayashi et al., 1993).

Part V
Management

Chapter 27
Genetic counselling for hearing impairment

ROBERT F MUELLER

Introduction

For most parents who have a child born with hearing impairment it occurs unexpectedly, in the absence of a family history of the disorder. When they begin to accept the short and longer term consequences for their child, they usually have two questions:

1. Why does their child have hearing impairment?
2. What is the chance for another child to be born similarly affected?

Genetic counselling is the process which provides answers to these questions. This requires consideration of the family history, the medical and obstetric history of the mother of the person with hearing impairment, along with a detailed assessment of the physical findings in the affected individual and specialist investigations and examinations.

It is also important for adults with hearing impairment to be given the opportunity to receive advice about the chances of their children having a hearing impairment. This can be particularly important since their partners frequently also have hearing impairment.

Before considering this process in more detail it is useful to outline the epidemiology of hearing impairment.

Epidemiology of hearing impairment

Surveys carried out over the last 4 decades in a number of different populations have shown that 1 in 1,000 to 2,000 children are born with, or present in early childhood with, profound hearing impairment (Parving, 1983; Newton, 1985).

Studies of the aetiology of hearing impairment have shown that they can be approximately equally split into the three main groups with hereditary causes being responsible in 20 – 60%, acquired causes in 20 – 40%, and unknown causes in the remaining 20 – 40% (Fraser, 1964; Newton, 1985; Parving, 1984). Of those with a genetic aetiology, various series have reported approximately two thirds (59 – 85%) as being due to an autosomal recessive gene, in the region of one third (15 – 33%) being due to an autosomal dominant gene, with the remainder (0 – 5%) due to an X-linked gene or mitochondrial inheritance (Chung and Brown, 1970; Fraser, 1976; Marazita et al., 1993).

There is a well recognised increase in the prevalence of hearing impairment with age (Morton, 1991), with the main acquired causes including infection and noise induced injury. Although a significant proportion of late-onset hearing impairment is genetic in origin, there are a limited number of formal genetic aetiological studies of this group (Cohen and Gorlin, 1995).

Aetiology

We shall consider the two causes of hearing impairment, genetic and acquired, in more detail.

Acquired causes

Although hearing impairment is often attributed to environmental causes, the evidence for this in many instances is circumstantial, e.g. an infection such as measles around the time a child is diagnosed as having a hearing impairment. Well recognised environmental causes include congenital infections such as rubella and cytomegalovirus, perinatal events such as prematurity and severe neonatal jaundice, and post-natal infection such as meningitis, mumps and measles.

Genetic causes

Hearing impairment due to a genetic cause can be separated into two main groups, occurring either in isolation, i.e. non-syndromal, or in association with other features, i.e. syndromal. The latter can occur due to chromosomal or single gene causes, while the former only occurs as a single gene disorder being due to either autosomal dominant, recessive, X-linked gene or mitochondrial inheritance.

Non-syndromal/syndromal hearing impairment

The presence of one or more major or minor congenital abnormalities in a child presenting with hearing impairment, means that he/she could have a recognised multiple malformation syndrome, many of which are associated with a significant risk of recurrence. 30% of persons with genetic hearing impairment have associated clinical features which allow diagnosis of a syndromal cause of hearing impairment (Reardon and Pembre, 1990; Arnos et al., 1992). There are 167 chromosomal disorders (Schinzel, 1994) and 396 syndromes of single gene or unknown aetiology (Winter and Baraitser, 1993) in which hearing impairment has been reported, occurring more commonly in some than in others.

Recognition of a syndromal cause of hearing impairment is important for two reasons. Firstly, the majority of the chromosomal and many of the single gene syndromes in which hearing impairment occurs are associated with developmental delay, i.e. the child is likely to have special educational needs, above and beyond that determined by the severity of the hearing impairment. Secondly, the diagnosis of a syndrome will have very different implications for recurrence risk advice in genetic counselling for the couple than if a child has isolated hearing impairment. As a consequence, a child with hearing impairment should be examined in detail for any associated features and, if these are present, should be referred to a specialist trained in the recognition of syndromes, or what is termed dysmorphology. This can be a paediatrician but will often be a clinical geneticist, either of whom can be greatly aided by use of texts such as that by Gorlin et al. (1995).

Evaluation of a person with hearing impairment

In order to provide genetic counselling, the assessment of a person with hearing impairment should involve the following four steps:

1. Taking a family history – including the maternal obstetric and medical history.
2. Audiometry – a detailed description of the type and severity of the hearing impairment.
3. Physical examination – looking for the presence/absence of associated abnormalities.
4. Investigations – specific investigations and/or specialist examinations.

Family history

This involves asking about individuals as distantly related as second degree relatives (i.e. grandparents, aunts and uncles) and their offspring. A family history of hearing impairment can often be obtained, but it is necessary to be sceptical and document the specific type in each instance since acquired causes of hearing impairment, such as conductive hearing impairment due to recurrent otitis media, industrial noise exposure or normal hearing loss with age, i.e. presbyacusis, are common.

If another individual in the family has a history of hearing impairment, it is important to ask about the developmental progress, general health and the presence of any abnormalities in these individuals, to pursue the possibility of a syndromal cause of hearing impairment.

Specific information about the physical characteristics of persons with hearing impairment in the family should include details about pigmentary alterations of the hair, skin or eyes, structural malformations of the external ears (e.g. tags or pits), eye disease (e.g. cataracts, retinitis pigmentosa, retinal detachment or glaucoma), other birth defects such as cleft lip and/or palate, congenital heart disease, kidney malformations and skeletal abnormalities, including a history of fractures.

The obstetric history of the mother of the individual with hearing impairment should include information about the health of the mother, medications taken during the pregnancy, antenatal infections and perinatal events. In addition, it is vital to enquire about childhood illnesses or infections, such as measles or meningitis, in the persons with hearing impairment. It is important to be sceptical of attributing the hearing impairment to these events, since the recognition of hearing impairment could have been coincidental.

Audiometry

A full neuro-otological assessment including pure tone audiometry, oto-admittance testing and vestibular evaluation of the proband should be carried out (see Chapter 8), including parents and siblings. This is particularly important if there is a suggestion of hearing impairment in any of them. This should include documentation of the age of onset, severity, site, laterality and symmetry if bilateral.

Physical examination

In addition to a formal otolaryngological evaluation, a detailed physical examination of the person with hearing impairment should be carried out. While the majority of people with hearing impairment will have non-syndromal hearing impairment, i.e. the absence of any other abnormalities, a significant proportion of those with hearing impairment have one or more other abnormalities as part of a syndrome. Some of the more commonly associated features which can be part of one of the more common syndromal causes of hearing impairment, the presence of which should specifically be looked for, include:

1. External ear abnormalities (ear pits or tags) – these occur in the Treacher Collins (Chapter 20), Goldenhar and branchio-oto-renal

(Chapter 19) syndromes. If the latter diagnosis is being considered, it is essential to carry out a renal ultrasound because of the association of renal anomalies.
2. Pigmentary – the presence of areas of depigmentation of the hair, or heterochromia irides and/or the presence of dystopia canthorum would suggest the possibility of the Waardenburg syndrome (Chapter 16).
3. Posterior cleft palate – a history of surgery for a posterior cleft palate or the presence of a submucous cleft of the hard palate would suggest the possibility of the Stickler syndrome. The presence of myopia and the characteristic facial features would also support this diagnosis.
4. Goitre – as part of Pendred syndrome. Thyroid function tests should be carried out including the perchlorate discharge test (Chapter 15).

Specialist examination/investigations

There are a number of specialist examinations and/or investigations which should be carried out routinely in the assessment of a child with non-syndromal sensorineural hearing impairment.

Ophthalmological examination

Formal ophthalmological assessment is indicated in a child with hearing impairment with associated eye findings such as retinal abnormalities or cataracts. In addition, in a child with isolated sensorineural hearing impairment, it is essential to look for the presence of retinitis pigmentosa as part of Usher syndrome (Chapter 14). The age of onset of the night blindness in type I Usher syndrome is usually in first decade or early second decade. In type II Usher syndrome, however, the age of onset of the night blindness is later, usually in adolescence or early adult life. A history of delay in walking or clumsiness in a child with hearing impairment suggests the possibility of abnormal vestibular function which could be part of type I Usher syndrome and should prompt formal eye examination. The diagnosis of Usher syndrome in the early stages of the disorder will require an electroretinogram.

Electrocardiogram

Cardiac arrhythmia occurs in the Jervell-Lange-Nielsen syndrome, the association of hearing impairment with a prolonged QT interval. It is a rare but well recognised cause of sudden death in people with hearing impairment, which can be treated with beta blockers. Although this syndrome is an uncommon syndromal cause of hearing impairment, an

ECG is a simple vital screening test to carry out in a child with hearing impairment, because suitable treatment can avoid a potentially fatal complication. A history of syncopal attacks would suggest the possibility of this diagnosis.

Urinalysis

This is to test for the presence of haematuria which would be suggestive of Alport syndrome (Chapter 17) and glycosuria as part of DID-MOAD (diabetes mellitus, diabetes insipidus, optic atrophy and hearing loss).

Serology

TORCH titres (toxoplasmosis, rubella, cytomegalovirus and herpes simplex) need to be done before the child with hearing impairment is 6 months of age in order to be diagnostic. If it is carried out after that age, the child can be sero-positive through post-natal infection. If maternal antenatal serum samples are available, specific maternal IgM levels can be assayed.

Cochlear computerised tomography

Although abnormalities of the cochlea are reported in some syndromes with hearing impairment, e.g. X-linked hearing impairment, the Treacher Collins, Pendred and the branchio-oto-renal syndromes (Phillips and Phelps, 1991), it is not always clear whether it is necessary to carry out this investigation as part of the diagnosis of the type and cause of hearing impairment, although many children will have it as part of the assessment for a cochlear implant.

Chromosomal analysis

If a child with hearing impairment presents with multiple malformations, it is possible that there will be a chromosomal cause. Therefore, the presence of any other congenital abnormality in a child with hearing impairment is an indication to consider taking blood for chromosomal analysis. The presence of non-specific findings such as pre- or post-natal growth retardation and/or developmental delay, would be further indications of the possibility of a chromosomal abnormality.

Other examinations or investigations

These would be indicated by the physical findings in the child with hearing impairment, e.g. a spine X-ray in a child with associated skeletal abnormalities such as in the Klippel-Feil syndrome, or assessment by a paediatric cardiologist in a child with a heart murmur.

The genetic counselling session

Although a multidisciplinary assessment of a child with hearing impairment should include a genetic evaluation, only a minority of couples who have had a child with hearing impairment receive formal advice about the chance of recurrence. There is, therefore, a need for a special session to be able to properly answer the questions 'Why did it happen?' and 'Will it happen again?', i.e. genetic counselling.

The timing of the genetic counselling session will depend on the individual couple and is mainly determined by when they are 'ready to hear' the answers to their questions. It is, therefore, often inappropriate and ineffective for this session to take place soon after the diagnosis of the hearing impairment in their child, when they are coming to terms with the implications for the future of their child.

The genetic counselling session should provide answers to the questions a couple has in terms which they can understand. The session should be non-directive in nature, i.e. providing information to the couple, pointing out the choices or options available and supporting them in the choices they make for themselves. In order to allow this, it is vital that sufficient time be set aside for the genetic counselling session.

Chance of recurrence of hearing impairment

For the single gene syndromes associated with hearing impairment and in families in which the hearing impairment has a clear pattern of Mendelian inheritance, it is possible to offer a precise chance of recurrence. Non-syndromal hearing impairment, in contrast, most commonly occurs sporadically, i.e. as an isolated case within the family. It is not possible to reliably discriminate between acquired and genetic causes of hearing impairment purely on clinical or audiological grounds, e.g. by age of onset, the severity of the hearing impairment or the shape of the audiogram, etc. (Taylor et al., 1975; Wildervanck, 1957). The chance of recurrence of hearing impairment in subsequent offspring in this situation is based on empirical figures, i.e. observed recurrences of hearing impairment in such families (Table 27.1) (Fraser, 1976; Newton, 1985; Majunder et al., 1989; Smith, 1991; Bieber and Nance, 1979).

Table 27.1 Chance of hearing impairment in a relative of person with hearing impairment.

Relative	Risk (%)
Sibling	1/10 – 1/5 (10 – 20%)*
Offspring	1/16 (6.25%)
Nephew/niece	1/130 (0.77%)
Offspring of hearing sibling	1/250 (0.4%)
Offspring of affected parent and child	2/5 (40%) **
Offspring of affected parent with affected sibling	1/100 (1%)

* if the parents are consanguineous, the risk is 1/4 (25%)
** although the chance of inheriting the gene is 1/2 (50%), the lower chance is due to incomplete penetrance of autosomal dominant disorders

The empirical recurrence figures used should be modified in certain situations, e.g. by the presence or absence of a family history of hearing loss (Table 27.2). In addition, if the parents of a sporadically affected child are consanguineous, the chance of recurrence for subsequent children is 1/4. Conversely, while the chance for a couple to have a subsequent child with hearing impairment after a second affected child is 1/4, the chances decrease the more normal hearing children a couple has (Table 27.2). In one study the more severe the sensorineural hearing impairment, the greater the chance of recurrence, with the chance of recurrence approaching 1/4 if the hearing impairment was greater than 80dB (Newton, 1989).

Segregation studies of the offspring of different types of matings, e.g. parents with normal hearing and parents with hearing loss, estimate that the number of genes responsible for non-syndromal sensorineural hearing impairment varies from 5 common genes (Chung and Brown, 1970; Stevenson and Cheeseman, 1956) to 36 or more loci (Chung et al., 1959). The numbers estimated from these studies will depend on the size of the survey and the genetic heterogeneity of the population studied, with fewer loci being likely to be responsible in populations in which inbreeding is prevalent (Morton, 1991). The demonstration of linkage, cloning and identification of the mutations in the genes responsible for a number of both non-syndromal as well as syndromal causes of inherited hearing impairment means that much more precise information on the chance of recurrence will be available in the future (Chapter 6).

Counselling adults with hearing impairment

Many adults with hearing impairment are often unaware that it could be due to a genetic cause despite (in some instances) a family history of hearing impairment, and the widespread availability of genetic counselling services (Nance, 1971; Israel, 1989; Lindhout et al., 1991; Arnos et al., 1992). In addition, it is common for a person with hearing impairment to have children with a partner who also has hearing impairment. In both situations there is a significant chance of hearing impairment in their offspring (Table 27.2). The chance of recurrence is, again, based on empirical data, as the genetics of the hearing impairment in any single family can be complex. For example, the chance of recurrence for hearing impairment in the offspring of two parents with hearing impairment who are consanguineous approaches 100%, since they are likely to be homozygous for the same autosomal recessive gene. However, most couples with sensorineural hearing impairment are likely to be homozygous at two different loci, in which case all their offspring would be heterozygous at those two loci, and will therefore probably have normal hearing. Similarly, if a parent with hearing impairment has a child with hearing impairment, although it is likely to be due to an autosomal dominant gene, it could be due to pseudodominance with the hearing partner being, by chance, a carrier for the same autosomal recessive gene.

Table 27.2 Chances of recurrence of hearing loss in various mating types (Nance, 1980).

Mating Types	Number of Deaf Offspring	Number of Tested Offspring					
		0	1	2	3	4	5
Hearing x Hearing							
Positive family history	1	NA	0.20	0.19	0.17	0.16	0.14
Negative family history	1	NA	0.10	0.08	0.07	0.05	0.04
Deaf x Hearing							
All hearing children	0	0.07	0.04	0.03	0.02	0.01	0.01
At least 1 deaf child	> 1	NA	0.41	0.41	0.41	0.41	0.41**
Deaf x Deaf*							
All hearing children	0	0.10	0.04	0.03	0.02	0.01	0.01
All deaf children		0.10	0.61	0.80	0.92	0.97	0.99
Deaf and hearing children		NA	NA	0.33	0.33	0.33	0.33

* if the parents are consanguineous, the risk is 100%
** although the chance of inheriting the gene is 1/2, the lower chance seen is due to reduced penetrance seen with autosomal dominant disorders

It is important to be aware that many members of the deaf community feel that genetic counselling has the hidden agenda of trying to eliminate hearing impairment, as they feel that society views hearing impairment as a disability. In contrast, the deaf community views hearing impairment as being part of human cultural and linguistic diversity (Jordan, 1991; Arnos, 1994). For these reasons, terms such as 'hearing' or 'deaf' and 'chance' should be used rather than 'normal' or 'abnormal' and 'risk' (Arnos et al., 1992). Despite these considerations, many adults with hearing impairment are still interested to know the cause of their hearing impairment and the probability that their child will have hearing impairment, even though they often feel that having a child with hearing impairment is not a special concern (Arnos et al., 1992). It is essential that genetic counselling of people with hearing impairment should include use of diverse communication methods such as counselling in sign language, special equipment for communication with deaf people and the use of specially prepared written and visual material.

Prenatal diagnosis

This is rarely asked for by couples identified as having an increased chance of having a child with hearing impairment. It is usually more appropriate to discuss screening in early infancy by auditory brainstem responses to enable early diagnosis of hearing impairment.

Chapter 28
Surgical problems in craniofacial deformities

LUIGI CLAUSER and CAMILLO CURIONI
This chapter is dedicated to Paul Tessier,
pioneer of craniofacial surgery
and still the undisputed leader of this speciality.

Craniofacial surgery – historical background

The techniques of modern craniofacial surgery were officially introduced by Paul Tessier at the 4th International Congress of Plastic and Reconstructive Surgery held in Rome in 1967. (Tessier, 1967; Tessier et al., 1967). Cases of Crouzon disease, Apert syndrome, hypertelorbitism, facial clefts, and Treacher Collins syndrome were brought to the audience's attention. Such malformations had been treated with a series of operations aimed at hiding the typical stigmata.

In the 1960s and 1970s, Tessier devoted his efforts to the correction of hypertelorbitism. He stressed the importance of moving the orbits behind the equator of the globe via the intra-extracranial route (Tessier et al., 1967; Tessier, 1971, 1974).

After the 1970s, other surgeons became interested in craniofacial surgery, introducing new ideas and innovations. Monasterio et al. (1978) described the frontofacial monobloc for the correction of Crouzon disease. Marchac and Renier (1979) introduced the 'floating forehead' technique as an early treatment for craniostenosis and craniofaciostenosis. van Der Meulen (1979) described the facial bipartition (medial faciotomy) as a radical corrective procedure in cases of hypertelorism associated with malocclusion.

General principles of techniques of craniofacial surgery

The craniofacial approach is the best method for the correction of malformations, even in the presence of a subtle orbito-cranial component.

The coronal approach is the preferred approach. It can be performed without hair shaving or with only a minimal shaving of 2 cm. The introduction of rigid fixation by means of plates, miniplates, microplates (Clauser et al., 1991; Curioni and Clauser, 1989; Jackson et al., 1986; Marchac, 1991) has undoubtedly simplified the reassembly of multifragmented bony segments.

When surgery requires either maxillo-mandibular or cranio-orbito-maxillary displacements, the intermaxillary fixation can be reduced or avoided with advantages both for the patient and for the neuromuscular system (Ellis and Carlson, 1989).

Over the past few years, several studies of the effects of rigid fixation on craniofacial development have been published. A remarkable growth reduction has been observed when the plate is positioned either across a suture or in the adjacent bones. Some authors have suggested plate removal after 4 – 5 months, in order to promote craniofacial growth (Marschall et al., 1991). The popularisation of cranial bone grafts has reduced the need for harvesting of bone from the iliac crest or from ribs (Laurie et al., 1984). The preferred source is the parietal bones (Tessier, 1982). The spectrum of cranial bone grafts includes: split cranial bones, full thickness, bone dust and bone flaps pedicled on the temporalis muscle or on the temporo-parietal fascia. There are specific indications for each technique.

The fronto-orbitofacial displacements are of great importance since they determine the position, relationship and functions of parts such as the canthi, eyelids, globes, nose, soft palate, lips, tongue. Careful repositioning of the facial mask to the facial skeleton after three dimensional movements is of paramount importance. In order to obtain an appearance as normal as possible, the soft tissues should heal on the new bone position.

General principles of treatments in craniosynostosis

During the first year of life, the brain 'explodes' in growth and triples its volume. In the early stenosis of the sutures, the surgeon's role is that of performing a kind of 'interceptive' surgery, which allows the brain to expand and the cranial base to develop (Marchac and Renier, 1979). In craniostenosis and craniofaciostenosis the goals of early surgery are:

• Opening the stenosed sutures.
• Increasing the intracranial volume.
• Correcting the position of bony segments.
• Introducing normal craniofacial growth.

The basic steps necessary to achieve these goals are:

• Removal of the frontal bone or of other cranial bones.
• Removal and reshaping of the frontal bandeau.
• Bending, advancement and repositioning of the bandeau.
• Remodelling of the frontal bone and, when necessary, of other cranial bones.

Plagiocephaly

In plagiocephaly, the orbit ipsilateral to the stenosis is higher and egg shaped. The side of the homolateral supraorbital ridge is recessed. On the opposite side, the roof and the supraorbital ridge are low. Therefore, the contralateral orbit seems in a lower position. However, when the orbital floors are compared, they appear at the same level. The difference lies more in the shape than in the horizontal position.

The nasoethmoidal complex is displaced and deviated to the opposite side. Generally, the axis of the upper jaw is unaffected and is used as a midline landmark for surgery.

In the most severe cases, there is a deviation of both the jaw and the mandible on the affected side. Other cases also present with hypertelorbitism. Such complex forms are unilateral forms of brachicephaly associated with hypertelorbitism. However, pure synostosis of the hemicoronal suture results in pure plagiocephaly.

Surgical Treatment

Since the effects of the monocoronal stenosis affect the whole forehead, plagiocephaly needs bilateral correction. The bilateral approach allows the normalisation of the orbital roof levels while introducing normal cranial growth (Marchac and Renier, 1979; Marchac, 1991). The whole supraorbital, orbital and cranial vault regions must be approached by the coronal route. The fragments creating the new forehead can be chosen either in a parietal or in a frontal area with normal bending. The nasal bones in children are not mobilised, although they are deviated. The normal fronto-orbital development often results in a better nasal position.

Brachicephaly and faciostenosis, Crouzon disease and Apert syndrome

In brachicephaly, the synostosis involves the coronal sutures and the anterior cranial base, with shortening of the sagittal axis. Over the past few years there have been various surgical approaches. Crouzon disease is characterised by craniosynostosis, shallow orbits, ocular proptosis, frequent strabismus and maxillary hypoplasia. Its prevalence is approximately 1 per 25,000 of the population.

The characteristic features of Apert syndrome are craniosynostosis, midfacial hypoplasia with retrusion, retromacrogenia, ocular proptosis, and symmetrical syndactyly of the hands and feet. Apert syndrome occurs in roughly 1 per 100,000 births.

A severe form of craniosynostosis is represented by the cloverleaf skull anomaly. The abnormal form of the cranium and face derives from multiple premature suture fusion in the calvaria and cranial base (Figure 28.1). Hydrocephalus is an associated defect. Other findings, sometimes incompatible with life, may be present.

Over the years, there have been various surgical approaches for correcting brachicephaly. The classical neurosurgical technique included linear craniectomy, which, however, did not change the frontal bar position. Another method included the horizontal advancing with Tessier-type (1967) lateral fixation. The outcomes appeared to be encouraging both from a morphological and a functional point of view.

In 1977 a new technique, named 'floating forehead', was introduced (Marchac and Renier, 1979). This method combines the total frontal advancement and the coronal craniectomy, fixing the forehead in an advanced position (1 – 2cm) only to the facial structures (nose and zygomas), leaving a wide posterior gap. The frontal bar detachment frees both the fronto-ethmoidal and the fronto-sphenoidal sutures. Therefore, the forehead is not fixed laterally and the brain's dynamic push ensures and maintains the advancement.

In the original concept, both the cranial base and the jaw should have benefited from such an approach. However, subsequently, it was demonstrated that in Crouzon disease and Apert syndrome this did not happen (Bachmayer et al., 1986). The lack of growth of the middle third of the face was also confirmed by Marchac (1991) in a paper reporting his experience with the 'floating forehead' method.

The surgical procedures to be performed at a later stage must be eclectic. They can include; le Fort III osteotomy, frontofacial monobloc, facial bipartition, monobloc associated with bipartition. When necessary, le Fort I osteotomy in association with mandibular osteotomies as an additional procedure can be performed.

Apert syndrome is a syndrome presenting true hypertelorbitism with euryprosopia associated with retrusion of the middle third of the face. The surgical treatment, performed at an age of 5 – 6 years, is an extensive procedure which includes:

- Advancement of the fronto-orbitomaxillary monobloc.
- Facial bipartition with central resection, derotation of orbits and of the two hemimaxilla, expansion of the part of the palate, bone grafts.
- Cranioplasty.

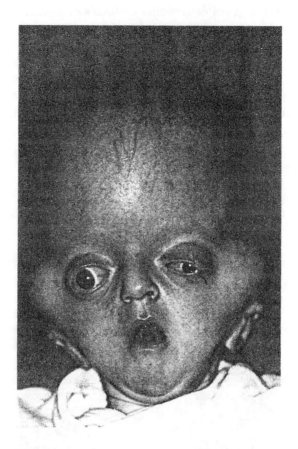

Figure 28.1 Cloverleaf Skull anomaly (pancraniofaciosynostosis). In this syndrome different sutures may be involved. Hydrocephaly is associated. Absent external auditory canals is often present. Note severe degree of exophthalmos and the ears that are displaced downward facing the shoulders.

If there is a relapse of maxillary retrusion, a le Fort I osteotomy can be scheduled after the age of 15. Early management of the hearing problems, occurring both in Crouzon disease and, particularly, in Apert syndrome, must be planned.

Mandibulofacial dysostosis

Mandibulofacial dysostosis, also known as Treacher Collins syndrome (1900), is a complex bilateral anomaly. Unlike hemifacial microsomia, mandibulofacial dysostosis is inherited as an autosomal dominant trait with variable expressivity (see Chapter 20).

In the complete form of Treacher Collins syndrome, all the stigmata are present; microtia, middle ear deformities with hearing loss, absence of zygoma and hypoplasia of the orbital skeleton, low eyelid colobomata, laxity and dystopia of the lateral canthus, maxillary hypoplasia with narrow palate and choanal atresia, together with severe micrognathia associated with macro-retrogenia. In the incomplete or abortive forms, the orbital area is generally more affected than the jaw and the mandible (Figures 28.2, 28.3).

Surgical treatment

The goals of the surgical treatment in Treacher Collins syndrome are twofold: aesthetic and functional. The surgical approach includes:

- Correction of coloboma.
- Orbito-malar reconstruction and beginning of orthodontic management.

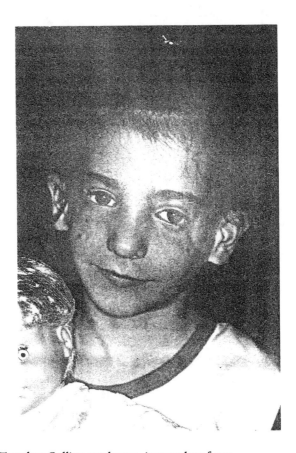

Figure 28.2 Treacher Collins syndrome, incomplete form.

- Reconstruction of middle ear deformities.
- Maxillo-mandibular osteotomy according to the severity of the malformation.
- Refinement surgery comprising further bone grafts, genioplasty, eyelid surgery, auricular correction.

The orbito-maxillary reconstruction is suggested for children of preschool age. The method was described by Tessier and Tulasne, (1987, 1989). The preferred bone source is the cranial vault. The two parietals can be harvested full thickness and split. Part of the split fragments will be repositioned in the donor site. The remainder will be used to reconstruct the zygomas and the orbits, and applied as 'onlay' both in the maxillary and in the superorbital regions.

Since, in Treacher Collins syndrome there is an absence of periosteum in the malar region, the resorption of bone grafts is greater than in other malformations. Therefore, in some cases, we have rotated two galeal pericranial flaps in order to furnish a vascularised supply cover-

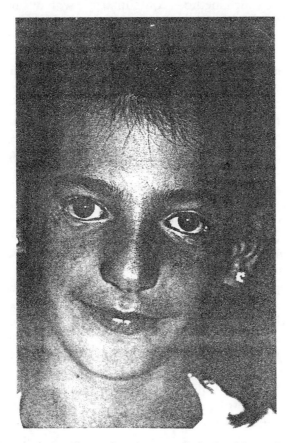

Figure 28.3 Result 4 years later after correction of orbital hypoplasia with cranial bone grafts and correction of lower eyelid coloboma.

ing the bone grafts. Lateral canthopexy and the re-fixation of soft tissues complete the surgical treatment. Additional iliac bone grafts should be planned after adolescence.

When necessary, maxillo-mandibular osteotomies can be performed later on, after the age of 14 – 16 years. The combined procedure includes a le Fort II osteotomy together with a reverse L-shaped osteotomy of the mandible (Tessier and Tulasne, 1987, 1989). Orthodontic treatment and ancillary procedures are the final steps for Treacher Collins syndrome correction.

Conclusions

Surgical reconstructions of the cranio-orbito-facial area for severe congenital malformations have become a reality after Tessier's first papers published at the end of the 1960s. However, for various reasons, such revolutionary techniques were applied only in adolescent or adult patients. They were considered too dangerous in early infancy and it was assumed that such methods could interfere with normal craniofacial growth and development. In the mid 1970s, these techniques were performed in patients under 5 years of age, for functional, growth and psychosocial reasons. The improvement of paediatric anaesthetic techniques, of post-operative monitoring along with the experience achieved by the craniofacial 'team', have also reduced the surgical risks in patients aged 6 – 7 months (McCarthy and Cutting, 1990).

There are still divergent opinions as to the effects of early surgery on growth. In simple craniostenosis, early surgery results in a global improvement of the cranio-orbital morphology (Marchac and Renier, 1979; Marchac, 1991).

The problem is more complex in the brachycephalic syndromes, Crouzon, Apert and Pfeiffer. It has been demonstrated that early surgery results in an improvement in the cranio-orbital morphology. The expected effects on development of the middle third of face has not been confirmed. Therefore, facial or craniofacial advancement osteotomies are often necessary.

The principle, 'correction in the pre-schooling age and refinement surgery in the following years', valid for other malformations, should also be considered in Treacher Collins syndrome. Over the last 20 years, studies have concentrated on achieving better understanding of the pathogenesis of the malformations, the choice of the type of surgery, the timing, the planning of osteotomies, the choice of bone grafts and discussion of the type of fixation.

Research is still evolving. In the future craniofacial surgeons will no longer need to harvest bone grafts. Research is aimed at the utilisation of a matrix (probably of a resorbable material) which, placed in the defect together with a biologic factor such as osteogenin, promotes bone formation (McCarthy, 1992). Fixation will be performed with resorbable materials.

The use of robotics in surgery is another science in the course of development. On the basis of computer studies, it will provide surgeons with guidance as to how to position osteotomised bony fragments.

New horizons are therefore opening in the field of cranio-orbito-facial surgery.

Chapter 29
Surgery for congenital conductive and mixed hearing loss without atresia of the ear canal

COR WRJ CREMERS

Introduction

Ear microsurgery underwent an enormous development through the introduction of stapes replacement surgery in 1958 by Shea. Previously, fixation of the stapes had been treated by fenestration of the horizontal semicircular canal or by mobilisation of the stapes using a hammer and chisel. Although stapes replacement found general application for the treatment of otosclerosis in the early 1960s, its adoption took much longer in the treatment of congenital stapes fixation. In many respects, the new technique of ear microsurgery met with great approval, but in the 1960s many surgeons still preferred to perform fenestration and stapes mobilisation for congenital stapes ankylosis (Shambaugh, 1952; Ombrédanne, 1959; House et al., 1958). This historical perspective is also applicable to stapes surgery for the treatment of non-isolated stapes anky- losis, i.e. stapes ankylosis with an associated ossicular chain anomaly.

In 1952 Shambaugh reported his success with the fenestration oper- ation in five cases of isolated congenital stapes ankylosis. In 1958, Howard House and co-workers described their attempts to mobilise the stapes footplate by needle and chisel techniques in 23 cases with con- genital footplate fixation. When no hearing improvement was achieved, an additional fenestration operation was performed. In 1969 Steele clearly described the results of exploratory tympanotomies performed by House in the 1960s for congenital stapes ankylosis. This indicates that House rarely performed stapedectomies for the condition at this time. Confidence gradually increased with the increasing success and safety of stapes interposition and stapedectomy procedures (e.g. Steele, 1969; House, 1969; Jahrsdörfer, 1980). This also led to the virtual abandonment of fenestration of the lateral semi-circular canal and stapes mobilisation. In this period stapes mobilisation was also used by others for congenital stapes ankylosis (e.g. Ombrédanne, 1966; Hough, 1958).

Ombrédanne's publications in the 1960s (e.g. 1959; 1966) show the success of stapes mobilisation and fenestration operations of the lateral semicircular canal in those cases where stapes mobilisation procedures did not result in a mobile stapes. In those days, stapes mobilisation was the procedure of choice. Partial stapedectomy with repositioning of the stapes on a vein graft and stapedectomy with interposition were considered to be second choice procedures, but appeared to be as effective as a successful stapes mobilisation. A series of publications confirmed the good results of stapedectomies with interposition using a prosthesis. The prosthesis was fixed to the long process of the incus or, where this was absent, to the long process of the malleus.

Fear of a perilymphatic gusher during stapes surgery and with the incidental occurrence of a dead ear may have influenced the continued choice of stapes mobilisation instead of a stapedectomy.

Congenital abnormalities of the middle ear are sporadic. In about one in every four ears with a congenital conductive hearing loss, the ear anomaly is part of a syndromal diagnosis. The syndromal diagnosis can be indicative about the type of anomaly to be found and the outcome of its surgery (Ombrédanne, 1966; Arslan and Giacomelli, 1963; Cremers, 1986).

Preoperative requirements

In the Nijmegen University ENT Department the following preoperative criteria have been developed:

- The patient must be at least 8 – 10 years of age.
- In children, a sufficiently long follow-up period must exclude intermittent periods of otitis media with effusion.
- Results of pure tone audiometry, speech audiometry and examination of the contralateral stapedial reflexes must be available.
- CT-scans of the petrous bones, particularly of the internal acoustic meatus and the inner ear must be performed.

The Nijmegen series – classification and results

The most up-to-date review of the literature regarding surgery for congenital middle ear surgery is given in the thesis by Teunissen (1992). He also showed the value of successful surgery for unilateral congenital hearing loss (Snik et al., 1994). He further presented the results of surgery in a consecutive series of 144 ears from the Nijmegen Department. In 127

of these 144, the exploratory tympanotomy was used to perform reconstructive surgery. The classification of these ears into four groups and
the results of surgery are shown in Tables 29.1 and 29.2 (Teunissen and
Cremers, 1993).

Table 29.1 Classification of minor congenital anomalies of the ear.

Class	Main Anomaly	Subclassification	No. of ears
I	Congenital stapes ankylosis		44
II	Stapes ankylosis associated with another congenital ossicular chain anomaly		55
III	Congenital anomaly of the ossicular	A. Discontinuity in ossicular chain	11
	chain but a mobile stapes footplate	B. Epitympanic fixation	20
IV	Congenital aplasia or severe dysplasia of the oval or round window	Aplasia	10
		Dysplasia:	
		Crossing facial nerve	3
		Persistent stapedial artery	1

Table 29.2 Air – bone gap 12 months after reconstructive surgery in 127 minor congenital ear anomalies.

Classification	No. of ears		Air-Bone Gap < 10 dB (%)	Air-Bone Gap 10 – 20 dB (%)	Air-Bone Gap > 20 dB (%)
	Per Class	Reconstructive Surgery			
Class I	44	41	20 (49%)	9 (22%)	12 (29%)
Class II	55	51	20 (39%)	17 (33%)	14 (27%)
Class III	31	31	9 (29%)	14 (45%)	8 (26%)
Class IV	14	4	1 (25%)	2 (50%)	1 (25%)

A survey of the results of the whole series showed that the most disappointing results occurred at the beginning of the series in the mid
1960s, in ears with severe mixed hearing losses. It appears that in later
years, the level of the sensorineural component of the hearing loss con-
stituted an additional selection criterion. Another interesting finding is
that almost all ears had a sensorineural hearing loss preoperatively and
postoperatively of 10 to 20 dB. It is important to realise this when predicting the degree of success of an operation.

Pitfalls

There are many pitfalls in the surgery of ears with congenital conductive
and mixed hearing losses, and the surgeon should be acquainted with

them. These problems include the X-linked recessive stapes gusher syndrome which may be recognised by preoperative audiometric features, CT-scanning and the family history. A syndromal diagnosis of those with craniosynostosis and the branchiogenic syndromes such as Treacher Collins syndrome and branchio-oto-renal syndrome can have a great impact on the findings and outcome of middle ear surgery. An aberrant facial nerve must be suspected, and a persistent stapedial artery is another interesting anomaly which can be found.

Conclusions

Surgery for congenital bilateral and unilateral conductive or mixed hearing losses can be very rewarding. More precautions must be taken than with routine stapes surgery for otosclerosis. The surgeon must take a special interest in the variations found in congenital middle ear anomalies and in the particular syndromes concerned. Extensive surgical experience in this field is beneficial to the outcome of this surgery.

Chapter 30
Rehabilitation of genetic hearing loss

SUSAN BELLMAN

Introduction

Genetic hearing impairment covers the whole spectrum of hearing abnormality. The degree of impairment can range from mild to total hearing loss, and it can be conductive, sensorineural or mixed in type. Although many of the more easily recognised forms of genetic hearing abnormality manifest themselves prenatally or in the early months of life, the onset of hearing impairment can be at any age, and the loss may be progressive in nature. The many different patterns of genetic hearing loss mean that rehabilitation strategies must vary from one individual to another. In addition some individuals have co-existing tinnitus or vestibular problems, which may also warrant rehabilitation. However there are some general rehabilitative needs applicable to early and postlingual onset of genetic hearing impairment, regardless of exact type and aetiology.

As a general principle, all children with hearing impairment will need appropriate help with education from suitably trained teachers, and input from a specialist speech and language pathologist. They and their families will also need both genetic counselling and long term general support and counselling. Many of the families will also need instruction in the appropriate sign language, if the child's hearing or general condition is such that reasonable language cannot be developed by the use of an aural/oral approach.

The needs of an older child or adult, who loses his or her hearing after the development of language, are slightly different, and their management can be broadly described by the rehabilitative management model first described by Goldstein and Stephens (1981). General and genetic counselling remain important, particularly if the loss is rapidly progressive, as can occur in some forms of early adult genetic disease. Acceptance of the hearing impairment can be particularly difficult when it occurs around the teenage years, for example in Alport syndrome. This is made even more difficult if the hearing loss is associated with a generally threatening condition, such as the renal failure seen in this condition. Rehabilitation may need to be directed towards the whole family, and not just at the affected individual, as communication strategies are developed. When severe to profound genetic hearing impairment occurs after the first decade, language may be maintained, but the quality of speech may deteriorate with time, as described by Plant (1984), and specialist help from a therapist will be helpful.

In addition to the various forms of personal amplification and devices discussed below, accessory devices and environmental aids to listening are also important. Most children use an FM or infra-red aid to improve the signal to noise ratio in classroom and other learning environments. These may also be applicable in college and university life, to enable a lecturer's voice to be heard more clearly. Group aids may also be used, particularly in schools for the deaf. Equipment to improve the quality of speech production includes the Speech Trainer, Laryngograph and an expanding number of computer program such as Visispeech. These are beginning to extend from the school situation to the home, as personal computers become more accessible.

Environmental aids include alerting devices, such as flashing light doorbells, vibrating or flashing alarms, and flashing light or adapted telephone bells. More recently hearing dogs have been trained to alert their owners to various sounds. There is a variety of different types of device for the television, including amplified earphones and subtitles. Some television programmes include signing support, but in general there is still insufficient input to provide access to all programmes for the more severely hearing impaired. Telephone listening aids include amplified handsets, Minicom systems and the developing videophone, which should enable some speechreading and signing to supplement residual hearing. Telephones include an induction loop for use with most personal aids. Induction loop systems or infra-red systems are available in many public buildings, for example concert halls, theatres and places of worship.

Rehabilitation, by definition, must include ensuring that individuals of any age are given access to equipment that helps them overcome their hearing disability and consequent handicap, in addition to optimal provision of their own personal worn device, discussed by Stephens (1984).

Conductive hearing loss

Middle ear effusions/otitis media

Some genetic conditions are associated with normal structural development of the middle ear, but there is an increased risk of persistent otitis media with effusion, sometimes associated with recurrent middle ear infections. These include Down syndrome, Turner syndrome, Marshall-Stickler's syndrome and some of the mucopolysaccharidoses. The sufferers are usually children, and the middle ear material may be viscous, and may contain abnormal substances related to the general condition.

The options for rehabilitation will depend on the overall condition of the child, and there is still controversy regarding the place of surgical intervention. In a fit child, particularly if there are recurrent infections, myringotomy and insertion of ventilation tubes may be the most appropriate first line of management. In an unfit child, for example with cardiac abnormalities, long term antibiotics to reduce infection, together with amplification may be a more acceptable form of management. In some children, the ventilation tubes may be associated with unmanageable otorrhoea and again amplification may be preferable. A few children will have a neurological deterioration to the extent that management may be limited to general support.

In a few of these children there may also be ossicular abnormalities, for example these are suggested to be present in 6% of individuals with Down syndrome. A co-existing sensorineural loss may also be present in any of these conditions, necessitating amplification. Under these circumstances ventilation tubes may provide better quality sound for the child, but any persistent otorrhoea which prevents hearing aid usage would preclude their use. In a small number of children with intractable middle-ear disease, an osseointegrated bone-anchored hearing aid may be the most satisfactory means of amplification, as long as the sensorineural hearing thresholds are adequate.

External/middle ear abnormalities

There are a number of forms of congenital genetic hearing loss where mild ossicular abnormalities are present, while the abnormalities in some of the cranio-facial syndromes may be far more extensive, involving not only severe middle ear deformities but also varying degrees of external atresia. Although the loss is usually conductive only, in a few individuals, particularly those with more severe malformations, there is a possibility of an additional sensorineural loss, sometimes associated with cochlear dysplasias. In addition there are some diseases of adult onset where there appears to be a genetic element to a progressive conductive hearing impairment. These include otosclerosis and Paget's disease, in both of which an additional sensorineural loss may develop.

Management can be broadly divided into reconstructive surgical techniques and provision of varying forms of amplification. There is still some controversy about the place of reconstructive surgery in these conditions, but experience has demonstrated the frequently disappointing outcomes of surgery for all but the most mild conditions. Even a well established technique such as stapedectomy has a recognised and measurable morbidity. The best results are obtained by surgeons who have specialised in this field and are carrying out sufficient operations to maintain their skills. There is no place for the general otolaryngologist carrying out occasional operations of this type.

To be useful, surgery must improve the hearing to a level where amplification is unnecessary, without undue complications. This may be feasible in a mild ossicular abnormality and may be the choice of an informed adult. CT scanning will demonstrate most abnormalities but it is still important to distinguish an apparent conductive loss due to splinting of the stapes on the oval window, seen for example in one form of X-linked hearing loss, where attempts at surgery may lead to a perilymph gusher. This complication of attempted reconstructive surgery has also been described in other conditions, such as oto-palatal-digital syndrome. In such conditions amplification remains the appropriate management.

For the more severe congenital abnormalities the possibility of corrective surgery will depend on the extent of abnormalities present. Techniques to create an external meatus in severe atresia are rarely reported to be successful, and the resulting canal frequently stenoses and becomes infected if an ear mould is regularly used. Reconstruction may be more successful where there is a thin atretic plate, but again the results will depend on the middle ear deformities, and any improvement in hearing may be insufficient to dispense with amplification.

As alternatives to reconstructive surgery become more acceptable, the timing of surgery is altering. Early surgery (two/three years) used to be common, but in view of the difficulties in confirming exact masked hearing thresholds, the general lack of co-operation in young children and the recognised complications, amplification is now the normal form of early management. Conventional postaural aids may be worn where an adequate meatus is present, and sufficient gain can be obtained without feedback, remembering that greater gain is needed for a conductive loss than a similar sensorineural loss. Where this is not possible a bone conduction vibrator can be driven by a postaural aid worn on a head band or equivalent. In the presence of a purely conductive loss these should provide good aided hearing, sufficient to develop normal language.

By 5 – 6 years of age the child should be able to carry out accurate audiometry and co-operate with any further imaging required. Reconstructive surgery could be considered at this stage, but many would consider that this should be deferred until the child can give fully informed consent. This is because surgery carries a risk of damage to both the hearing and facial nerve, and amplification may still be necessary. Amplification, on the other hand, ensures excellent hearing thresholds with no risk, the only problem being the cosmetic acceptance of a hearing aid. Children with adequate meati can be fitted with in-the-ear aids when felt appropriate, but alternative aids are visible and may be rejected at times by young adults, particularly if they feel they draw attention to other cosmetic deformities.

At this age the other option to be considered is the use of an osseointegrated bone conductor device. The two systems available at the present time are the Xomed system and the Branemark system. The former has the advantage of having a subcutaneous placement, as opposed to the bone-anchored Branemark system with its percutaneous abutment and thus potential for infection and direct damage. However, in practice these are not significant problems as long as the device is adequately monitored. The gain in hearing is greater with the percutaneous device, so that a head-worn instrument is sufficient to give excellent results with a quality of sound preferred to that of a conventional BC aid as demonstrated by Cremers, Snik and Beyon (1992), and Abramson, Fay, Kelly et al. (1989). It is also possible to use this device when there is a mild sensorineural loss, although a more powerful bodyworn aid may be needed to drive the device. The superior hearing results obtained have led to this being the more widely used device. For children (and adults) with severe abnormalities or absence of the pinna, osseointegrated bone-anchored prosthesis based on the Branemark system can also be provided, with excellent cosmetic results, shown by Jacobsson, Tjellstrom, Fine and Jansson (1992). In many centres the use of these osseointegrated devices has replaced the more risky and less effective forms of reconstructive surgery.

Sensorineural hearing loss

The severity and configuration of sensorineural hearing impairment in genetic disease varies enormously, as already noted. For the majority of individuals a satisfactory degree of amplification can be provided from within the range of conventional behind-the-ear aids with appropriately modified moulds and tubing. Mini aids are available to suit all but the more profound hearing losses or those with particularly difficult configurations, and the range is extending all the time. These aids may have a number of modifications to make wearing easier under different circumstances. For example peak clipping and automatic gain control prevent tolerance problems due to recruitment, and the signal can be divided into channels that are treated independently, to improve discrimination. Programmable aids can be used for difficult configurations and can have more than one programme available for use under different listening conditions (for example a quiet situation and a situation with marked background noise). There are many reviews of the ever updating situation in this field.

When there is insufficient residual hearing to access speech sounds with a conventional aid, more specialised devices can be considered.

The first of these devices is the High Frequency Transposition Aid. Various devices have been used successfully on an experimental basis in the past, but there is only one device, the Transonic, which is currently available commercially. This is suitable where there is usable aided hearing up to around 1 kHz but the aided hearing falls outside the speech range for the higher frequencies. The incoming signal is divided by the aid into 'low' and 'high' frequency bands, and these are individually transposed downwards by an amount calculated from the actual audiogram. High frequency sounds are thus transposed to the audible frequencies for the individual. This gives the wearer access to sounds of a wider range of frequencies, and the lower frequency sound produces less feedback, resulting in a greater degree of gain for the low/mid frequencies. An improved response to sound is noticed immediately, but time is needed to get used to this very different signal as far as understanding of speech is concerned.

For a very few individuals with genetic hearing impairment, the residual hearing is insufficient to access speech sounds, even when the most powerful aids are used. Some of these individuals may benefit from cochlear implantation, although a detailed assessment and counselling are required to ensure that this is the most appropriate form of management. The benefits of cochlear implantation in this group are most evident in young congenitally deaf children, particularly those under eight years of age, and preferably those under five years of age. Among older individuals with a genetic hearing loss, most with a congenital profound/total loss do not benefit greatly from implantation and many eventually reject the device. However, those with a progressive genetic loss, and with reasonable oral language and some memory of sound often make very good use of the electrically produced signal.

There are a number of different devices available, and comparison of these demonstrates the superiority of the multi-channel devices over the earlier single channel devices. Most individuals with genetic loss who undergo implantation fall into the young age group, and the majority at the present time are implanted with a nucleus/cochlear device, which has FDA approval for use in children. There are many articles and reviews of aspects of cochlear implantation, and these are being updated regularly. One of the most wide ranging of these was edited by Tyler (1993), with a particularly relevant chapter on speech perception by children. Overall the results of cochlear implantation are very promising, with many children developing good oral language.

Potential implantees with genetic hearing loss often differ from individuals with an acquired loss, who may identify strongly with the hearing world. When counselling the genetically hearing impaired and their families, it must be remembered that for many cochlear implantation is seen as a threat to their deaf community and culture. This is particularly so where there are other affected family members. Implantation may be seen as an attempt to cure hearing loss, with the implication that the culturally deaf are inferior to the hearing majority. For these individuals, signing is the normal means of communication, and they see no advantage, and possibly some disadvantages, in learning oral language. Refusal of a cochlear implant is a perfectly valid option for any individual or family, for whom all other forms of rehabilitation may be acceptable. A rehabilitation programme must always be flexible enough to support this. It must also be remembered that an implanted individual remains deaf, and many will choose to use sign language in addition to their developing oral language, so that they can remain part of both the deaf and hearing communities.

A very few individuals with genetic hearing loss will have severe dysplasias of the inner ear, extending to aplasia and absence of the eighth nerve. In these cases conventional hearing aids and cochlear implants will not be applicable. Experimental brain stem implants are being tried on a few adults with acquired damage to the eighth nerve, but this technique is not yet suitable for young congenitally deaf children. Signing will be the main means of developing language in these children, but vibrotactile devices may give an awareness of not only environmental sounds, but also of the stress patterns of speech to aid lip reading. A few children may develop greater degrees of discrimination using some of the more complicated devices. A comparison of some of the vibrotactile aids is provided by Thornton and Phillips (1992). Vibrotactile aids may also be of help to hearing aid users, as they provide additional auditory information.

Conclusions

It can be seen from the above brief account that the range of rehabilitative strategies is very broad, and that these need to be tailored to the individual. For this reason auditory rehabilitation is best carried out within multi-disciplinary teams, where the client can obtain help from a variety of professionals. It is also important to offer long term support, as the rehabilitative needs of an individual, particularly a child, may alter and extend over time.

Glossary

ABUTMENT – An anchorage fixed to the skull for the attachment of a bone anchored hearing aid or an artificial pinna.

ACOUSTIC REFLEX THRESHOLD (ART) – The lowest intensity of acoustical stimulation for a specified stimulus which will result in a measurable contraction of the stapedius muscle.

ALLELE (Allelomorph) – One of several possible forms of a particular gene.

ALLELIC ASSOCIATION – Allele A_1 at locus A and allele B_1 at locus B are associated if the frequency of B_1 is significantly different in people carrying A_1 than in the general population. This may indicate that the A and B loci are close together on the same chromosome.

AMINOGLYCOSIDE – One of a group of antibiotics, derived from various species of Streptomyces, which interfere with the function of bacterial ribsosomes, and which are generally ototoxic.

ANKYLOSIS – Immobility of a joint, for example involving the ossicular chain of the middle ear.

ANTICIPATION – The tendency of a dominantly inherited condition to become more severe, or to show earlier age of onset, in successive generations. Many variable diseases show apparent anticipation, but in most cases this is caused by biased ascertainment; true anticipation is seen in only a handful of conditions (e.g. myotonic dystrophy).

ANTIMONGOLOID – Downward slanting of the palpebral fissures (opposite to one of the characteristics of Down syndrome).

APLASIA – The lack of development of an organ or tissue.

AUDIOGRAM – A plot of subjective hearing sensitivity for pure tones by frequency.

AUDIOSCAN – An audiometer developed by Meyer-Bisch (1990) which is programmed to scan across frequencies at an iso-hearing level, covering up to 64 frequencies per octave, and which highlights subtle abnormalities of the auditory threshold.

AUDITORY BRAINSTEM RESPONSE (ABR) – The averaged evoked response obtained from the cochlear nerve and brainstem to click or tonal stimulation of the ear, and which is recorded by far field electrodes. It is sometimes known as Brainstem Evoked Response (BSER).

AUTOSOME – A chromosome other than a sex chromosome.

AUTOZYGOSITY MAPPING – A method of mapping recessive characters in inbred families by looking in affected people for chromosomal segments that are identical on the maternal and paternal chromosomes. Much used for recessive non-syndromal hearing loss.

BASE PAIR (bp) – The basic unit of the DNA double helix, used as a measure of the length of a piece of DNA.

BÉKÉSY AUDIOMETRY – A technique of semi-automatic audiometry sweeping across a set frequency range, developed by George von Békésy (1947).

CALORIC TEST – A test of function of the lateral semicircular canals which are stimulated by hot and cold air or water.

CARRIER – A phenotypically normal person who is heterozygous for a recessive condition.

cDNA – A synthetic DNA complementary to a messenger RNA molecule.

CENTIMORGAN (cM) – In genetic mapping, loci 1 cM apart show 1% recombination.

CENTROMERE – A region of a chromosome to which spindle traction fibres attach during meiosis and mitosis.

CHROMATIDS – The daughter strands of a duplicated chromosome joined by a single centromere.

CLONES – Identical copies of an organism, cell or DNA sequence.

COCHLEAR IMPLANT – A device consisting of a microphone, signal processor and electrode system capable of stimulating the cochlear nerve fibres directly, and used in cases of profound and total deafness.

COHORT – A group of individuals of similar age within a population.

COLOBOMA – A defect of ocular tissue usually due to failure of a part of the foetal tissue to close.

CONCORDANCE – The occurrence of a given trait in both members of a twin pair.

CONDUCTIVE HEARING LOSS – A hearing loss arising from a disease or abnormality of the outer or middle ear.

CONSANGUINEOUS – Of spouses, having a genetic relationship closer than usual in the population.

CONTIG – An ordered set of DNA clones containing between them a contiguous stretch of DNA sequence.

CO-SEGREGATE – Alleles at two loci co-segregate if they are inherited together from a parent more often than by chance (normally because they are physically close on the same chromosome).

COSMID – A vector designed for cloning large (45 kb) fragments of DNA.

CpG ISLAND – A specialised DNA sequence often found close to genes, and so providing a means of recognising genes in genomic DNA.

DELETION – The loss of a segment of the genetic material from a chromosome.

DENATURING – The loss of the native 3-dimensional configuration of a macromolecule (protein or DNA usually) through heat treatment, extreme pH etc.

DISABILITY – The consequences of an impairment on the functional performance and activity of an individual, i.e. the hearing difficulties experienced, e.g. hearing in noisy places.

DNA – Deoxyribonucleic acid.

DOMINANT – A phenotype which is manifest when present in the heterozygous state.

DOMINANT NEGATIVE MUTATION – A mutant allele whose product is not only non-functional itself, but also in a heterozygote inhibits the function of the product of the normal allele.

DYNAMIC POSTUROGRAPHY – A technique which aims to control the relative contributions of visual, somatosensory and vestibular inputs required for balance and assess their effect on equilibrium by measurement of body sway or changes in the centre of gravity.

DYSPLASIA – An abnormality of development.

ELECTROCARDIOGRAM (ECG) – A technique, using far field electrodes placed on the chest, for recording the electrical activity of the heart.

ELECTROCOCHLEOGRAPHY (ECochG) – A technique for recording the electrical activity of the cochlea and cochlear nerve usually performed with a needle electrode passed through the tympanic membrane on to the bony promontory, or with an electrode in the external auditory canal.

ELECTRONYSTAGMOGRAPHY (ENG)/ELECTRO-OCULOGRAPHY (EOG) – A technique for recording eye movements using electrodes placed on either side of the eyes (and sometimes above and below the eyes) and based on measures of the corneo-retinal potential.

ELECTRORETINOGRAM (ERG) – A technique for measuring the electrical response of the retina to light stimulation.

EUKARYOTIC – Organisms whose cells have nuclei enclosed by membranes; these include all animals and plants, but not bacteria, which are prokaryotic.

ENVIRONMENTAL AIDS (ASSISTIVE LISTENING DEVICES) – Devices to help hearing impaired people understand electronic speech (e.g. TV, telephone) and to be aware of alerting/warning signals. They may entail altering the acoustical signal or adding a different sensory modality (e.g. vibratory alarm).

EPIDEMIOLOGY – The study of the relationships of various factors determining the frequency and distribution of disease.

EXON – A segment of a gene that becomes part of the mature messenger RNA after splicing out of introns.

EXPRESSED SEQUENCE TAG (EST) – A short partial cDNA sequence, supposed to be sufficient to define a gene uniquely. Techniques exist to identify ESTs on a very large scale.

EXPRESSIVITY – The range of phenotypes expressed by a given genotype under any given set of environmental conditions.

FENESTRATION – The former surgical treatment for otosclerosis involving the creation of a new opening in the lateral semi-circular canal.

FETOSCOPY – Viewing the foetus in utero by means of an endoscope.

FISH (Fluorescence *in situ* hybridisation) – A gene mapping technique in which a fluorescently-labelled DNA clone is used to pick out its cognate sequence in a spread of chromosomes under the microscope.

FRAMESHIFT MUTATION – A mutation that changes the reading frame of nucleotide triplets read by ribosomes from messenger RNA, by inserting or deleting a number of nucleotides that is not an exact multiple of 3.

FREQUENCY TRANSPOSITION AID – A digital hearing aid in which sound frequencies from one band are shifted to another (usually lower) within the range of the individual's hearing range.

FUNCTIONAL APPROACH – In gene cloning, cloning a gene through knowing its function or knowing the aminoacid sequence of the protein it encodes.

GENETIC MAPPING – Working out the order and spacing of genes along a chromosome by observing the frequency of genetic recombination between loci in breeding experiments or human pedigrees. Genetic map distances are measured in centimorgans (q.v.).

GENETIC MARKER – Any genetic character that is Mendelian and polymorphic. In practice, almost always DNA polymorphisms.

GENOME – All the genes carried by a single gamete.

GENOMIC DNA – DNA as it occurs in the genome of an organism, complete with all the non-coding sequences.

GENOTYPE – The genetic constitution of an organism.

GESTALT – The overall appearance of a patient, an important part of syndrome recognition.

HANDICAP – The effect of an impairment or disability on the individual's life, e.g. social withdrawal.

HAPLOINSUFFICIENCY – The unusual situation where half the normal quantity of the product of a particular gene is not sufficient to produce a normal phenotype, so that people heterozygous for a loss of function mutation are abnormal.

HETEROPLASMY – Having two or more genetically different clones of mitochondria.

HETEROZYGOUS – Having two dissimilar alleles at a locus.

HOMOPLASMY – Having all mitochondria genetically identical (normal or abnormal).

HOMOZYGOUS – Having identical alleles at a locus.

HUMAN GENOME PROJECT – The international research effort to map and characterise all human genes and ultimately define the complete DNA sequence of the human genome.

HYBRIDISATION – In DNA technology, allowing two complementary DNA or RNA strands to form a double helix.

IgM – Human immunoglobulin M.

IMPAIRMENT – An abnormality of function as a result of a disease or malformation, e.g. elevated auditory threshold.

INDUCTION LOOP – A wire carrying an electrical current output from a sound source which induces an electromagnetic field which can be picked up by a sensitive coil in a hearing aid.

INSERTION – The addition of one or more base pairs into a DNA molecule.

INTRON – In split genes, a segment that is transcribed into nuclear RNA, but is subsequently removed from within the transcript and rapidly degraded.

KILOBASE (kb) – 1,000 base pairs, a measure of the size of a piece of DNA.

LARYNGOGRAPH – An electrical device for recording movements of the vocal cords.

LEIOMYOMATOSIS – Affected by a leiomyoma, a benign tumour derived from smooth muscle.

LIBRARIES – In molecular genetics, collections of random genomic DNA or cDNA fragments cloned into a vector.

LINKAGE – Two loci are linked if alleles at the loci tend more often than by chance to co-segregate into gametes.

LINKAGE ANALYSIS – Typing individuals in a pedigree or breeding experiment for alleles at two or more loci to check whether they are co-segregating.

LINKAGE DISEQUILIBRIUM – A common cause of allelic association (q.v.). Linkage disequilibrium is seen between alleles at two loci when the chromosomal segment carrying them in apparently unrelated people is in fact often derived intact from a common ancestor.

LOCUS – The position that a gene occupies on a chromosome.

LOD SCORE – A statistical measure (logarithm of the odds for or against linkage) which is the outcome of linkage analysis.

LYONIZATION – The inactivation of all but one of the X chromosomes in most cells of all mammals, as first described by Dr Mary Lyon.

MANUAL COMMUNICATION – Communication by the use of sign language.

MATRILINEAL – The transmission of an entity or character only by the mother, and not by the father. Typical of mitochondria and characters they determine.

mRNA – Messenger RNA.

MEGABASE (Mb) – 1 million bases (a measure of size of DNA fragments).

MELANOCYTE – A pigment cell containing melanin granules.

MENIÈRE'S DISORDER – Idiopathic endolymphatic hydrops with fluctuant low frequency hearing loss, tinnitus, pressure sensation and episodic vertigo.

MICRODELETION – A chromosomal deletion at or below the limit of visibility under the microscope.

MICROSATELLITES – Genetic markers consisting of variable length runs of a simple tandemly repeated sequence, typically CACACACA ... For technical reasons microsatellites are the most widely used markers in human genetic mapping.

MINICOM – A text telephone system operated by a keyboard.

MISSENSE MUTATION – A mutation in which a mRNA codon is changed to one specifying a different amino acid, such as the GAG (glutamic acid) → GUG (valine) mutation causing sickle cell disease.

MONDINI APLASIA – A developmental abnormality of the inner ear in which the normal coils of the cochlea fail to develop.

MULTIFACTORIAL – Governed by many factors, which may include genetic and environmental factors.

MUTATION – The process by which a gene undergoes a structural alteration.

NEURO-OTOLOGY – That part of audiological medicine concerned with the diagnosis and medical treatment of hearing and balance disorders.

NON-PENETRANCE – The situation when a person does not manifest a character despite having a genotype that normally produces that character. Typically seen when a dominant disease skips a generation.

NON-SYNDROMAL – (In relation to hearing loss) a loss unaccompanied by any other abnormalities.

NONSENSE MUTATION – A mutation that converts a mRNA codon for an amino acid into a chain terminating codon (UAA, UAG or UGA).

NORTHERN BLOT – A technique for examining mRNA present in a given tissue sample.

NYSTAGMUS – Involuntary rapid movements of the eyeball.

OLIGOGENIC – A character governed by the combined effects of a small number of genes.

ORAL COMMUNICATION – Communication by means of speech and hearing.

OSSEOINTEGRATED BONE CONDUCTION DEVICE – A type of hearing aid fixed to the skull by an abutment, and which converts sound waves into mechanical vibrations stimulating the inner ear. Also known as a bone anchored hearing aid (BAHA).

OSEOTOMY – Incision or transection of a bone.

OTITIS MEDIA WITH EFFUSION (OME) – Non-purulent inflammation of the middle ear, associated with an accumulation of serous or mucoid fluid, caused by obstruction of the Eustachian tube. Sometimes known as glue ear or secretory otitis media.

OTOACOUSTIC EMISSIONS (OAEs) – Acoustical emissions emanating from the active processes of the outer hair cells and which may be recorded by a microphone in the ear canal. They may be spontaneous or evoked.

OTOADMITTANCE – The measurement of the amount of sound absorbed by the ear and how it is influenced by the pressure applied to the tympanic membrane and contraction of the middle ear muscles. Also known as impedance testing.

PCR (POLYMERASE CHAIN REACTION) – A technique for producing unlimited numbers of copies of a short segment of DNA. PCR is the key technique in much of molecular genetics.

PEDIGREE – A family; the family tree.

PENETRANCE – The proportion of individuals of a specified genotype that show the expected phenotype under a given set of environmental conditions.

PERCHLORATE TEST – An assessment of radio-iodine discharge by the thyroid gland in response to perchlorate challenge. The test is designed to unmask organification defects in the thyroid gland by provoking the discharge of inorganic iodide.

PHYSICAL MAP – A map showing the physical locations of genes or sequences on chromosomes or cloned DNA fragments. Physical map distances are measured in base pairs, kilobases, megabases etc., or in terms of the chromosomal bands recognised by cytogeneticists.

POLYGENIC – A character dependent on the interaction of a number of genes (strictly, a very large number of genes, each with a very small effect).

POLYMORPHISM – The existence of two or more genetically different classes in the same interbreeding population at frequencies such that the rarest could not be maintained simply by recurrent mutation. A common working definition is that at least two alleles should have frequencies above 1% in the population.

POLYTOMOGRAPHY – Radiographic tomography performed in several predetermined planes.

POSITIONAL CANDIDATE APPROACH – In cloning disease genes, a strategy in which a candidate chromosomal region is defined by linkage analysis, and then genes already known to map to this region are tested to see if they cause the disease.

POSITIONAL CLONING APPROACH – Cloning a gene using only knowledge of its approximate chromosomal location. A difficult task.

POSTNATAL – Occurring after birth.

PRENATAL – Occurring before birth.

PRIMER – A short synthetic piece of DNA used to initiate DNA synthesis at a defined point on a template strand, particularly in PCR.

PROBE – In molecular genetics, a piece of DNA or RNA labelled with a radioactive isotope or tagged in other ways, used to pick out sequences to which it can hybridise.

PROKARYOTIC – Organisms whose cells lack a membrane-bound nucleus containing chromosomes. The group comprises all bacteria, but not animals or plants.

PROTO-ONCOGENE – A cellular gene that functions in controlling the proliferation of cells and that, when abnormally activated, can contribute to the development of cancer.

RECESSIVE – A character that is manifest only in the homozygous state, not in heterozygotes.

RECOMBINANT – Of an individual or a gamete, having a combination of alleles different from the combination inherited by the parent. Of DNA, a sequence made by joining two previously separate sequences.

RETROCOCHLEAR – Occurring rostral to the cochlea. In general clinical practice it usually refers to the cochlear nerve and conditions affecting it.

RFLP – Restriction fragment length polymorphism, a type of DNA polymorphism used as a genetic marker (but now largely superseded by microsatellites, q.v.).

RNA – Ribonucleic acid.

SENSITIVITY – The ability of a test to detect those individuals showing a particular abnormality.

SEX LINKED – A gene, or character determined by a gene, located on the X (or sometimes the Y) chromosome; the pedigree pattern resulting therefrom.

SHORT TANDEM REPEAT POLYMORPHISMS (STRP) – Microsatellites, q.v.

SIGN LANGUAGE – A linguistic system based on communication by the use of gestures.

SOMATIC CELL HYBRIDS – Hybrid human-rodent cells grown in the laboratory and used to help map genes to specific chromosomal locations.

SPECIFICITY – The ability of a test to categorise the normal individuals as being normal.

SPORADIC – Of a character, not obviously running in the family.

STAPEDECTOMY – The treatment of otosclerosis by removal of the stapes and its replacement with a prosthesis connecting the incus to the oval window.

STEREOCILIA – Motile cilia of the cochlear and vestibular hair cells.

STRINGENCY OF HYBRIDISATION – The degree to which imperfectly matching DNA sequences are able to hybridise in a given experiment, which the experimenter controls by choosing the temperature and salt concentration.

STS (SEQUENCE-TAGGED SITE) – A short defined and recognisable DNA sequence, unique in the genome. STS markers are widely used to help recognise clones and build contigs (q.v.).

SYNDROMAL – (In relation to hearing loss) a loss accompanied by other abnormalities. Some would describe pure hearing loss, but with a strikingly characteristic audiogram or age of onset, as syndromal.

TORCH – A screening test for congenital infections, testing for toxoplasma, rubella, cytogmegalovirus and herpes simplex infections.

TRACHEOTOMY – Incision of the trachaea through the skin and muscles of the neck.

TRANSCRIPTION – The formation of a mRNA molecule upon a DNA template by complementary base pairing.

TRANSCRIPTION FACTORS – Cellular proteins that regulate transcription of specific genes.

TRANSLATION – The formation of a protein directed by a specific mRNA molecule.

TUMOUR SUPPRESSOR GENE – A class of genes controlling cell proliferation, in which complete loss of function (by mutation or loss of both copies) can lead to cancer.

TYMPANOMETRY – The aspect of otoadmittance testing concerned with the effect of the pressure applied to the ear canal on the sound absorbed by the ear.

VECTOR – A DNA molecule able to survive and replicate in cells, into which DNA sequences to be cloned can be incorporated.

VESTIBULAR AQUEDUCT – A part of the bony labyrinth running from the labyrinth to the posterior surface of the petrous bone containing one or more small veins and the endolymphatic duct.

VIBROTACTILE AID – A device which detects sounds and converts them into tactile stimuli. Different systems are available which can be single or multichannel and which have different processing strategies.

VIDEOPHONE – A telephone including a visual image.

VISISPEECH – A computer-based speech display system used to provide the patient with feedback on the overall pitch, intonation, voice quality, timing and distinction between voiced and voiceless phonemes.

VISUAL RESPONSE AUDIOMETRY (VRA) – A hearing test used in young children in which a correct response to the auditory stimulus is reinforced by the presentation of visual stimulus, such as an illuminated toy.

VNTR (VARIABLE NUMBER OF TANDEM REPEATS) – A class of DNA polymorphism, including microsatellites, widely used as genetic markers.

YEAST ARTIFICIAL CHROMOSOME (YAC) – A cloning vector that can be propagated in yeast cells. Larger DNA fragments can be cloned in YACs than in any other current vector.

References

Aase JM (1990) Diagnostic Dysmorphology. New York and London: Plenum Medical Book Company.

Abramowicz MJ, Targovnik HM, Varela V et al. (1992) Identification of a mutation in the coding sequence of the human thyroid peroxidase gene causing congenital goiter. Journal of Clinical Investigation 90: 1200-04.

Abramson M, Fay TH, Kelly JP et al. (1989) Clinical results with a percutaneous bone-anchored hearing aid. Laryngoscope 99: 707-10.

Abs R, Berhelst J, Schoofs E et al. (1991) Hyperfunctioning metastatic follicular thyroid carcinoma in Pendred's syndrome. Cancer 67: 2191-3.

Agarwal N, Hsieh C-L, Sills D et al. (1991) Sequence analysis, expression and chromosomal localisation of a gene, isolated from a subtracted human retina cDNA library, that encodes an insulin-like growth factor binding protein (IGFBP2). Experimental Eye Research 52: 549-61.

Akbarnia BA, Bowen JR, Dougherty J (1979) Familial arthrogrypotic-like hand abnormality and sensorineural deafness. American Journal of Diseases in Children 133: 403-5.

Albrecht W (1922) Uber die Vererbung der konstitutionell sporadischen Taubstummheit, der hereditären Labyrinhschwerhörigkeit und der Otosclerose. Archiv fur Ohr-Nase und Kehlk Heilkunde 110: 15-48.

Albrecht W (1933) Die Veränderungen der Schnecke bei hereditärer Innenohrschwerhörigkeit. Zeitschrift der Hals, Nase und Ohrenheilkunde 34: 261-5.

Alcolado JC, Majid A, Brockington M et al. (1994) Mitochondrial gene defects in patients with NIDDM. Diabetologia 37: 372-6.

Almeida F, Temporal A, Cavalcanti N et al. (1974) Pendred's syndrome in an area of endemic goitre in Brazil. In Dunn JT, Medeiros-Neto GA (Eds) Endemic goitre and cretinism: continuing threats to world health. Pan American Health Organisation 292, Washington DC. pp167-71.

Almqvist C, Haugan H (1992) Audiometric notches - an indication of recessive genetic deafness. Preclinical Dissertation Lund.

Al-Shihabi BA (1994) Childhood sensorineural hearing loss in consanguineous marriages. Journal of Audiological Medicine 3: 151-9.

Althous P (1994) Fast tracks to disease genes. Science 265: 2008-10.

Altmann F, Glasgold A, McDuff JP (1967) The incidence of otosclerosis as related to race and sex. Annals of Otology, Rhinology and Laryngology 76: 377-92.

Anderson H, Wedenberg E. (1968) Audiometric identification of normal hearing carriers of genes for deafness. Acta Otolaryngologica 65: 535-54.

Anderson H, Wedenberg E (1976) Identification of normal hearing carriers of genes for deafness. Acta Otolaryngologica 82: 245-8.

Annas GJ, Elias S (1992) Gene Mapping – Using Law and Ethics as Guides. New York: Oxford University Press.

Antignac C, Zhou J, Sanak M et al. (1992) Alport syndrome and diffuse leiomy-omatosis: deletions in the 5' end of the *COL4A5* collagen gene. Kidney International 42: 1178-83.

Aran JM (1978) Contribution of electrocochleography to diagnosis in infancy: an eight year survey. In Gerber SA, Mencher GT (Eds) Early Diagnosis of Hearing Loss. New York: Grune and Stratton.

Arcand P, Desrosiers M, Dubé J, Abela A (1991) The large vestibular aqueduct syndrome and sensorineural hearing loss in the pediatric population. Journal of Otolaryngology 20: 247-50.

Arias S (1971) Genetic heterogeneity in the Waardenburg syndrome. Birth Defects: Original Article Series 7: 87-101.

Arias S, Mota M (1978) Apparent non-penetrance for dystopia in Waardenburg syndrome type I with some hints on the diagnosis of dystopia canthorum. Journal de Génétique Humain 26: 101-31.

Arias S, Penchaszadeh VB, Pinto Cisterna J, Larrauri S (1980) The IVIC syndrome: a new autosomal dominant complex pleiotropic syndrome with radial ray hypoplasia, hearing impairment, external ophthalmoplegia and thrombocytopenia. American Journal of Medical Genetics 6: 25-9.

Arn PH, Mankinen C, Jabs EW (1993) Mild mandibulofacial dysostosis in a child with a deletion of 3p. American Journal of Medical Genetics 46: 534-6.

Arnaudo E, Dalakas M, Shanske S, Moraes CT, Dimauro S, Schon EA (1991) Depletion of muscle mitochondrial DNA in AIDS patients with Zidovudine-induced myopathy. Lancet 337: 508-10.

Arnaudo E, Hirano M, Seelan RS et al. (1992) Tissue-specific expression and chromosome assignment of genes specifying two isoforms of subunit VIIa of human cytochrome c oxidase. Gene 119: 299-305.

Arnold W, Friedmann I (1987) Presence of viral specific antigens (measles, rubella) around the active otosclerotic focus. Annals of Rhinology and Laryngology 66: 167-71.

Arnold W, Friedmann I (1990) Immunohistochemistry of otosclerosis. Acta Otolaryngologica Supplement 470: 124-9.

Arnold WJ, Laissue JA, Friedmann I, Naumann HH (1987) Diseases of the Head and Neck. An Atlas of Histopathology. New York: Thieme Medical Publishers.

Arnos K, Israel J, Devlin L, Wilson M (1992) Genetic counselling for the deaf. Otolaryngologic Clinics of North America 25: 953-71.

Arnos K, Cunningham M, Israel J, Marazita M (1992) Innovative approach to genetic counselling services for the deaf population. American Journal of Medical Genetics 44: 345-51.

Arnos K (1994) Hereditary hearing loss. New England Journal of Medicine 331: 469-70.

Arnvig J (1955) Vestibular function in deafness and severe hard of hearing. Acta Otolaryngologica 45: 283-8.

Arslan E, Conti G, Prosser S (1986) Electrocochleography and brainstem response: threshold assessment. In Gallai V (Ed) Maturation of CNS and Evoked Potentials. Amsterdam: Elsevier Science Publishers.

Arslan E, Lupi G, Turrini M, Orzan E (1995) Comparison between auditory brainstem response and electrocochleography in infant hearing threshold assessment. Paper presented at the British Society of Audiology Short Papers Meeting on experimental studies of hearing and deafness. Oxford, Sept 1995.

Arslan E, Prosser S, Conti G, Michelini S (1983) Electrocochleography and brainstem potentials in the diagnosis of the deaf child. International Journal of Pediatric

Otorhinolaryngology 5: 251-9.

Arslan M, Giacomelli F (1963) Considérations cliniques sur l'ankylose stapédio-vestibulaire congenitale. Annales d'Otolaryngologie (Paris) 80: 13-28.

Ascherson FM (1832) De Fistulis Colli Congenitis. Berolini.

Atkin CL, Gregory MC, Border WA (1988) In Scher RW, Gottschalk CW (Eds) Diseases of the Kidney. 4th edn. Boston: Little, Brown and Co. pp617-41.

Attardi G, Schatz G (1988) Biogenesis of mitochondria. Annual Reviews of Cell Biology 4: 289-333.

Avraham KB, Hasson T, Steel KP et al. (1995) The mouse *Snell's waltzer* deafness gene encodes an unconventional myosin required for structural integrity of inner ear hair cells. Nature Genetics 11: 369-75.

Bach I, Brunner HG, Beighton P et al. (1992) Microdeletions in patients with X-linked progressive mixed deafness and perilymphatic gusher during stapes surgery (*DFN3*). American Journal of Human Genetics 50: 38-44.

Bachmayer DL, Ross RB, Munro IR (1986) Maxillary growth following le Fort III advancement surgery in Crouzon Apert and Pfeiffer Syndrome. American Journal of Orthodontics and Dentofacial Orthopedics 90: 420.

Bacino C, Prezant TR, Bu X, Fournier P, Fischel-Ghodsian N (1995) Susceptibility mutations in the mitochondrial small ribosomal RNA gene in aminoglycoside induced deafness. Pharmacogenetics 5: 165-72.

Baldwin CT, Hoth CF, Amos JA, da-Silva EO, Milunsky A (1992) An exonic mutation in the HuP2 paired domain gene causes Waardenburg's syndrome. Nature 355: 637-8.

Baldwin CT, Weiss S, Farrer LA et al. (1995) Linkage of congenital, recessive deafness (*DFNB4*) to chromosome 7q31 and evidence for genetics heterogeneity in the Middle Eastern Druze population. Human Molecular Genetics 4: 1637-42.

Baldwin D, King TT, Chevretton E, Morrison AW (1991) Bilateral cerebellopontine angle tumours in neurofibromatosis type II. Journal of Neurosurgery 74: 910-5.

Balestrazzi P, Baeteman MA, Mattei MG, Mattei JF (1983) Franceschetti syndrome in a child with a *de novo* balanced translocation (5;13)(q11;p11) and significant decrease of hexosaminidase B. Human Genetics 64: 305-8.

Balkany T, Telischi FF, McCoy MJ, Lonsbury-Martin BL, Martin GK (1994) Otoacoustic emissions in otologic practice. American Journal of Otology 15 (suppl 1): 29-38.

Ballinger SW, Shoffner JM, Hedava EV et al. (1992) Maternally transmitted diabetes and deafness associated with a 10.4 kb mitochondrial deletion. Nature Genetics 1: 11-15.

Ballinger SW, Wallace DC (1995) Maternally transmitted diabetes and deafness. The Endocrinologist 5: 104-21.

Bamford J, McSporran E (1993) Visual reinforcement audiometry. In McCormick (Ed) Paediatric Audiology 0-5 years. London: Whurr.

Barker DF, Hostikka SL, Zhou J (1990) Identification of mutations in the *COL4A5* collagen gene in Alport Syndrome. Science 248: 1224-7.

Baschieri L, Benedetti G, de Luca F et al. (1963) Evaluation and limitations of the perchlorate test in the study of thyroid dysfunction. Journal of Clinical Endocrinology and Metabolism 23: 786-91.

Baser ME, Ragge N, Riccardi V, Ganz B, Janus T, Pulst S (1995) Neurofibromatosis 2 in monozygotic twins. American Journal of Human Genetics 57 (suppl): A54.

Batsakis JG, Nishiyama RH, Schmidt RW (1963) Sporadic goitre syndrome. A clinicopathologic analysis. American Journal of Clinical Pathology 39: 241-51.

Bauer J, Stein C (1925) Vererbung und Konstitution bei Ohrenkrankheiten. Zeitschrift der Gesellschaft für Anatomie 10: 483.

Bauham TM (1966) Congenital columella type stapes. Journal of Laryngology 80: 98-100.

Bax GM (1966) Typical and atypical cases of Pendred's syndrome in one family. Acta Endocrinologica 53: 264-70.

Becker MA, Smith PR, Taylor W, Mustafi R, Switzer RL (1995) The genetic and functional basis of purine nucleotide feedback - resistant phosphoribosy/pyrophosphate synthetase superactivity. Journal of Clinical Investigation 96: 2133-2141.

Beisel KW, Kennedy JE (1994) Identification of novel alternatively spliced isoforms of the tropomyosin-encoding gene, TM*nm*, in the rat cochlea. Gene 143: 251-6.

Beighton P, Horan F, Hamersma H. (1977) A review of the osteopetroses. Postgraduate Medical Journal 53: 507-15.

Beighton P, Hamersma H, Horan F (1979) Craniometaphyseal dysplasia: variability of expression within a large family. Clinical Genetics 15: 252-8.

Beighton P, Hamersma H, Raad M. (1979) Oculodento-osseous dysplasia: heterogeneity or variable expression? Clinical Genetics 16: 169-77.

Beighton P, Cremin B (1980) Sclerosing Bone Dysplasias. Berlin: Springer Verlag.

Beighton P, Hamersma H (1980) Frontometaphyseal dysplasia: autosomal dominant or X-linked? Journal of Medical Genetics 17: 53-6.

Beighton P, Sellars S (1982) Genetics and Otology. Edinburgh: Churchill Livingstone.

Beighton P (1988a) Sclerosteosis. Journal of Medical Genetics 25: 200-03.

Beighton P (1988b) Inherited Disorders of the Skeleton. 2nd edn. Edinburgh: Churchill Livingstone.

Beighton P (1990) Hereditary Deafness. In Emery AEH and Rimoin DL (Eds) Principles and Practice of Medical Genetics. 2nd edn. Edinburgh: Churchill Livingstone. pp 733-48.

Beighton P, De Paepe A, Hall JG et al. (1992) Molecular nosology of heritable disorders of connective tissue. American Journal of Medical Genetics 42: 431-48.

Békésy G von (1947) A new audiometer. Acta Otolaryngologica 53: 411-22.

Bell AG (1883) Upon the formation of a deaf variety of the human race. Memoirs of the National Academy of Sciences 2: 177.

Bell J (1933) Retinitis pigmentosa and allied diseases. In Treasury of Human Inheritance. Vol.2. London: Cambridge University Press.

Bellus GA, McIntosh I, Smith EA et al. (1995) A recurrent mutation in the tyrosine kinase domain of fibroblast growth factor receptor 3 causes hypochondroplasia. Nature Genetics 10: 357-9.

Ben Arab S, Bonaïti-Pellié C, Belkahia A (1990) An epidemiological and genetic study of congenital profound deafness in Tunisia (governorate of Nabeul). Journal of Medical Genetics 27: 29-33.

Ben Arab S, Bonaïti-Pellié C, Belkahia A (1993) A genetic study of otosclerosis in a population living in the north of Tunisia. Annals of Genetics 36: 111-6.

Ben-Yoseph Y, Baylerian MS, Nadler HL (1984) Radiometric assays of N-acetylglucosaminyl phosphotransferase and L-N-acetylglucosaminyl phosphodiesterase with substrates labelled in the glucosamine moeity. Analytical Biochemistry 142: 297-304.

Berger W, Meindl A, van de Pol TJR et al. (1992) Isolation of a candidate gene for Norrie disease by positional cloning. Nature Genetics 1: 199-203.

Berger W, van de Pol D, Warburg M (1992) Mutations in the candidate gene for Norrie disease. Human Molecular Genetics 1: 461-5.

Bergstrom LV, Neblett LM, Hemenway WG (1972) Otologic manifestations of acrocephalosyndactyly. Archives of Otolaryngology 96: 117-23.

Bernes SM, Bacino C, Prezant TR et al. (1993) Identical mitochondrial DNA deletion in mother with progressive external ophthalmoplegia and son with Pearson marrow-pancreas syndrome. Journal of Pediatrics 123: 598-602.

Bernstein L (1966) Congenital absence of the oval window. Archives of Otolaryngology 83: 533-7.

Berry GA (1889) A note on a congenital defect (?coloboma) of the lower lid. Royal London Ophthalmic Hospital Reports 12: 255-7.

Beutler E, Grabowski GA (1995) Gaucher's disease. In Scriver C, Beaudet A, Sly W, Valle D (Eds) The Metabolic and Molecular Basis of Inherited Disease. New York: McGraw Hill. p 2651.

Biancalana V, Marec B, Odent S, van den Hurk JAMJ, Hanauer A (1991) Oto-palato-digital syndrome type I: further evidence for assignment of the locus to Xq28. Human Genetics 88: 228-30.

Bieber F, Nance W (1979) Hereditary hearing loss. In Jackson C, Schimke N (Eds) Clinical Genetics: A Course Book for Physicians. New York: John Wiley and Sons. pp 443-61.

Bikker H, Denhartog MT, Baas F et al. (1994) 20-base pair duplication in the human thyroid peroxidase gene results in a total iodide organification defect and congenital hypothyroidism. Journal of Clinical Endocrinology and Metabolism 79: 248-52.

Bikker H, Vulsma T, Baas F et al. (1995) Identification of 5 novel inactivating mutations in the human thyroid peroxidase gene by denaturing gradient gel–electrophoresis. Human Mutation 6: 9-16.

Billerbeck AEC, Cavaviere H, Goldberg AC et al. (1994) Clinical and genetic studies in Pendred's syndrome. Thyroid 4: 279-84.

Binghong Bu, Kaban L, Vargervik K (1989) Effect of Le Fort III osteotomy in patients with Crouzon and Apert syndromes. Journal of Oral and Maxillofacial Surgery 47: 666-71.

Bishop JO, Morton JG, Rosebach M, Richardson M (1974) Three abundant classes in HeLa cell messenger RNA. Nature 250: 199-204.

Bixler D, Spivack J, Bennett J, Christian JC (1971) The ectrodactyly-ectodermal dysplasia-clefting (EEC) syndrome. Clinical Genetics 3: 43-51.

Blegvad B and Hvidegaard T (1983) Hereditary dysfunction of the brain stem auditory pathways as the major cause of speech retardation. Scandinavian Audiology 12: 179-87.

Bock GR, Steel KP (1983) Inner ear pathology in the deafness mutant mouse. Acta Otolaryngologica (Stockholm) 96: 39-47.

Bogard B, Lieber E (1977) Males with deafness, nasal bone abnormalities and hand contractures in three generations. Birth Defects: Original Article Series 13: 226 only.

Bonafede RP, Beighton P (1979) Autosomal dominant inheritance of scalp defects with ectrodactyly. American Journal of Medical Genetics 3: 35-41.

Bonné-Tamir B, DeStefano AL, Briggs CE, Adair R, Franklyn B, Weiss S et al (1996). Linkage of congenital recessive deafness (gene DFNB10) to chromosome 21q22.3. American Journal of Human Genetics, 58, 1254-1259.

Borg E, Canlon B, Engström B (1995) Noise-induced hearing loss – literature review and experiments in rabbits. Scandinavian Audiology 24: Suppl. 40.

Botstein D, White RL, Skolnick M, Davis RW (1980) Construction of a genetic linkage map in man using restriction fragment length polymorphisms. American Journal of Human Genetics 32: 314-31.

Boughman JA, Vernon M, Shaver KA (1983) Usher syndrome: definition and estimate of prevalence from two high risk populations. Journal of Chronic Diseases 36: 595-603.

Bourn D, Carter SA, Mason S, Evans DGR, Strachan T (1994) Germline mutations in the neurofibromatosis type II tumour suppressor gene. Human Molecular Genetics 5: 813-6.

Bowen P, Bierderman B, Hoo JJ (1985) The critical segment for the Langer-Giedon syndrome. Annales de Génétique 28: 224-7.

Brain WR (1927) Heredity in simple goitre. Quarterly Journal of Medicine 20: 303-19.

Brake B, Braghetta P, Banting G, Bressan G, Luzio JP, Stanley KK (1990) A new recombinant DNA strategy for the molecular cloning of rare membrane proteins. Biochemical Journal 267: 631-7.

Brown KA, Sutcliffe MJ, Steel KP, Brown SDM (1992) Close linkage of the olfactory marker protein gene to the mouse deafness mutation *shaker-1*. Genomics 13: 189-93.

Brown Kelly HD (1960) Observations on stapes mobilisation. Journal of Laryngology 74: 37-41.

Brown SDM (1994) Integrating maps of the mouse genome. Current Opinions in Genetics and Development 4: 389-94.

Brown SDM, Steel KP (1994) Genetic deafness – progress with mouse models. Human Molecular Genetics 3: 1453-6.

Brownstein Z, Friedlander Y, Peritz E and Cohen T (1991) Estimated number of loci for autosomal recessive severe nerve deafness within the Israeli Jewish population, with implications for genetic counseling. American Journal of Medical Genetics 41: 306-12.

Brunner HG, van Bennekom CA, Lambermon EMM et al. (1988) The gene for X-linked progressive mixed deafness with perilymphatic gusher during stapes surgery (*DFN3*) is linked to PGK. Human Genetics 80: 337-40.

Brunner HG, Smeets B, Smeets D, Nelen M, Cremers CWRJ, Ropers HH (1990) Molecular genetics of X-linked hearing impairment. In Ruben RJ, van der Water TR, Steel KP (Eds) Genetics of hearing impairment. Annals of New York Academy of Science 630: 176-90.

Brunner HG, van Beersum SEC, Warman ML, Olsen BJ, Ropers HH, Mariman ECM (1994) A Stickler syndrome gene is linked to chromosome 6 near the *Col11A2* gene. Human Molecular Genetics 3: 1561-4.

Bu X, Yang HY, Shohat M, Rotter JI (1992) Two-locus mitochondrial and nuclear gene models for mitochondrial disorders. Genetic Epidemiology 9: 27-44.

Bu X, Rotter JI (1993) Wolfram Syndrome: a mitochondrially-mediated disorder? Lancet 342, 598-600.

Budarf ML, Collins J, Gong W, Roe B, Wang Z, Bailey LC et al. (1995) Cloning a balanced translocation associated with DiGeorge syndrome and identification of a disrupted candidate gene. Nature Genetics 10: 269-278.

Buhler EM, Beutler C, Buhler UK, Fessler RA. (1987) A final word on the tricho-rhinopharyngeal syndromes. Clinical Genetics 31: 273-5.

Buhler EM, Malik NJ (1984) The tricho-rhino-pharyngeal syndromes: chromosome 8 long arm deletion: is there a shortest region of overlap between reported cases? Are they separate entities? American Journal of Medical Genetics 19: 113-9.

Bujia J, Alsalameh S, Jerez R, Sittinger M, Wilmes E, Burmester G (1994) Antibodies to the minor cartilage collagen type IX in otosclerosis. American Journal of Otology 15: 222-4.

Buran DJ, Duvall AJ (1967) The Oto-Palato-Digital syndrome (OPD). Archives of Otolaryngology 85: 394-9.

Burrow GN, Spaulding SW, Alexander NM et al. (1973) Normal peroxidase activity in Pendred's syndrome. Journal of Clinical Endocrinology and Metabolism 36: 522-8.

Buyse ML (1990) Birth Defect Encyclopedia. Center for Birth Defects Information Services Inc, Dover MA.

Byers PH, Wallis GA, Willing MC (1991) Osteogenesis imperfecta: translation of mutation to phenotype. Journal of Medical Genetics 28: 433-42.

Cable J, Barkway C, Steel KP (1992) Characteristics of stria vascularis melanocytes of viable dominant spotting (W^v/W^v) mouse mutants. Hearing Research 64: 6-20.

Cable J, Huszar D, Jaenisch R, Steel KP (1994) Effects of mutations at the W locus (c-kit) on inner ear pigmentation and function in the mouse. Pigment Cell Research 7: 17-32.

Carmi R, Binshtock M, Abeliovich D, Bar-Ziv J (1983) The branchio-oto-renal (BOR) syndrome: report of bilateral renal agenesis in three sibs. American Journal of Medical Genetics 14: 625-7.

Caronni EP (1985) Craniofacial Surgery. Boston: Little Brown.

Causse JR, Causse JB (1984) Otospongiosis as a genetic disease. American Journal of Otology 5: 211-23.

Cave WT Jr, Dunn JT (1975) Studies on the thyroidal defect in an atypical form of Pendred's syndrome. Journal of Clinical Endocrinology and Metabolism 41: 590-9.

Cawthorne T (1955) Otosclerosis. Journal of Laryngology and Otology 69: 437-56.

Ceuterick C, Martin JJ, Foulard M (1986) Nieman-Pick disease type C: skin biopsies in parents. Neuropediatrics 17: 111-2.

Chabot B, Stephenson DA, Chapman VM, Besmer P, Bernstein A (1988) The proto-oncogene c-kit encoding a transmembrane tyrosine kinase receptor maps to the mouse W locus. Nature 335: 88-9.

Chaib H, Lina-Granade G, Guïford P et al. (1994) A gene responsible for a dominant form of neurosensory non-syndromic deafness maps to the NSRD1 recessive deafness gene interval. Human Molecular Genetics 3: 2219-22.

Chaïb H, Dode C, Place C et al. (1995) The chromosomal localisation and cloning of human genes involved in sensorineural, non-syndromic recessive deafness. In Proceedings of 2nd International Conference on The Molecular Biology of Hearing and Deafness, Bethesda. p 22.

Chaïb H, Place C, Salem N et al. (1996) A gene responsible for a sensorineural non-syndromic recessive deafness maps to chromosome 2p22-23. Human Molecular Genetics 5: 155-8.

Chaïb H, Place C, Salem N, Chardenoux S, Vincent C, Weissenbach J et al. (1996a) A gene responsible for a sensorineural non-syndromic recessive deafness maps to chromosome 2p22-23. Human Molecular Genetics 5: 155-158.

Chaïb H, Place C, Salem N, Dodé C, Chardenoux S, Weissenbach J et al. (1996b) Mapping of DFNB12, a gene for a non-syndromal autosomal recessive deafness to chromosome 10q21-22. Human Molecular Genetics 5: 1061-1064.

Chang B, Heckenlively JR, Hawes NL, Roderick TH (1993) New mouse primary retinal degeneration (rd-3) Genomics 16: 45-49.

Cheatham MA, Dallos P (1993) Longitudinal comparisons of IHC ac and dc receptor potentials recorded from the guinea pig cochlea. Hearing Research 68: 107-14.

Chen A, Francis M, Ni L et al. (1995a) Phenotypic manifestations of branchio-oto-renal syndrome. American Journal of Medical Genetics (in press).

Chen AH, Li N, Fukushima K et al. (1995) Linkage of a gene for dominant non-syndromic deafness to chromosome 19. Human Molecular Genetics 4: 1073-6.

Chen H, Thalmann I, Adams JC et al. (1995) cDNA cloning, tissue distribution, and chromosomal localization of Ocp2, a gene encoding a putative transcription-associated factor predominantly expressed in the auditory organs. Genomics 27: 389-98.

Chen ZY, Hendriks RW, Jobling MA et al. (1992) Isolation and characterization of a candidate gene for Norrie disease. Nature Genetics 1: 204-8.

Chevance LG, Bretlau P, Jorgensen MB, Causse J (1970) Otosclerosis. An electron microscopic and cytochemical study. Acta Otolaryngologica Supplement (Stockholm) 272: 1-44.

Chevance LG, Causse J, Jorgensen MB, Bergés J (1972) Hydrolytic activity of the perilymph in otosclerosis. A preliminary report. Acta Otolaryngologica (Stockholm) 74: 23-28.

Chitayat D, Hodgkinson KA, Chen M-F, Haber GD, Nakishma S, Sando I (1992) Branchio-oto-renal syndrome: further delineation of an underdiagnosed syndrome. American Journal of Medical Genetics 43: 970-5.

Chole RA (1993) Differential osteoclast activation in endochondral and intramembranous bone. Annals of Otology, Rhinology and Laryngology 102: 616-9.

Christiansen JB (1991) Sociological implications of hearing loss. In Ruben RJ, van der Water TR, Steel KP (Eds) Genetics of hearing impairment. Annals of New York Academy of Science 630: 230-5.

Chung C, Robison O, Morton N (1959) A note on deaf mutism. Annals of Human Genetics 23: 357-66.

Chung C, Brown K (1970) Family studies of early childhood deafness ascertained through Clarke school for the deaf. American Journal of Human Genetics 22: 630-44.

Clauser L, Curioni C. (1990) Orbital hypertelorism: Details of surgical technique. Abstracts 10th Congress EACMFS, Brussels, p 146 bis.

Clauser L, Baciliero U, Nordera P, Curri D, Pinna V, Curioni C, (1991) Frontoethmoidal meningoencephalocele. A one-stage correction, reconstruction and plating by means of the microsystem. Journal of Craniofacial Surgery 1: 2-8.

Coakley JC, Keir EH, Connelly JF (1992) The association of thyroid dyshormonogenesis and deafness (Pendred syndrome): experience of the Victorian neonatal thyroid screening programme. Journal of Paediatrics and Child Health 28: 398-401.

Cohen MM Jr (1975) An etiologic and nosologic overview of the craniosynostosis syndromes. Birth Defects 22: 137-89.

Cohen MM, Kreiborg S (1992) Upper and lower airway compromise in the Apert syndrome. American Journal of Medical Genetics 44: 90-93.

Cohen M, Gorlin R (1995) Epidemiology, etiology, and genetic patterns. In Gorlin R, Toriello H, Cohen M (Eds) Hereditary Hearing Loss and its Syndromes. Oxford: Oxford University Press. pp 9-21.

Cohen M, Francis M, Luxon LM, Bellman S, Coffey R, Pembrey M (1995) Dips on Békésy or Audioscan fail to identify carriers of autosomal recessive non-syndromic hearing loss. Acta Otolaryngologica (in press).

Collins C, Schappert K, Hayden MR (1992) The genomic organization of a novel regulatory myosin light chain (MYL5) that maps to chromosome 4p16.3 and shows different patterns of expression between primates. Human Molecular Genetics 1: 727-33.

Collins FS (1992) Positional cloning: let's not call it reverse any more. Nature Genetics 1: 3-6.

Collins FS (1995) Positional cloning moves from perditional to traditional. Nature Genetics 9: 347-50.

Collins RL, Fuller JL (1968) Audiogenic seizure prone (asp): a gene affecting behavior in linkage group VIII of the mouse. Science 162: 1137-9.

Collins RL (1970) A new genetic locus mapped from behavioral variation in mice:

audiogenic seizure prone (ASP). Behavior Genetics 1: 99-109.

Connor JM, Evans DAP (1982) Genetic aspects of fibrodysplasia ossificans progressiva. Journal of Medical Genetics 19: 35-9.

Connor JM, Ferguson Smith (1994) Essential Medical Genetics. Oxford: Blackwell

Copeland NG, Jenkins NA, Gilbert DJ et al. (1993) A genetic linkage map of the mouse: Current applications and future prospects. Science 262: 57-66.

Corral-Debrinski M, Horton T, Lott MT et al. (1992) Mitochondrial DNA deletions in human brain: Regional variability and increase with advanced age. Nature Genetics 2: 324-9.

Costeff H, Dar H (1980) Consanguinity analysis of congenital deafness in Northern Israel. American Journal of Human Genetics 32: 64-8.

Coucke P, van Camp G, Djoyodiharjo B et al. (1994) Linkage mapping of a form of autosomal dominant hearing loss to the short arm of chromosome 1. New England Journal of Medicine 331: 425-31.

Cox GR, Green ED, Lander ES, Cohen D, Myers RM (1994) Assessing mapping progress in the human genome project. Science 265: 2031-2.

Coyle B, Coffey R, Armour JAL et al. (1996) Pendred Syndrome (goitre and sensorineural hearing loss) Maps to chromosone 7 in the region containg the nonsyndromic deafness gene DFNB4. Nature Genetics 12, 421-423

Cremers CWRJ (1979) Autosomal recessive non-syndromal progressive sensorineural deafness in childhood: a separate, clinical and genetic entity. International Journal of Pediatric Otorhinolaryngology 1: 193-9.

Cremers CWRJ, Fikkers-van Noord M (1980) The ear-pits-deafness syndrome: clinical and genetic aspects. International Journal of Pediatric Otorhinolaryngology 2: 309-22.

Cremers CWRJ, Thijssen HOM, Fischer AJEM, Marres EHMA (1981) Otological aspects of the earpits-deafness syndrome. Oto-Rhino-Laryngology 43: 223-39.

Cremers CWRJ, Hombergen GCJH, Wentges RThR (1983) Perilymphatic gusher and stapes surgery. A predictable complication? Clinical Otolaryngology 8: 235-40.

Cremers CWRJ, Huygen PLM (1983) Clinical features of female heterozygotes in the X-linked mixed deafness syndrome (with perilymphatic gusher during stapes surgery). International Journal of Pediatric Otorhinolaryngology 6: 179-85.

Cremers CWRJ, Hoogland GA, Kuypers W (1984) Hearing loss in the cervico-oculoacoustic (Wildervanck) syndrome. Archives of Otolaryngology 110: 54-7.

Cremers CWRJ (1985) Audiological features of the X-linked progressive mixed deafness syndrome with perilymphatic gusher during stapes surgery. American Journal of Otology 6: 243-6.

Cremers CWRJ (1985) Osteogenesis imperfecta tarda en stapeschirurgie. Nederlandse Tijdschrift van Geneeskunde 129: 888-90.

Cremers CWRJ, Hombergen GCHJ, Scaff JJ, Huygen PLM, Volkers WS, Pinckers AJLG (1985) X-linked progressive mixed deafness with perilymphatic gusher during stapes surgery. Archives of Otolaryngology 111: 249-54.

Cremers CWRJ, Theunissen E, Kuijpers W (1985) Proximal symphalangia and stapes ankylosis. Archives of Otolaryngology 111: 765-7.

Cremers CWRJ (1986) Genetic aspects in neuro-otology. In House J, O'Connor AF (Eds) Handbook of Neurological Diagnosis. New York: Marcel Dekker.

Cremers CWRJ, Snik AFM, Beyon AJ (1992) Hearing with the bone-anchored hearing aid (BAHA HC 2000) compared to a conventional bone-conduction hearing aid. Clinical Otolaryngology 17: 275-9.

Cremers CWRJ, Brown SDM, Steel KP, Brunner HG, Read AP, Kimberling WJ (1995) Gene linkage and genetic deafness. Proceedings of International Journal of

Pediatric Otorhinolaryngology, Rotterdam 32: S167-S174.

Cremers FPM (1989) Choroideremia and deafness with stapes fixation: a contiguous gene deletion syndrome in Xq21. American Journal of Human Genetics 45: 415-9.

Cremers FPM, van de Pol TJR, van Kerkhoff EPM, Wieringa B, Ropers HH (1990) Cloning of a gene that is rearranged in patients with choroideremia. Nature 347: 674-7.

Crowe FW, Schull WJ, Neel JV (1956) A Clinical Pathological and Genetic Study of Multiple Neurofibromatosis. Springfield, Illinois: Charles C Thomas.

Curioni C, Clauser L (1989) Rigid skeletal fixation in craniomaxillofacial surgery for trauma, tumors, deformities. Paper presented at Symposium and Workshop – Cranio-maxillofacial Surgery and Rigid Skeletal Fixation. London 9-10 June.

Cyr D, Moore G, Möller C (1988) Clinical application of computerized dynamic posturography. Ear Nose and Throat Journal (suppl) 36-47.

Dallapiccola B, Mingarelli R, Novelli G (1995) The link between cytogenetics and mendelism. Biomed Pharmacotherapy 49: 83-93.

Dallos P (1986) Neurobiology of cochlear inner and outer hair cells: intracellular recordings. Hearing Research 22: 185-98.

Dallos P, Cheatham MA (1976) Production of cochlear potentials by inner and outer hair cells. Journal of the Acoustical Society of America 60: 510-12.

Dallos P, Schoeny ZG, Cheatham MA (1972) Cochlear summating potentials: descriptive aspects. Acta Otolaryngologica Supplement 302: 1-46.

Daniilidis J, Maganaris T, Dimitriadis A, Iliades T, Manolidis L (1978) Stapes gusher and the Klippel Feil syndrome. Laryngoscope 88: 1178-83.

Das VK (1987) Pendred's syndrome with episodic vertigo, tinnitus and vomiting and normal bithermal caloric responses. Journal of Laryngology and Otology 101: 721-2.

Davenport CB, Milles BL, Frink LB (1933) The genetic factor in otosclerosis. Archives of Otolaryngology 17: 135-70, 340-83, 503-48.

Davenport SLH, Omenn GS (1977) The heterogeneity of Usher syndrome. Publication no. 426. Amsterdam Excerpta Medica Foundation. International Congress Series abst. 215: 87-8.

David DJ, Poswillo D, Simpson D. (1982) The Craniosynostoses. Berlin: Springer Verlag.

Davidson J, Hyde ML, Alberti PW (1988) Epidemiology of hearing impairment in childhood. Scandinavian Audiology 30: 13-20.

Davis A. (1989) The prevalence of hearing impairment and reported hearing disability among adults in Great Britain. International Journal of Epidemiology 18: 911-7.

Davis A (1995) Hearing in Adults. London: Whurr.

Davis A, Parving A (1994) Towards appropriate epidemiology data on childhood hearing disability: a comparative European study of birth-cohorts 1982-1988. Journal of Audiological Medicine 3: 35-47.

Davis A, Wood S (1992) The epidemiology of childhood hearing impairment; factors of relevance to planning of services. British Journal of Audiology 26: 77-90.

Davis JG, Oberholtzer C, Burns FR, Greene MI (1995) Molecular cloning and characterization of an inner ear-specific structural protein. Science 267: 1031-4.

De Kleyn A (1915) Familiaire binnenoordoofheid. Nederlandse Tijdschrift van Geneeskunde 59: 1843.

De Kok YJM, van der Maarel SM, Bitner-Glindwiez M et al. (1995) Association between X-linked mixed deafness and mutations in the POU domain gene POU3F4. Science 267: 685-8.

Declau F (1991) Morfologische organisatie van het beenweefsel in het otische kapsel van de humane foetus. Ph.D Thesis. University of Antwerp, Belgium.

Demeester-Mirkine N, van Sande J, Corvilain B et al. (1975) Benign thyroid nodule with normal iodide trap and defective organification. Journal of Clinical Endocrinology and Metabolism 41: 1169-71.

Deol MS (1954) The anomalies of the labyrinth of the mutants *Varitint-waddler, Shaker-2* and *Jerker* in the mouse. Journal of Genetics 52: 562-94.

Deol MS (1956) The anatomy and development of the mutants *pirouette, shaker-1* and *waltzer* in the mouse. Proceedings of the Royal Society of London Series B 145: 206-13.

Deol MS (1966) Influence of the neural tube on the differentiation of the inner ear in the mammalian embryo. Nature 209: 219-20.

Deol MS (1980) Genetic malformations of the inner ear in the mouse and in man. Birth Defects 16: 243-61.

Deol MS, Kocher W (1958) A new gene for deafness in the mouse. Heredity 12: 463-6.

Deol MS, Robbins MW (1962) The spinner mouse. Journal of Heredity 53: 133-6.

Di George AM, Olmsted RW, Harley RD (1960) Waardenburg's syndrome. Journal of Pediatrics 57: 649-69.

Dias O, Andrea M (1990) Childhood hearing impairment and deafness in Portugal – etiological factors and diagnosis of hearing loss. International Journal of Pediatric Oto-Rhino-Laryngology 18: 247-55.

Diefendorf AO, Bull MJ, Casey-Harvey D et al. (1995) Down's syndrome – a multi-disciplinary perspective. Journal of the American Academy of Audiology 6: 39-46.

Dietrich WF, Miller JC, Steen RG et al. (1994) A genetic map of the mouse with 4,006 simple sequence length polymorphisms. Nature Genetics 7: 220-45.

Dixon MJ, Read AP, Donnai D, Colley A, Dixon J, Williamson R (1991a) The gene for Treacher Collins syndrome maps to the long arm of chromosome 5. American Journal of Human Genetics 49: 17-22.

Dixon MJ, Haan E, Baker E et al. (1991b) Association of Treacher Collins syndrome and translocation 6p21.31;16p13.11: exclusion of the locus from these candidate regions. American Journal of Human Genetics 48: 274-80.

Dixon MJ, Dixon J, Raskova D et al. (1992) Genetic and physical mapping of the Treacher Collins syndrome locus: refinement of the localization to chromosome 5q32-33.2. Human Molecular Genetics 1: 249-53.

Dixon MJ, Marres HAM, Edwards SJ, Dixon J, Cremers CWRJ (1994) Treacher Collins syndrome: correlation between clinical and genetic linkage studies. Clinical Dysmorphology 3: 96-103.

Dobin SM, Daniel CA (1988) Further delineation of the natural history of Kniest syndrome. Paper presented at March of Dimes Clinical Genetics Conference, Baltimore, July 1988.

Dolnick E (1993) Deafness as culture. Atlantic Monthly, September: 37-53.

Driscoll DA, Budarf ML, Emanuel BS (1992) A genetic etiology for DiGeorge syndrome: consistent deletions and microdeletions of 22q11. American Journal of Human Genetics 50: 924-33

Dryja TP, McGee TL, Reichel E et al. (1990) A point mutation of the rhodopsin gene in one form of retinitis pigmentosa. Nature 343: 364-6.

Eberwine J, Yeh H, Miyashiro K et al. (1992) Analysis of gene expression in single live neurons. Proceedings of the National Academy of Sciences of the USA 89: 3010-4.

Edery P, Manach Y, Le Merrer M et al. (1994) Apparent genetic homogeneity of the

Treacher Collins-Franceschetti syndrome. American Journal of Medical Genetics 52: 174-7.

Edwards SJ, Fowlie A, Cust MP, Liu DTY, Young ID, Dixon M (1996) Prenatal diagnosis in Treacher Collins syndrome using combined linkage analysis and ultrasound imaging. Journal of Medical Genetics (in press).

Elgoyhen AB, Johnson DS, Boulter J, Vetter DE, Heinemann S (1994) a9: an acetylcholine receptor with novel pharmacological properties expressed in rat cochlear hair cells. Cell 79: 705-15.

Ellis E. III, Carlson DS (1989) The effects of mandibular immobilization on the masticatory system: a review. Clinics in Plastic Surgery 16: 133-46.

Elman DS (1958) Familial association of nerve deafness with nodular goiter and thyroid carcinoma. New England Journal of Medicine 259: 219-23.

Engström H (1939) On the frequency of otosclerosis. Acta Otolaryngologica 27: 608-14.

Enlow DH (1957) Facial Growth. Philadelphia: Saunders.

Epstein CJ, Sahud MA, Piel CF et al. (1972) Hereditary macrothrombocytopenia, nephritis and deafness. American Journal of Medicine 52: 299-310.

Epstein DJ, Vekemans M, Gros P (1991) Splotch (Sp^{2H}), a mutation affecting development of the mouse neural tube, shows a deletion within the paired homeodomain of Pax3. Cell 67: 767-74.

Ernfors P, El Shamy WM, van De Water T, Loring J, Jaenisch R (1995) A crucial role of BDNF and NT-3 in vestibular and auditory development and their protective effects in the adult. In Proceedings of 2nd International Conference on The Molecular Biology of Hearing and Deafness, Bethesda. p 5.

Evans DGR, Huson SM, Donnai D et al. (1992a) A clinical study of type II neurofibromatosis. Quarterly Journal of Medicine 84: 603-18.

Evans DGR, Huson SM, Donnai D et al. (1992b) A genetic study of type II neurofibromatosis in the United Kingdom. I: Prevalence, mutation rate, fitness and confirmation of maternal transmission effect on severity. Journal of Medical Genetics 29: 841-6.

Evans DGR, Huson SM, Donnai D et al. (1992c) A genetic study of type II neurofibromatosis in the United Kingdom. II: Guidelines for genetic counselling. Journal of Medical Genetics 29: 847-52.

Evans DGR, Ramsden R, Huson SM, Harris R, Lye R, King TT. (1993) Type II neurofibromatosis: the need for supraregional care. Journal of Laryngology and Otology 107: 401-6.

Evans DGR, Bourn D, Wallace A, Ramsden RT, Mitchell JD, Strachan T (1995a) Diagnostic issues in a family with late onset type II neurofibromatosis. Journal of Medical Genetics 32: 470-4.

Evans DGR, Blair V, Strachan T, Lye RH, Ramsden RT (1995b) Variation in expression of the gene for type II neurofibromatosis: absence of a gender effect on vestibular schwannoma. Journal of Laryngology and Otology (in press).

Evans EF (1975) The sharpening of frequency selectivity in the normal and abnormal cochlea. Audiology 14: 419-42.

Evans KL, Fantes J, Simpson C et al. (1993) Human olfactory marker protein maps close to tyrosinase and is a candidate gene for Usher syndrome type I. Human Molecular Genetics 2: 115-8.

Everberg G (1957) Hereditary unilateral deafness. Acta Otolaryngologica 47: 303-11.

Ezoe K, Holmes SA, Ho L et al. (1995) Novel mutations and deletions of the KIT (steel factor receptor) gene in human piebaldism. American Journal of Human Genetics 56: 58-66.

Fargnoli J, Holbrook NJ, Forance AJ Jr (1990) Low-ratio hybridisation subtraction. Analytical Biochemistry 187: 364-73.

Farrar GJ, Kenna P, Jordan SA et al. (1991) A three-base-pair deletion in the peripherin-RDS gene in one form of retinitis pigmentosa. Nature 354: 478-80.

Farrer LA, Grundfast KM, Amos J et al. (1992) Waardenburg syndrome (WS) type I is caused by defects at multiple loci, one of which is near ALPP on chromosome 2: first report of the WS Consortium. American Journal of Human Genetics 50: 902-13.

Farrer LA, Arnos KS, Asher JH et al. (1994) Locus heterogeneity for Waardenburg syndrome is predictive of clinical subtypes. American Journal of Human Genetics 55: 728-37.

Fay EA (1898) Marriages of the Deaf in America. Washington, DC: Volta Bureau.

Feingold J, Bois E, Chompret A, Broyer M, Gubler MC, Grünfeld JP (1985) Genetic heterogeneity of Alport syndrome. Kidney Ant. 27: 672-7.

Feinmesser M, Tell L, Levi H (1990) Decline in the prevalence of childhood deafness in the Jewish population of Jerusalem. Ethnic and genetic aspects. Journal of Laryngology and Otology 104: 675-7.

Fisch L (1955)The aetiology of congenital deafness and audimetric patterns. Journal of Laryngology and Otology 69: 479-93.

Fisch L (1959) Deafness as part of an hereditary syndrome. Journal of Laryngology 73: 355-82.

Fischel-Ghodsian N, Prezant TR, Bu X, Öztas S (1993) Mitochondrial ribosomal RNA gene mutation associated with aminoglycoside ototoxicity. American Journal of Otology 14: 399-403.

Fischel-Ghodsian N, Prezant TR, Chaltran W et al. (1996) Mitochondrial gene mutations are a common predisposing factor in aminoglycoside ototoxicity. American Journal of Otolaryngology (in press).

Fischel-Ghodsian N, Prezant TR, Bu X, Öztas S (1993) Mitochondrial ribosomal RNA gene mutation associated with aminoglycoside ototoxicity. American Journal of Otology 14: 399-403.

Fishman GA (1979) Usher's syndrome: visual loss and variations in clinical expressivity. Perspectives in Ophthalmology 3: 99-103.

Fishman GA, Kumar A, Joseph ME, Torok N, Anderson RJ (1983) Usher's syndrome: ophthalmic and neuro-otologic findings suggesting genetic heterogeneity. Archives of Ophthalmology 110: 1367-74.

Fitch N, Srolovitz H (1976) Severe renal dysgenesis produced by a dominant gene. American Journal of Diseases in Children 130: 1356-7.

Forge A (1991) Structural features of lateral wall in mammalian cochlear outer hair cells. Cell and Tissue Research 265: 473-83.

Fourman P, Fourman J (1955) Hereditary deafness in family with ear-pits (fistula auris congenita) British Medical Journal 2: 1354-6.

Fox RM, Wood MH, Royse-Smith D, O'Sullivan WJ (1973) Hereditary orotic aciduria: Types I and II. American Journal of Medicine 55: 791-8.

Fox S, Eicher EM, Reynolds S (1978) Mouse Newsletter 59: 50.

Foy C, Newton VE, Wellesley D, Harris R, Read AP (1990) Assignment of WS I locus to human 2q37 and possible homology between Waardenburg syndrome and the *Splotch* mouse. American Journal of Human Genetics 46: 1017-23.

France EA, Stephens SDG (1995) The all Wales audiology and genetic service for hearing impaired young adults. Journal of Audiological Medicine 4: 67-84.

Franceschetti A, Klein D (1949) Mandibulo-facial dysostosis: new hereditary syndrome. Acta Ophthalmologica 27: 143-224.

Frank U, Lasson U (1985) Ophthalmoplegic neurolipidosis storage cells in heterozygotes. Neuropediatrics 16: 3-6.

Fraser FC, Ling D, Clogg D, Nogrady B (1978) Genetic aspects of the BOR syndrome – branchial fistulas, ear pits, hearing loss and renal anomalies. American Journal of Medical Genetics 2: 241-52.

Fraser FC, Sproule JR, Halal F (1980) Frequency of the branchio-oto-renal (BOR) syndrome in children with profound hearing loss. American Journal of Medical Genetics 7: 341-9.

Fraser FC, Aymé S, Halal F, Sproule J (1983) Autosomal dominant duplication of the renal collecting system, hearing loss, and external ear anomalies: a new syndrome? American Journal of Medical Genetics 14: 473-8.

Fraser GR, Morgans ME, Trotter WR (1960) The syndrome of sporadic goitre and congenital deafness. Quarterly Journal of Medicine 29: 279-95.

Fraser GR (1964) In Fisch L (Ed) Research in Deafness in Children. Oxford: Blackwell. pp 10-13.

Fraser GR (1965) Sex-linked recessive congenital deafness and the excess of males in profound childhood deafness. Annals of Human Genetics 29: 171-96.

Fraser GR (1965) Association of congenital deafness with goitre (Pendred's syndrome). Annals of Human Genetics 28: 201-48.

Fraser GR (1976) The Causes of Profound Deafness in Childhood. Baltimore: Johns Hopkins University Press.

Friedmann I (1974) Pathology of the Ear. Oxford: Blackwell.

Friedman TB, Liang Y, Weber JL et al. (1995) A gene for congenital, recessive deafness DFNB3 maps to the pericentromeric region of chromosome 17. Nature Genetics 9: 86-91.

Friis J (1987) The perchlorate discharge test with and without supplement of potassium iodide. Journal of Endocrinological Investigation 10: 581-4.

Fryns JP, van den Berghe H (1986) 8q24.1 interstitial deletion in the tricho-rhino-pharyngeal syndrome type I. Human Genetics 74: 188-9.

Fukushima K, Ramesh A, Srisailapathy CRS et al. (1995a) Consanguineous nuclear families used to identify a new locus for recessive non-syndromic hearing loss on 14q. Human Molecular Genetics 4: 1643-8.

Fukushima K, Ramesh A, Srisailapathy CRS et al. (1995b) An autosomal recessive non-syndromic form of sensorineural hearing loss maps to 3p-DFNB6. Genome Research 5: 305-8.

Funasaka S (1979) Congenital ossicular anomalies without malformations of the external ear. Archives of Otorhinolaryngology 224: 231-40.

Furusho T, Yasuda N (1973) Genetic studies on inbreeding in some Japanese populations. XIII. A genetic study of congenital deafness. Japanese Journal of Human Genetics 18: 47-65.

Gale JE, Ashmore JA (1995) Microsecond resolution of patch movement and associated charge displacement in the lateral membrane of guinea-pig outer hair cells. Journal of Physiology (in press).

Gapany-Gapanavicius B (1975) Otosclerosis: Genetics and Surgical Rehabilitation. Jerusalem: Keter.

Gardner WJ, Frazier CH (1930) Bilateral acoustic neurofibromas: a clinical study and field survey of a family of five generations with bilateral deafness in thirty eight members. Archives of Neurology and Psychiatry 23: 266-302.

Garruba V, Grandori F, Lamoretti M, Nicolai P, Zanetti D, Antonelli AR (1991) Electric response audiometry in infants and preschool children. Long term control of the result. Acta Otolaryngologica Supplement 482: 36

Gausden E, Armour JAL, Coyle B et al. (1996) Thyroid peroxidase : evidence for disease gene exclusion in Pendred syndrome. Clinical Endocrinology (in press).

Geissler EN, Ryan MA, Housman DE (1988) The dominant white spotting (*W*) locus of the mouse encodes the *c-kit* proto-oncogene. Cell 55: 185-92.

Gerhardt HJ, Otto HD (1970) Steigbügelmissbildungen. Acta Otolaryngologica 70: 35-44.

Gershoni-Baruch R, Baruch Y, Viener A, Lichtig C (1988) Fechtner syndrome: clinical and genetic aspects. American Journal of Medical Genetics 31: 357-67.

Giacoia JP, Klein SW (1969) Waardenburg's syndrome with bilateral cleft lip. American Journal of Diseases of Childhood 117: 344-8.

Gibson F, Walsh J, Mburu P et al. (1995) A type VII myosin encoded by the mouse deafness gene *shaker-1*. Nature 374: 62-4.

Gillies H, Millard DR (1957) The Principles and Art of Plastic Surgery. Boston: Little Brown.

Gimsing S, Dyrmose J (1986) Branchio-oto-renal dysplasia in three families. Annals of Otology, Rhinology and Laryngology 95: 421-6.

Glasscock ME (1973) The stapes gusher. Archives of Otolaryngology 98: 82-91.

Gold M, Rapin I (1994) Non-Mendelian mitochondrial inheritance as a cause of progressive genetic sensorineural hearing loss. International Journal of Pediatric Oto-Rhino-Laryngology 30: 91-104.

Goldberg MF (1966) Waardenburg's syndrome with fundus and other anomalies. Archives of Ophthalmology 76: 797-809.

Goldberg R, Motzkin B, Marion R, Scambler PJ, Shprintzen RJ (1993) Velo-cardio-facial syndrome: a review of 120 cases. American Journal of Medical Genetics 45: 313-9.

Goldstein DP, Stephens SDG (1981) Audiological rehabilitation: management model I. Audiology 20: 432-52.

Gordon MA (1989) The genetics of otosclerosis: a review. American Journal of Otology 10: 426-38.

Gordon MA, McPhee JR, van De Water TR, Ruben RJ (1992) Aberration of the tissue collagenase system in association with otosclerosis. American Journal of Otology 13: 398-407.

Gorga MP, Neely ST, Bergman BM, Beauchaine KL, Kaminsky JR, Liu Z (1994) Towards understanding the limits of distortion product otoacoustic emission measurements. Journal of the Acoustical Society of America 96: 1494-500.

Gorlin RJ, Meskin LH, Geme JWS (1963) Oculodentodigital dysplasia. Journal of Pediatrics 63: 69-75.

Gorlin RJ, Poznanski AK, Hendon I (1973) The otopalatodigital (OPD) syndrome in females: heterozygote expression of an X-linked trait. Oral Surgery 35: 218-24.

Gorlin RJ, Cohen MM. Levin SL (1990) Syndromes of the Head and Neck. 3rd edn. New York, Oxford: Oxford University Press.

Gorlin RJ, Toriello HV, Cohen MM (Eds) (1995) Hereditary Hearing Loss and its Syndromes. Oxford: Oxford University Press.

Gorlin RJ (1995) Genetic hearing loss with no associated abnormalities. In Gorlin RJ, Toriello HV, Cohen MM (Eds) Hereditary Hearing Loss and its Syndromes, pp43-61. Oxford: Oxford University Press.

Goto Y, Nonaka I, Horai S (1990) A mutation in the tRNA[Leu(UUR)] gene associated with the MELAS subgroup of mitochondrial encephalomyopathies. Nature 348: 651-3.

Green ED, Cox DR, Myers RM (1995) The human genome project and its impact on the study of human diseases. In Scriver CR et al. (Eds) The Metabolic Bases of Inherited Disease. 7th edn. New York: McGraw-Hill.

Greenberg CR, Trevenen CL, Evans JA (1988) The BOR syndrome and renal agenesis – prenatal diagnosis and further clinical delineation. Prenatal Diagnosis 8: 103-8.

Gristwood RE, Venables WN (1983) Pregnancy and otosclerosis. Clinics in Otolaryngology 8: 205-10.

Grondahl J (1986) Tapeto-retinal degeneration in four Norwegian counties. I. Diagnostic evaluation of 89 probands. Clinical Genetics 29: 1-16.

Gubler U, Hoffman BJ (1983) A simple and very efficient method for generating cDNA libraries. Gene 25: 263-9.

Guild SR (1944) Histologic otosclerosis. Annals of Otology, Rhinology and Laryngology 53: 246-67.

Guilford P, Ayadi H, Blanchard S et al. (1994a) A human gene responsible for neurosensory, non-syndromic recessive deafness is a candidate homologue of the mouse *sh-1* gene. Human Molecular Genetics 3: 989-93.

Guilford P, Ben Arab, S, Blanchard S et al. (1994b) A non-syndromic form of neurosensory, recessive deafness maps to the pericentromeric region of chromosome 13q. Nature Genetics 6: 24-8.

Guilford P, Dode C, Crozet F et al. (1995) A YAC contig and an EST map in the pericentromeric region of chromosome 13 surrounding the loci for neurosensory nonsyndromic deafness (*DFNB1* and *DFNA3*) and limb-girdle muscular dystrophy type IIC (*LGMD2C*). Genomics 29: 163-9.

Gulley RL, Reese TS (1977) Regional specialisation of hair cell plasmalemma in organ of Corti. Anatomical Record 189: 109-24.

Gundersen T (1967) Congenital malformations of the stapes footplate. Archives of Otolaryngology 85: 171-6.

Haan EA, Hull YJ, White S, Cockington R, Charlton P, Callen DF (1989) Tricho-rhino-phalangeal and branchio-oto-renal syndromes in a family with an inherited rearrangement of chromosome 8q. American Journal of Medical Genetics 32: 490-4.

Haber DA, Buckler AJ, Glaser T et al. (1990) An internal deletion within an 11p13 zinc finger gene contributes to the development of Wilms' tumor. Cell 61: 1257-69.

Hageman M, Delleman J (1977) Heterogeneity in Waardenburg syndrome. American Journal of Human Genetics 29: 468-85.

Hageman M, Oosterveld WJ (1977) Vestibular findings in 25 patients with Waardenburg syndrome. Acta Otolaryngologica 103: 648-52.

Hall JG (1974) Otosclerosis in Norway. A geographical and genetical study. Acta Otolaryngologica Supplement 324: 1-20.

Hall JG, Froster-Iskenius UG, Allanson JE (1989) Handbook of Normal Physical Measurements. Oxford: Oxford Medical Publication.

Hall JW III, San Agustin TB, Lesperance MM, Wilcox ER, Bess FH (1995) Autosomal dominant nonsyndromic low frequency hearing loss in five generations. In Proceedings of 2nd International Conference on The Molecular Biology of Hearing and Deafness, Bethesda. p 105.

Hallgren B (1959) Retinitis pigmentosa combined with congenital deafness; with vestibulo-cerebellar ataxia and mental abnormality in a proportion of cases. A clinical and genetico-statistical study. Acta Psychiatrica Scandinavica 34 (supplement 138): 5-101.

Hammerschlag V (1905) Zur Frage der Vererbbarkeit der 'Otosklerose'. Wiener

Klinische Rundschau 19: 5-7.

Hartmann A (1880) Taubstummenheit und Taubstummenbildung nach den vorhandenen Quellen, sowie beiliegenen Beobachtungen und Erfahrungen. Stuttgart.

Harvey D, Steel KP (1992) The development and interpretation of the summating potential response. Hearing Research 61: 137-46.

Hasson T, Mooseker M (1995) Molecular motors, membrane movements and physiology: emerging roles for myosins. Current Opinion in Cell Biology 7: 587-94.

Hastbacka J, Sistonen P, Kaitila I, Weiffenbach B, Kidd KK, de la Chapelle A (1991) A linkage map spanning the locus for diastrophic dysplasia (DTD). Genomics 11: 968-73.

Hastbacka J, de la Chapelle A, Mahtami MM et al. (1994) The diastrophic dysplasia gene encodes a novel sulfate transporter: positional cloning by fine-structure linkage disequilibrium mapping. Cell 78: 1073-87.

Hedrick S, Cohen DI, Nielsen EA, Davis MM. (1984) Isolation of cDNA clones encoding T-cell-specific membrane-associated proteins. Nature 308: 149-53.

Heidet L, Dahan K, Zhou J et al. (1995) Deletions of both α5(IV) and α6(IV) collagen genes in Alport syndrome and in Alport syndrome associated with smooth muscle tumours. Human Molecular Genetics 4: 99-108.

Heimler A, Lieber E (1986) Branchio-oto-renal syndrome: reduced penetrance and variable expressivity in four generations of a large kindred. American Journal of Medical Genetics 25: 15-27.

Hernandez-Orozco F, Courtney GT (1964) Genetic aspects of clinical otosclerosis. Annals of Otology, Rhinology and Laryngology 73: 632-44.

Hernden JH, Steinberg D, Uhlendorf BW (1969) Refsum's disease: defective oxidation of phytanic acid in tissue cultures derived from homozygotes and heterozygotes. New England Journal of Medicine 281: 1034-8.

Herrmann J (1974) Symphalangism and brachydactyly syndromes. Report of the WL symphalangism-brachydactyly syndrome. Birth Defects: Original Article Series 10: 23-53.

Heusinger CF (1864) Hals-Kiemen-Fisteln von noch nicht beobachteter Form. Virchows Archive der Anatomie 29: 358-80.

Higashi K (1989) Unique inheritance of streptomycin-induced deafness. Clinical Genetics 35: 433-6.

Hirsch, A (1988) Hearing loss and associated handicaps in pre-school children. Scandinavian Audiology, Supplementum 30: 31-64.

Hodgkinson CA, Moore KJ, Nakayama A et al. (1993) Mutations at the mouse microphthalmia locus are associated with defects in a gene encoding a novel basic helix-loop-helix zipper protein. Cell 74: 395-404.

Hoeksema PE (1967) Congenital deformation of the middle ear. Practica ORL (Basel) 29: 143-4.

Holmgren L (1958) Mobilizing in a case of congenital fixed stapes. Acta Otolaryngologica Supplement 140: 152-9.

Horan FT, Beighton P (1978) Osteopathia striata with cranial sclerosis: an autosomal dominant entity. Clinical Genetics 13: 201-6.

Hough J (1958) Malformations and anatomical variations seen in the middle ear during the operation for mobilization of the stapes. Laryngoscope 68: 1337-79.

House HP, House WF, Hildyard VH (1958) Congenital stapes footplate fixation: a preliminary report of twenty-three operated cases. Laryngoscope 63: 932-51.

House HP (1969) Congenital fixation of the stapes footplate. In Hearing loss-problems in diagnosis and treatment. Otolaryngological Clinics of North America 35-51.

House JW, Sheehy JL, Antunez JC (1980) Stapedectomy in children. Laryngoscope 90: 1804-9.

Hovnanian A, Duquesnoy P, Blanchet-Bardon C et al. (1992) Genetic linkage of recessive dystrophic epidermolysis bullosa to the type VII collagen gene. Journal of Clinical Investigation 90: 1032-6.

Howell N (1994) Mitochondrial gene mutations and human diseases: a prolegomenon. American Journal of Human Genetics 55: 219-24.

Hu DN, Qiu WQ, Wu BT et al. (1987) Prevalence and genetic aspects of deaf mutism in Shanghai. Journal of Medical Genetics 24: 589-92.

Hu DN, Qui WQ, Wu BT et al. (1991) Genetic aspects of antibiotic induced deafness: mitochondrial inheritance. Journal of Medical Genetics 28: 79-83.

Hudson BG, Kalluri R, Gunwar S et al. (1992) The pathogenesis of Alport syndrome involves type IV collagen molecules containing the α3(IV) chain; evidence from anti-GBM nephritis after renal transplantation. Kidney Ant. 42: 179-87.

Hudspeth AJ, Gillespie PG (1994) Pulling springs to tune transduction: adaptation by hair cells. Neuron 12: 1-9.

Hueb MM, Goycoolea MV, Paparella MM, Oliveira JA (1991) Otosclerosis: the University of Minnesota temporal bone collection. Otolaryngology and Head and Neck Surgery 105: 396-405.

Hughes AE, Newton VE, Liu XZ, Read AP (1994) A gene for Waardenburg syndrome type II maps close to *MITF*, the human homologue of the mouse *microphthalmia* gene, at chromosomal location 3p12-pl4.1. Nature Genetics 7: 509-12.

Huson SM, Compston DAS, Harper PS (1989) A genetic study of von Recklinghausen neurofibromatosis in South East Wales. II: Guidelines for genetic counselling. Journal of Medical Genetics 26: 704-11.

Hutchin T, Haworth I, Higashi K et al. (1993) A molecular basis for human hypersensitivity to aminoglycoside antibiotics. Nucleic Acids Research 21: 4174-9.

Hutchin T, Cortopassi G. (1995) A molecular and cellular model for aminoglycoside-induced deafness. Hereditary Deafness Newsletter 10: 37.

Hutchinson JC, Calderelli DD, Valvassori GE, Pruzansky S, Parris PJ (1977) The otologic manifestations of mandibulofacial dysostosis. Transactions of the American Academy of Ophthalmology and Otolaryngology 84: 520-29.

Huygen PL, Verhagen WIM, Noten JFP (1994) Auditory abnormalities, including 'precocious presbyacusis' in myotonic dystrophy. Audiology 33: 73-84.

Hvidberg-Hansen J, Balslev Jorgensen M (1968) The inner ear in Pendred's syndrome. Acta Otolaryngologica 66: 129-35.

Hyde ML, Riko K, Malizia K (1990) Audiometric accuracy of the click ABR in infants at risk for hearing loss. Journal of the American Academy of Audiology 1: 59-66.

HYP Consortium (1995) A gene (*PEX*) with homologies to endopeptidases is mutated in patients with X-linked hypophosphatemic rickets. Nature Genetics 11: 130-6.

Illum P, Kiaer HW, Hvidberg-Hansen J et al. (1972) Fifteen cases of Pendred's syndrome. Archives of Otolaryngology 96: 297-304.

Ishikiriyama S, Tonoki H, Shibuya Y et al. (1989) Waardenburg syndrome type I in a child with de novo inversion (2) (q35q37.3). American Journal of Medical Genetics 33: 505-7.

ISO 7029 (1984) Acoustics – Threshold of Hearing by Air Conduction as a Function of Age and Sex for Otologically Normal Persons. Geneva: International Organization for Standardization.

Israel J (1989) Counselling in deaf/hearing impaired adult populations. Perspectives in Genetic Counselling 22: 1-4.

Jaber L, Shohat M, Bu X et al. (1992) Sensorineural deafness inherited as a tissue specific mitochondrial disorder. Journal of Medical Genetics 29: 86-90.

Jabs EW, Coss CA, Hayflick SJ et al. (1991a) Chromosomal deletion 4p15.32-p14 in a Treacher Collins syndrome patient: Exclusion of the disease locus from and mapping of anonymous DNA sequences to this region. Genomics 11: 188-92.

Jabs EW, Li X, Coss CA, Taylor EW, Meyers DA, Weber JL (1991b) Mapping the Treacher Collins syndrome locus to 5q31.3-q33.3. Genomics 11: 193-8.

Jabs EW, Li X, Lovett M et al. (1993) Genetic and physical mapping of the Treacher Collins syndrome locus with respect to loci in the chromosome 5q3 region. Genomics 18: 7-13.

Jackson IT, Somers PC, Kjar JG (1986) The use of Champy miniplates for osthesynthesis in craniofacial deformities. Plastic and Reconstructive Surgery 77: 729-36.

Jacobson JT (1995) Nosology of deafness. Journal of American Academy of Audiology 6: 15-27.

Jacobsson M, Tjellstrom A, Fine L, Jansson K (1992) An evaluation of auricular prostheses using osseointegrated implants. Clinical Otolaryngology 17: 482-6.

Jahrsdörfer R (1980) Congenital malformations of the ear. Analysis of 94 operations. Annals of Otology and Laryngology 89: 348-52.

Jain PK, Deshmukh D, Thomas E et al. (1995) Non-syndromic recessive hearing impairment gene maps to chromosome 9q11-q13. In Proceedings of 2nd International Conference on The Molecular Biology of Hearing and Deafness, Bethesda. p 24.

Jain PK, Fukushima K, Deshmukh D et al. (1995) A human recessive neurosensory nonsyndromic hearing impairment locus is a potential homologue of the murine deafness (dn) locus. Human Molecular Genetics 4: 2391-4.

James WH (1991) Sex ratios in otosclerotic families. Journal of Laryngology and Otology 103: 1036-9.

Johnsen S (1954) Some aetiological aspects of high tone perceptive deafness in children. Acta Otolaryngologica 44: 175, 205.

Johnsen T, Balslev Jorgensen M, Johnsen S (1986) Mondini cochlea in Pendred's syndrome. Acta Otolaryngologica 102: 239-47.

Johnsen T, Larsen C, Friis J et al. (1987) Pendred's syndrome: acoustic, vestibular and radiological findings in 17 unrelated patients. Journal of Laryngology and Otology 101: 1187-92.

Johnsen T, Sorensen MS, Feldt-Rasmussen U et al. (1989a) The variable intrafamiliar expressivity in Pendred's syndrome. Clinical Otolaryngology 14: 395-9.

Johnsen T, Videbaek H, Olsen KP (1989b) CT-Scanning of the cochlea in Pendred's syndrome. Clinical Otolaryngology 14: 389-93.

Johnstone JR, Alder VA, Johnstone BM, Robertson D, Yates GK (1979) Cochlear action potential threshold and single unit thresholds. Journal of the Acoustical Society of America 65: 254-7.

Jones KL (1988) Smith's Recognizable Patterns of Human Malformation. Philadelphia: WB Saunders.

Jordan IK (1991) Ethical issues in the genetic study of deafness. Annals of the New York Academy of Sciences 630: 236-9.

Jorgensen MB, Kristensen HK (1967) Frequency of histological otosclerosis. Annals of Otology, Rhinology and Laryngology76: 83-8.

Kaback MM, Nathan TJ, Greenwald S (1977) Tay-Sachs disease: Heterozygote screening and prenatal diagnosis – U.S. experience and world perspective. In Kaback MM (Ed): Tay-Sachs Disease: Screening and Prevention. New York: Liss. p 13.

Kabat C (1943) A family history of deafness. Journal of Heredity 34: 377-8.

Kacser H, Burns JA. (1981) The molecular basis of dominance. Genetics 97: 639-66.

Kadowaki T, Kadowaki H, Mori Y et al. (1994) A subtype of diabetes mellitus associated with a mutation of mitochondrial DNA. New England Journal of Medicine 330: 962-8.

Kaiser-Kupfer MI, Freidlin V, Datiles MB et al. (1989) The association of posterior capsular lens opacities with bilateral acoustic neuromas in patients with neurofibromatosis type II. Archives of Ophthalmology 107: 541-4.

Kajiwara K, Hahn LB, Mukai S, Travis GH, Berson EL, Dryja TP (1991) Mutations in the human retinal degeneration slow gene in autosomal dominant retinitis pigmentosa. Nature 354: 480-3.

Kajiwara K, Berson EL, Dryja TP (1994) Digenic retinitis pigmentosa due to mutations at the unlinked peripherin/*RDS* and *ROM1* loci. Science 264: 1604-8.

Kalluri R, van den Heuvel LP, Smeets HJM et al. (1995) A *COL4A3* gene mutation and post-transplantantion-α3(IV) collagen alloantibodies in Alport syndrome. Kidney International 47: 1199-204.

Kankkunen A (1982) Pre-school children with impaired hearing. Acta Otolaryngologica Supplementum 391: 59-99.

Kanter WR, Eldridge R, Fabricant R, Allen JC, Koerber T (1980) Central neurofibromatosis with bilateral acoustic neuroma: Genetic, clinical and biochemical distinctions from peripheral neurofibromatosis. Neurology 30: 851-9.

Kaplan J, Gerbers G, Bonneau D et al. (1991) Probable location of Usher type I gene on chromosome 14q by linkage with D14S13 (MLJ14 probe). Cytogenetics and Cell Genetics 58: 1988.

Kaplan J, Gerbers G, Bonneau D et al. (1992) A gene for Usher syndrome type I (USH1A) maps to chromosome 14q. Genomics 14: 979-87.

Karjalainen S, Pakarinen L, Terasvirta M, Kaariainen H, Vartiainen E. (1989) Progressive hearing loss in Usher's syndrome. Annals of Otology, Rhinology and Laryngology 38: 863-6.

Kashtan C, Fish AJ, Kieppel MM, Yoshioka K, Michael AF (1986) Nephritogenic antigen determinant in epidermal and renal basement membranes of kindreds with Alport-type familial nephritis. Journal of Clinical Investigation 78: 1035-44.

Katagiri H, Asano T, Ishihara H et al. (1994) Mitochondrial diabetes mellitus: prevalence and clinical characterization of diabetes due to mitochondrial tRNA[Leu(UUR)] gene mutation in Japanese patients. Diabetologia 37: 504-10.

Kay ED, Kay CN (1989) Dysmorphogenesis of the mandible, zygoma, and middle ear ossicles in hemifacial microsomia and mandibulofacial dysostosis. American Journal of Medical Genetics 32: 27-31.

Keats BJB, Nouri N, Huang J-M, Money M, Webster DB, Berlin CI (1995) The *deafness* locus (*dn*) maps to mouse chromosome 19. Mammalian Genome 6: 8-10.

Keith RW (1973) Impedance audiometry with neonates. Archives of Otolaryngology and Head and Neck Surgery 97: 465-7.

Kelemen G, Alonso A (1980) Penetration of the cochlear endost by the fibrous component of the otosclerotic focus. Acta Otolaryngologica 89: 453-8.

Kemp DT (1978) Stimulated acoustic emissions from within the human auditory system. Journal of the Acoustical Society of America 64: 1386-91.

Kiang NYS, Watanabe T, Thomas EC, Clark LF (1965) Discharge Patterns of Single Fibers in the Cat's Auditory Nerve. (Res. Monograph No. 35) Cambridge: M.I.T. Press.

Kimberling W J (1993) Difficulties and opportunities in the study of genetic deafness. Paper given at the Royal Society of Medicine Symposium on Molecular

Genetics in Hearing Impairment. London.

Kimberling WJ, Smith SD, Ing PS, Tinley S (1989) A comment on the analysis of families with prelingual deafness. American Journal of Human Genetics 45: 157-8.

Kimberling WJ, Weston MD, Möller C et al. (1990) Localization of Usher syndrome type II to chromosome 1q. Genomics 7: 245-9.

Kimberling WJ, Möller CG, Davenport S et al. (1992) Linkage of Usher syndrome type I gene (USH1B) to the long arm of chromosome 11. Genomics 14: 988-94.

Kimberling WJ, Weston, MD, Möller C et al. (1995) Gene mapping of Usher syndrome type IIa: localization of the gene to a 2.1-cM segment on chromosome lq41. American Journal of Human Genetics 56: 216-23.

Kimura S, Hong YS, Kotani T et al. (1989) Structure of the human thyroid peroxidase gene: comparison and relationship to the human myeloperoxidase gene. Biochemistry 28: 4481-9.

Kirschhofer K, Hoover DM, Kenyon JB et al. (1995) Localisation of a gene responsible for an autosomal dominant non-syndromic sensorineural hearing loss to chromosome 15. In Proceedings of 2nd International Conference on The Molecular Biology of Hearing and Deafness, Bethesda. p 100.

Klein D (1983) Historical background and evidence for dominant inheritance of the Klein-Waardenburg syndrome (type III). American Journal of Medical Genetics 14: 231-9.

Kleppel MM, Kashtan CE, Butkowski RJ, Fish AJ, Michael AF (1987) Alport familial nephritis: absence of 28 kilodalton non-collagenous monomers of type IV collagen in glomerular basement membrane. Journal of Clinical Investigation 80: 263-6.

Kleppel MM, Fan WW, Cheong HI, Michael AF (1992) Evidence for separate networks of classical and novel basement membrane collagen. Characterization of α 3(IV)-Alport antigen heterodimer. Journal of Biological Chemistry 267: 4137-42.

Kloepfer HW, Laguaite JK, McLaurin JW (1966) The hereditary syndrome of congenital deafness and retinitis pigmentosa (Usher's syndrome). Laryngoscope 76: 850-62.

Knowlton RG, Weaver EJ, Struyk AF et al. (1989) Genetic linkage analysis of hereditary arthro-ophthalmopathy (Stickler syndrome) and the type II procollagen gene. American Journal of Human Genetics 45: 681-8.

Kobayashi S, Amikura R, Okada M (1993) Presence of mitochondrial large ribosomal RNA outside mitochondria in germ plasm of Drosophila melanogaster. Science 260: 1521-4.

Københavns Statistiske Årbog (1975; 1993) Copenhagen: Copenhagen Statistical Department.

Koch MC, Steinmeyer K, Lorenz C et al. (1992) The skeletal muscle chloride channel in dominant and recessive human myotonia. Science 257: 797-800.

Konigsmark BW, Gorlin RJ (1976) Genetic and Metabolic Deafness. Philaldelphia: Saunders.

Körner O (1905) Das Wesen der Otosklerose im Lichte der Vererbungslehre. Zeitschrift fur Ohrenheilkunde 50: 98.

Kraus N, Ozdamar O, Stein L, Reed N (1984) Absent auditory brain stem response: peripheral hearing loss or brainstem dysfunction? Laryngoscope 94: 400-6.

Kreiborg S (1981) Crouzon syndrome. Scandinavian Journal of Plastic and Reconstructive Surgery Supplement 18: 1-198.

Kumar S, Kimberling WJ, Kenyon JB, Smith RJH, Marres HAM, Cremers CWRJ (1992) Autosomal dominant branchio-oto-renal syndrome – localization of a disease gene to chromosome 8q by linkage in a Dutch family. Human Molecular Genetics 7: 491-5.

Kumar S, Kimberling W, Conolly C, Tinley S, Marres H, Cremers C (1994) Refining the region of branchio-oto-renal syndrome and defining the flanking markers on chromosome 8q by genetic mapping. American Journal of Human Genetics 55: 1188-94.

Lalwani AK, Brister JR, Fex J et al. (1994) A new nonsyndromic X-linked sensorineural hearing impairment linked to Xp21.2. American Journal of Human Genetics 55: 685-94.

Lander ES, Botstein D (1987) Homozygosity mapping: a way to map human recessive traits with the DNA of inbred children. Science 236: 1567-70.

Lander ES, Schork NJ (1994) Genetic dissection of complex traits. Science 265: 2037-48.

Lane PW, Deol MS (1974) Mocha, a new coat color and behavior mutation on chromosome 10 of the mouse. Journal of Heredity 65: 362-4.

Lane W, Robson M, Lowry RB, Lenny AKC (1994) X-linked recessive nephritis with mental retardation, sensorineural hearing loss, and macrocephaly. Clinical Genetics 45: 314-7.

Langenbeck B (1935) Das Symmetriegesetz der erblichen Taubheit. Zeitschrift für Ohrenheilkunde 223: 261.

Langenbeck B (1938) Symmetriesymptome, Symmetrieregel und Symmetriegesetz. Zeitschrift fur Hals, Nase und Ohrenheilkunde 43: 370-86.

Larsson A (1960) Otosclerosis: a genetic and clinical study. Acta Otolaryngologica Supplement 154: 1-86.

Laurie SWS, Kaban LB, Mulliken JB, Murray JE (1984) Donor-site morbidity after harvesting rib and iliac bone. Plastic and Reconstructive Surgery 73: 933-7.

Le Fort R (1901) Etude expérimentale sur les fractures de la machoire supérieure. Revue de Chirurgie 23: 208, 360, 479.

Le Guern E, Couillin P, Oberlé I, Ravise N, Boué AJ (1990) More precise localization of the gene for Hunter syndrome. Genomics 7: 358-62.

Lenardt M (1981) Childhood central auditory processing disorder with brainstem evoked response verification. Archives of Otolaryngology 107: 623-5.

Lenzi A, Zaghis A (1988) Incidence of genetic factors in the causation of deafness in childhood. Scandinavian Audiology Supplementum 30: 37-41.

Leon PE, Bonilla JA, Sanchez JR et al. (1981) Low frequency hereditary deafness in man with childhood onset. American Journal of Human Genetics 33: 209-14.

Leon PE, Raventos H, Lynch'E, Morrow J, King M-C (1992) The gene for an inherited form of deafness maps to chromosome 5q31. Proceedings of the National Academy of Sciences of the USA 89: 5181-4.

Leppert MF, Lewis RA (1991) Human genetic mapping and inherited deafness syndromes. In Ruben RJ, van der Water TR, Steel KP (Eds) Genetics of hearing impairment. Annals of New York Academy of Science 630: 38-48.

Leske MC (1981) Prevalence estimates of communicative disorders in the U.S. Language, hearing and vestibular disorders. American Speech and Hearing Association 23: 229-37.

Lesperance MM, Hall JW, Bess FH et al. (1995) A gene for autosomal dominant nonsyndromic hereditary hearing impairment maps to 4p16.3. Human Molecular Genetics 4: 1967-72.

Levin G, Fabian P, Stahle J (1988) Incidence of otosclerosis. American Journal of Otology 9: 299-301.

Lewin B (1987) Genes III. New York: John Wiley. p 382.

Lewis RA et al. (1990) Mapping recessive ophthalmic diseases: linkage of the locus for Usher syndrome type II to a DNA marker on chromosome 1q. Genomics 7: 250-6.

Liberman MC (1982) The cochlear frequency map for the cat: labelling auditory-nerve fibers of known characteristic frequency. Journal of the Acoustical Society of America 72: 1441-9.

Lidenov H (1945) The etiology of deaf-mutism with special reference to heredity. Opera ex Domo Biologicae Hereditariae Humanae Universitatis Hafniensis 8: 1-268.

Lindhout D, Frets P, Niermeijer M (1991) Approaches to genetic counselling. In Ruben RJ, van der Water TR, Steel KP (Eds) Genetics of hearing impairment. Annals of the New York Academy of Science 630: 223-9.

Lindsay EA, Goldberg R, Juredic V et al. (1995) Velo-cardio-facial syndrome: frequency and extent of 22q11 deletions. American Journal of Medical Genetics 57: 514-22.

Lindsay JR, Beal DD (1966) Sensorineural deafness in otosclerosis: observations on histopathology. Annals of Otology, Rhinology and Laryngology 75: 436-57.

Linthicum FH (1967) Pathology and pathogenesis of sensorineural deafness in otosclerosis. EENT Digest 29: 51-6.

Linthicum FH, Filipo R, Brody S (1975) Sensorineural hearing loss due to cochlear otospongiosis: theoretical considerations of etiology. Annals of Otology, Rhinology and Laryngology 85: 544-51.

Liu X, Xu L, Zhang S, Xu Y (1993) Prevalence and aetiology of profound deafness in a general population of Sichuan, China. Journal of Laryngology and Otology 107: 990-3.

Liu X, Xu L (1994) Non-syndromic hearing loss. An analysis of audiograms. Annals of Otology, Rhinology and Laryngology 103: 428-33.

Liu X, Xu L, Newton V (1994) Audiometric configuration in non-syndromic genetic hearing loss. Journal of Audiological Medicine 3: 99-106.

Liu XZ, Newton VE, Read AP (1995) Waardenburg syndrome type II: phenotypic findings and diagnostic criteria. American Journal of Medical Genetics 55: 95-100.

Livan M (1961) Contributo alla conoscenza delle sordità ereditaria. Archive Italiani di Otologia 72: 331-9.

Lloyd GAS, Phelps PD (1979) Radiology of the ear in mandibulo-facial dysostosis-Treacher Collins syndrome. Acta Radiologica: Diagnosis 20: 233-40.

Loebell H (1938) Zur Erbtaubheit 2. Teil: Erbgesundheitsgutachter. Zeitschrift für den Hals, Nase und Ohrenarzt 29 (supplement).

Loftus SK, Edwards SJ, Scherpbier-Heddema T, Buetow KH, Wasmuth JJ, Dixon MJ (1993) A combined genetic and radiation hybrid map surrounding the Treacher Collins syndrome locus on chromosome 5q. Human Molecular Genetics 2: 1785-92.

Loftus SK, Dixon J, Koprivnikar K, Dixon MJ, Wasmuth JJ (1996) Transcriptional Map of the Treacher Collins Candidate Gene Region. Genome Research 6: 26-34.

Lonsbury-Martin BL, Martin GK, McCoy MJ, Whitehead ML (1994) Otoacoustic emissions testing in young children: middle ear influences. American Journal of Otology 15 (suppl 1): 13-20.

Lonsbury-Martin BL, Martin GK, McCoy MJ, Whitehead ML (1995) New approaches to the evaluation of the auditory system and a current analysis of otoacoustic emissions. Otolaryngology and Head and Neck Surgery 112: 50-62.

Luhr HG (1990) Indications for use of a microsystem for internal rigid fixation in craniofacial surgery. Journal of Craniofacial Surgery 1: 35-52.

Lumb KM (1981) Prevalence of hearing loss in children of Asian origin. In Proceedings of the Scientific Meeting of the British Association of Audiological Physicians and Community Pediatric Group, Manchester.

Lundborg H (1912) Über die Erblichkeitsverhältnisse der konstitutionellen (hereditären) Taubstummheit und einige Worte über die Bedeutung der Erblichkeitsforschung für die Krankheitslehre. Archive der Rassen- und Gesundheits Biologie 9: 133.

Lundborg H (1920) Hereditary transmission of genotypical deaf-mutism. Hereditas (Lund) 1: 35.

Lynch ED, Raventos H, Morrow I, Leon PE, King MC (1992) Closing in on a gene for inherited primary deafness on 5q31. American Journal of Human Genetics 51: A194.

Lyon MF, Rastan S, Brown SDM (1995) Genetic Variants and Strains of the Laboratory Mouse. Oxford: Oxford University Press.

Lyon MF, Searle AG (1989) Genetic variants and strains of the laboratory mouse. Oxford: Oxford University Press.

McCarthy JG, Cutting CB (1990) The timing of surgical intervention in craniofacial anomalies. Clinics in Plastic Surgery 17: 161-82.

McCarthy JG (1992) The role of research in craniofacial surgery. In Montoya A (Ed) Proceedings of the Fourth Meeting of The International Society of Craniofacial Surgery: Bologna: Monduzzi.

MacCollin M, Mohney T, Troffater J, Wertelecki W, Ramesh V, Gusella J (1993) DNA diagnosis of neurofibromatosis II. Altered coding sequence of the merlin tumor suppressor in an extended pedigree. Journal of the American Medical Association 270: 2316-20.

MacCollin M, Ramesh V, Jacoby LB et al. (1994) Mutational analysis of patients with neurofibromatosis II. American Journal of Human Genetics 55: 314-20.

McCormick (1993) Behavioural hearing tests, 6 months to 3;6 years. In McCormick (Ed) Paediatric Audiology 0-5 years. London: Whurr. pp 102-23.

McCormick (1995) The Medical Practitioner's Guide to Paediatric Audiology. Cambridge: Cambridge University Press.

McKenna M, Mills BG (1990) Ultrastructural and immunohistochemical evidence of measles virus in active otosclerosis. Acta Otolaryngologica (Stockholm) Supplement 470: 130-40.

McKusick VA, Francomano CA, Antonorakis SE, Pearson P (1994) Mendelian Inheritance in Man, a catalog of human genes and genetic disorders. Baltimore: Johns Hopkins University Press.

McLaughlin ME, Sandberg MA, Berson EL, Dryja TP (1993) Recessive mutations in the gene encoding the b-subunit of rod phosphodiesterase in patients with retinitis pigmentosa. Nature Genetics 4: 130-3.

MacPherson RI (1974) Craniodiaphyseal dysplasia, a disease or group of diseases? Journal of Canadian Association of Radiology 25: 22-3.

Mair IWS (1973) Hereditary deafness in the white cat. Acta Otolaryngologica Supplement 314: 1-48.

Majumder P, Ramesh A, Chinnappan D (1989) On the genetics of prelingual deafness. American Journal of Human Genetics 44: 86-99.

Malcolm S, Emery AEH (1995) Introduction to Recombinant DNA 2nd edn. New York: John Wiley.

Manolidis L, Daniilidis T, Moser M (1972) Über isolierte Missbildungen des Mittelohres. HNO 20: 176-179.

Marazita M, Ploughman L, Rawlings B, Remington E, Arnos K, Nance W (1993) Genetic epidemiological studies of early-onset deafness in the U.S. school-age population. American Journal of Medical Genetics 46: 486-91.

Marchac D, Renier D (1979) Le front flotant. Traitment précoce de craniostenoses. Annales de Chirurgie Plastique 24: 121-6.

Marchac D (1991) Evaluation of 11 years of experience in surgery of craniosynostosis (405 patients). In Pfeifer G (Ed) Craniofacial Abnormalities and Clefts of the Lip, Alveolus and Palate. Thieme Verlag. pp66-8.

Marcus RE (1968) Vestibular function and additional findings in Waardenburg's syndrome. Acta Otolaryngologica Supplement. 229: 1-30.

Marres HAM, Cremers CWRJ (1989) Autosomal recessive non-syndromal profound childhood deafness in a large pedigree. Archives of Otolaryngology and Head and Neck Surgery 115: 591-5.

Marres HAM, Cremers CWRJ, Dixon MJ, Huygen PLM, Joosten FBM (1995) The Treacher Collins syndrome: a clinical, radiological and genetic linkage study on two pedigrees. Archives of Otolaryngology 121: 509-14.

Marschall MA, Chidyllo SA, Figueroa AA, Cohen M (1991) Long-term effects of rigid fixation on the growing craniomaxillofacial skeleton. Journal of Craniofacial Surgery 2: 63-8.

Martin JAM, Bentzen O, Colley JRT et al. (1981) Childhood deafness and hearing impairment in the European Community. Scandinavian Audiology 10: 165-74.

Martini A, Mazzoli M, Rosignoli M, Prosser S (1996a) Audiometric patterns of genetic non syndromic sensorineural hearing loss: Journal of Audiological Medicine (in press).

Martini A, Prosser S, Milani M, Rosignoli M (1996b) Contribution of age-related factors to the progression of non-syndromic hereditary hearing loss (in press).

Matthijs G, Claes S, Longo-Mbenza B, Cassiman JJ (1994) Teenage-onset non-syndromic deafness associated with a mutation and a polymorphism in the mitochondrial 12S ribosomal RNA gene in a large Zairese pedigree. American Journal of Human Genetics 55: A231.

Mauk GW, Behrens TR (1993) Historical, political and technological context associated with early identification of hearing loss. Seminars in Hearing 14: 1-17.

Maurizi M, Conti G, Galli J (1992) Metodiche diagnostiche: impedenzometria. In Le Ipoacusie Neurosensoriali dell'Infanzia. Relazione ufficiale al XII Congresso della Societá italiana di ORL pediatrica, S. Tecla-Acireale

Maw MA, Allen-Powell DR, Goodey RJ, Stewart IA, Nancarrow DJ, Hayward NK et al. (1995) The contribution of the DFNB1 locus to neurosensory deafness in a Caucasian population. American Journal of Human Genetics 57: 629-35.

Meizner I, Carmi R, Katz M (1991) Prenatal ultrasonic diagnosis of mandibulofacial dysostosis (Treacher Collins syndrome). Journal of Clinical Ultrasound 19: 124-7.

Melnick M, Bixler D, Silk K, Yune H, Nance WE (1975) Autosomal dominant branchio-oto-renal dysplasia. Birth Defects Original Article Series XI: 121-8.

Melnick M, Bixler D, Nance WE, Silk K, Yune H (1976) Familial branchio-oto-renal dysplasia: a new addition to the branchial arch syndromes. Clinical Genetics 95: 25-34.

Melnick M, Hodes ME, Nance WE, Yune H, Sweeney A (1978) Branchio-oto-renal dysplasia and branchio-oto dysplasia: two distinct autosomal dominant disorders. Clinical Genetics 13: 425-42.

Mendel G (1865) Versuche über Pflantzenhybriden. Brünn: Verhandlungen des Naturvorschenden Vereins.

Mendoza D, Rius M, De Stefani E, Leborgne F Jr (1969) Experimental otosclerosis.

Its causation by ionizing radiations. Acta Otolaryngologica 67: 9-16.

Mengel MC, Konigsmark BW, Berlin CI, McKusick VA (1967) Recessive early-onset neural deafness. Acta Otolaryngologica (Stockholm) 64: 313-26.

Ménière P (1846) Recherches sur l'origine de la surdi-mutité. Gazette Medicale de Paris 3: 223.

Ménière P (1856) Du mariage entre parents considéré comme cause de la surdi-mutité congénitale. Gazette Médicale de Paris 3: 303-6.

Meredith R (1991) Audiometric identification of carriers of non-manifesting genes for deafness. MSc dissertation, University of Southampton.

Meredith R, Stephens D, Meyer-Bisch C, Reardon W, Sirimanna T (1992) Audiometric detection of carriers of Usher's Syndrome type II. Journal of Audiological Medicine 1: 11–19.

Merel P, Hoang-Xuan K, Sanson M et al. (1995) Screening for germline mutations in the NF2 gene. Genes, Chromosomes and Cancer 12: 117-27.

Merin S, Abraham FA, Auerbach E (1974) Usher's and Hallgren's syndrome. Acta Genet. Med. Gemellologica 23: 49-55.

Meyer WJ III, Migeon BR, Migeon CJ (1975) Focus on human X chromosome for dihydrotestosterone receptor and androgen insensitivity. Proceedings of the National Academy of Sciences of the USA 72: 1469-72.

Meyer-Bisch (1990) Audiometrie automatique de dépistage préventif: le balayage fréquential asservi (audioscan). Cahiers de notes documentaires 130: 335-45.

Michaels L (1987) Ear, Nose and Throat Histopathology. London: Springer.

Michel O, Breunsbach J, Matthias R (1991) Das angeborene Liquordrucklabyrinth. HNO 39: 486-90.

Milligan DA, Harlass FE, Duff P, Kopelman JN (1994) Recurrence of Treacher Collins syndrome with sonographic findings. Military Medicine 159: 250-2.

Mochizuki T, Lemmink HH, Mariyama M et al. (1994) Identification of mutations in the α3 (IV) and α4 (IV) collagen genes in autosomal recessive Alport syndrome. Nature Genetics 8: 77-82.

Mohn KL, Laz TM, Hsu JC, Melby AE, Bravo R, Taub R (1991) The immediate-early growth response in regenerating liver and insulin-stimulated H-35 cells: comparison with serum-stimulated 3T3 cells and identification of 41 novel immediate-early genes. Molecular and Cell Biology 11: 381-90.

Mohr J, Mageroy K. (1960) Sex-linked deafness of a possibly new type. Acta Geneticae Statisticae Medicae (Basel) 10: 54-62.

Möller C, Odkvist L (1989) The plasticity of compensatory eye movements in bilateral vestibular loss. Acta Otolaryngologica 108: 345-54.

Möller C, Kimberling W, Davenport S et al. (1989) Usher syndrome: An otoneurologic study. Laryngoscope 99: 73-9.

Monasterio FO, Fuente del Campo A, Carillo A (1978) Advancement of the orbits and the midface in one piece, combined with frontal repositioning for the correction of Crouzon's deformity. Plastic and Reconstructive Surgery 61: 507-13.

Moraes CT, Dimauro S, Zeviani M et al. (1989) Mitochondrial DNA deletions in progressive external ophthalmoplegia and Kearns-Sayre syndrome. New England Journal of Medicine 320: 1293-9.

Morgans ME, Trotter WR (1957) Defective organic binding of iodide by the thyroid in Hashimoto's thyroiditis. Lancet i: 553-5.

Morgans ME, Trotter WR (1958) Association of congenital deafness with goitre. The nature of the thyroid defect. Lancet i: 607-9.

Morimitsu T, Matsumoto I, Takahashi M, Komuwe S (1980) Vestibular fenestration and stapedoplasty in congenital stapes and vestibular window anomaly. Archives of Otorhinolaryngology 226: 27-33.

Morrison AW (1967) Genetic factors in otoslerosis. Annals of the Royal College of Surgeons of England 41: 202-37.

Morrison AW, Bundey SE (1970) The inheritance of otosclerosis. Journal of Laryngology and Otology 84: 921-32.

Mortier GR, Wilkin DJ, Wilcox WR et al. (1995) A radiographic, morphologic, biochemical and molecular analysis of a case of achondrogenesis type II resulting from substitution for a glycine residue (Gly 691→Arg) in the type II collagen trimer. Human Molecular Genetics 4: 285-8.

Morton CC, Skvorak A, Yin Y, Weremovicz S, Bieber FR, Robertson NG (1995) Cloning genes involved in hearing: a tissue specific library approach. In Proceedings of 2nd International Conference on The Molecular Biology of Hearing and Deafness, Bethesda.

Morton NE (1958) Segregation analysis in human genetics. Science 127: 79.

Morton NE (1960) The mutational load due to detrimental genes in man. American Journal of Human Genetics 12: 348-64.

Morton NE (1991) Genetic epidemiology of hearing impairment. In Ruben RJ, van der Water TR, Steel KP (Eds) Genetics of hearing impairment. Annals of New York Academy of Science, 630: 16-31.

Morton NE, Chung CS (1959) Are the MN blood groups maintained by selection? American Journal of Human Genetics 11: 237.

Muchnik C, Hildesheiner M, Rubinstein M, Gleitman Y (1989) Validity of tympanometry in cases of confirmed otosclerosis. Journal of Laryngology and Otology 103: 36-8.

Mueller RF, Young ID (1995) Emery's Elements of Medical Genetics. 9th edn. Edingburgh; Churchill Livingstone.

Nager F (1939) Zur klinishen und pathologischen Anatomie der Otosklerose. Acta Oto-laryngologica 27: 542.

Nagley P, Zhang C, Martinus RD, Vaillant F, Linnane AW (1993) Mitochondrial DNA mutation and human ageing: molecular biology, bioenergetics, and redox therapy. In DiMauro S, Wallace DC, (Eds) Mitochondrial DNA in Human Pathology. New York: Raven Press.

Nance WE (1971) Genetic counseling for the hearing impaired. Audiology 10: 222-3.

Nance WE (1977) Genetic counseling of hereditary deafness: an unmet need. Childhood Deafness 211-6.

Nance WE (1980) The genetic analysis of profound prelingual deafness. Birth Defects Original Article Series 16: 263-9.

Nance WE, Setieff R, McLeod T, Sweeney A, Cooper C, McConnell F (1971) X-linked mixed deafness with congenital fixation of the stapedial footplate and perilymphatic gusher. Birth Defects: Original Article Series 7: 64-9.

Nance WE, Rose SP, Conneally PM, Miller JZ (1977) In Lubs HA, de la Cruz F (Eds),Genetic Counseling. New York: Raven Press. pp 307-331.

Narod SA, Martuza R, Frohtali M, Haines J, Gusella JF, Rouleau GA (1992) Neurofibromatosis type II appears to be a genetically homogeneous disease. American Journal of Human Genetics 51: 486-96.

National Institutes of Health Consensus Development Conference (1988) Neurofibromatosis Consensus Statement. Archives of Neurology 45: 575-8.

Neame JH (1962) Anomalies of the ossicular chain. Journal of Laryngology and Otology 76: 596-600.

Nelson RA (1992) Auditory Brainstem Implant. In Tos M, Thomsen J (Eds) Acoustic

Neuroma (Proceeding of First International Conference on Acoustic Neuroma Copenhagen 1991) Amsterdam/New York: Kugler Publications. pp 869-72.

Nemansky J, Hageman MJ (1975) Tomographic findings of the inner ears of 24 patients with Waardenburg syndrome. American Journal of Roentgenology 124: 250-5.

Neufeld EF, Muenzer J (1995) The Mucopolysaccharidoses. In Scriver C, Beaudet A, Sly W, Valle D (Eds) The Metabolic and Molecular basis of Inherited Disease. New York: McGraw Hill. p 2482.

New MI, Lorenzen F, Lerner AJ et al. (1983) Genotyping steroid 21-hydroxylase deficiency: Hormonal reference data. Journal of Clinical Endocrinology and Metabolism 57: 320-6.

Newton VE (1985) Aetiology of bilateral sensorineural hearing loss in young children. Journal of Laryngology and Otology (Supplement) 10: 1-57.

Newton VE (1989) Genetic counselling for isolated hearing loss. Journal of Laryngology and Otology 103: 12-15.

Newton VE (1989) Waardenburg's syndrome: a comparison of biometric indices used to diagnose lateral displacement of the inner canthi. Scandinavian Journal of Audiology 18: 221-3.

Newton VE, Liu XZ, Read AP (1994) The association of sensorineural hearing and pigmentation abnormalities in Waardenburg syndrome. Journal of Audiological Medicine 3, 69–77.

Ni L, Wagner MJ, Kimberling WJ et al. (1994) Refined localization of the branchiootorenal syndrome gene by linkage and haplotype analysis. American Journal of Medical Genetics 51: 176-84.

Nicolaides KH, Johansson D, Donnai D, Rodeck CH (1984) Prenatal diagnosis of mandibulo-facial dysostosis. Prenatal Diagnosis 4: 201-5.

Norton SJ (1994) Emerging role of evoked otoacoustic emissions in neonatal hearing screening. American Journal of Otology 15 (suppl1): 4-12.

Northern JL, Downs MP (1991) Hearing in Children. Baltimore: Williams and Wilkins.

Nyhan WL, Sakati NA (1987) Diagnostic Recognition of Genetic Disease. Philadelphia: Lea and Febiger.

Oka Y, Katagiri H, Yazaki Y, Murase T, Kobayashi T (1993) Mitochondrial gene mutation in islet-cell-antibody-positive patients who were initially non-insulin-dependent diabetics. Lancet 342: 527-8.

Okumura T, Takahashi H, Honjo I, Takagi A, Mitamura K (1995) Sensorineural hearing loss in patients with large vestibular aqueduct. Laryngoscope 105: 289-94.

Olson NR, Lehman RH (1968) Cerebrospinal fluid otorrhea and the congenitally fixed stapes. Laryngoscope 78: 352-9.

O Mahoney CF, Luxon LM, Chew SL et al. (1996) When the triad of congenital hearing loss, goitre and perchlorate positive is not Pendred's syndrome. Journal of Audiological Medicine (in press).

Ombrédanne M (1959) Les surdités congénitales par malformations ossiculaires: leur traitement surgical. Annales d'Otolaryngologie et Chirurgie Cervicofaciale 76: 424-54.

Ombrédanne M (1960) Chirurgie des surdités congénitales par malformations ossiculaires de 10 nouveaux cas. Annales d'Otolaryngologie (Paris) 77: 423-49.

Ombrédanne M (1962) Chirurgie des surdités congénitales par malformations ossiculaires. Trente-quatre nouveaux cas d'aplasies mineures opérées. Annales d'Otolaryngologie (Paris) 79: 485-518; 637-62.

Ombrédanne M (1964) Chirurgie des aplasies mineures. Ses résultats dans les grandes surdités congénitales par malformations ossiculaires. Annales d'Otolaryngologie (Paris) 81: 201-22.

Ombrédanne M (1966) Transposition d'osselets dans certaines 'aplasies mineures'. Annales d'Otolaryngologie (Paris) 83: 273-80.

Ombrédanne M (1966) Malformations des osselets dans les embryopathies de l'oreille. Acta Otolaryngologica Belgiae 20: 623-52.

Omenn GS, McKusick VA (1979) The association of Waardenburg syndrome and Hirschsprung megacolon. American Journal of Medical Genetics 3: 217-23.

Osako S, Hilding DA (1971) Electron microscopic studies of capillary permeability in normal and Ames waltzer deaf mice. Acta Otolaryngologica 71: 365-76.

Ostri B, Johnsen T, Bergmann I (1991) Temporal bone findings in a family with branchio-oto-renal syndrome (BOR). Clinical Otolaryngology 16: 163-7.

Paget J (1877) Cases of branchial fistulae on the external ears. Lancet ii: 804.

Paget J (1878) Cases of branchial fistulae in the external ears. Medical and Chirurgical Transactions 61: 41-50.

Palmer AR (1995) Neural signal processing. In Moore BCJ (Ed) Hearing: Handbook of Perception and Cognition. 2nd edn. London: Academic Press. pp 75-112.

Pantke OA, Cohen MM (1971) The Waardenburg syndrome. Birth Defects Original Article Series VII, 147-52.

Parahy CH, Linthicum FH (1983) Otosclerosis: relationship of spiral ligament hyalinization to sensorineural hearing loss. Laryngoscope 93: 717-20.

Parry DM, Eldridge R, Kaiser-Kupfer MI, Bouzas EA, Pikus A, Patronas N (1994) Neurofibromatosis II: clinical characteristics of 63 affected individuals and clinical evidence for heterogeneity. American Journal of Medical Genetics 52: 450-1.

Parving A (1978a) Reliablity of Békésy threshold tracing in identification of carriers of genes for an X-linked disease with deafness. Acta Otolaryngologica 85: 40-4.

Parving A (1978b) Hearing disorders in Norrie's syndrome. Advances in Audiology 3: 52-7.

Parving A (1983) Epidemiology of hearing loss and aetiological diagnosis of hearing impairment in childhood. International Journal of Pediatric Otorhinolaryngology 5: 151-65.

Parving A (1984) Aetiologic diagnosis in hearing-impaired children – clinical value and application of a modern programme. International Journal of Pediatric Otorhinolaryngology 7: 29-38.

Parving A (1988) Longitudinal study of hearing disabled children – a follow-up investigation. International Journal of Pediatric Oto-Rhino-Laryngology 15: 223-44.

Parving A (1993a) Congenital hearing disability – epidemiology and identification: a comparison between two health authority districts. International Journal of Pediatric Oto-Rhino-Laryngology 27: 29-46.

Parving A (1993b) Hearing disability in childhood – a cross-sectional and longitudinal investigation of causative factors. International Journal of Pediatric Oto-Rhino-Laryngology 27: 101-11.

Parving A (1995) Factors causing hearing impairment – some perspectives from Europe. Journal of the American Academy of Audiology (in press).

Parving A, Schwartz M (1991) Audiometric tests in gene carriers of Norrie's disease. International Journal of Pediatric Oto-Rhino-Laryngology 21: 103-11.

Parving A, Hauch A-M (1994) The causes of profound hearing impairment in a school for the deaf – a longitudinal study. British Journal of Audiology 28: 63-9.

Parving A, Christensen B (1995) Epidemiology of permanent hearing impairment in childhood in relation to costs of a health surveillance program. International

Journal of Pediatric Oto-Rhino-Laryngology (in press).

Parving A, Newton V (1995) Editorial: Guidelines for description of inherited hearing loss. Journal of Audiological Medicine 4, ii-v.

Parving A, France EA, Stephens SDG (1996) Factors causing hearing impairment in identical birth-cohorts in Denmark and Wales – brief communication. Journal of Audiological Medicine (in press).

Parving A, Ostri B, Poulsen G, Gyntelberg F (1983) Epidemiology of hearing impairment in male adult subjects at 49-69 years of age. Scandinavian Audiology 12: 191-6.

Parving A, Hein HO, Suadicani P, Ostri B, Gyntelberg F (1993) Epidemiology of hearing disorders. Some factors affecting hearing. The Copenhagen male study. Scandinavian Audiology 22: 101-7.

Patuzzi RB, Yates GK, Johnstone BM (1989) The origin of the low-frequency microphonic in the first cochlear turn of guinea pig. Hearing Research 39: 177-88.

Pearson RD, Kurland LT, Cody DTR (1974) Incidence of diagnosed clinical otosclerosis. Archives of Otolaryngology 99: 288-91.

Peck JE (1984) Hearing loss in Hunter's syndrome, mucopolysaccharidosis II. Ear and Hearing 5: 243-6.

Pedersen KE (1990) Presbyacusis. An epidemiological study. Dissertation, University of Göteborg.

Pedersen U (1985) Osteogenesis imperfecta: hearing loss and stapedectomy. Acta Otolaryngologica Supplement 145: 1-36.

Pelletier LP, Tanguay RB (1975) X-linked recessive inheritance of sensorineural hearing loss expressed during adolescence. American Journal of Human Genetics 27: 609-13.

Pendred V (1896) Deaf mutism and goitre. Lancet ii: 532.

Peterson LC, Rao KV, Crosson JT, White JG (1985) Fechtner syndrome: a variant of Alport's syndrome with leucocyte inclusions and macrothrombocytopenia. Blood 65: 397-406.

Petrovic A, Shambaugh GE Jr (1966) Promotion of bone calcification by sodium fluoride: short-term experiments on newborn rats using tetracycline labeling. Archives of Otolaryngology 83: 104-22.

Phelps PD, Poswillo D, Lloyd GAS (1981) The ear deformities in mandibulofacial dysostosis. Clinical Otolaryngology 6: 15-28.

Phelps PD, Lloyd GAS (1990) Diagnostic Imaging of the Ear. 2nd edn. London: Springer.

Phelps PD, Reardon W, Pembrey M, Bellman S, Luxon L (1991) X-linked deafness, stapes gushers and a distinctive defect of the inner ear. Neuroradiology 33: 326-330.

Phillips R, Phelps P (1991) Imaging in congenital deafness. Archives of Diseases in Childhood 66: 1372-4.

Pickles JO (1982) An Introduction to the Physiology of Hearing. London: Academic Press.

Pickles JO, Comis SD, Osborne MP (1984) Cross-links between stereocilia in the guinea pig organ of Corti, and their possible relation to sensory transduction. Hearing Research 15: 103-12.

Pickles JO, Corey DP (1992) Mechanoelectrical transduction by hair cells. Trends in Neurosciences 15: 254-9.

Pieke Dahl S, Kimberling WJ, Gorin MB et al. (1993) Genetic heterogeneity of Usher syndrome type II. Journal of Medical Genetics 30: 843-8.

Piel CF, Biava CG, Goodman JR (1982) Glomerular basement membrane alternation in familial nephritis and 'benign' hematuria. Journal of Pediatrics 101: 358-65.

Pizzuti A, Novelli G, Mari A et al. (1996) The human homologue of the Drosophila *dishevelled* polarity gene is deleted in DiGeorge syndrome. American Journal of Human Genetics (in press).

Plant G (1984) The effects of an acquired profound hearing loss on speech production. British Journal of Audiology 18: 39-48.

Plester D (1971) Congenital malformations of the middle ear. Acta Otolaryngologica Belgica 25: 877-84.

Politzer A (1882) Lehrbuch der Ohrenheilkunde für Praktische Ärzte und Studierende. II Band. Stuttgart: Ferdinand Enke.

Politzer A (1894) Uber primäre Erkrankung der Knochernen Labyrinthkapsel. Zeitschrift fur Ohrenheilkunde 25: 309.

Polymeropoulos MH, Swift RG, Swift M (1994) Linkage of the gene for Wolfram syndrome to markers on the short arm of chromosome 4. Nature Genetics 8: 95-7.

Popkin JS, Polomeno RC (1974) Stickler's syndrome (hereditary progressive arthro-ophthalmopathy). Canadian Medical Association Journal 111: 1071-6.

Poswillo DE (1975) The pathogenesis of the Treacher Collins syndrome (mandibulofacial dysostosis). British Journal of Oral Surgery 13: 1-26.

Poswillo DE (1989) Myths, masks and mechanisms of facial deformity: Friel memorial lecture. European Journal of Orthodontics 11: 1-9.

Pou JW (1963) Congenital absence of the oval window. Laryngoscope 73: 384-91.

Prezant TR, Agapian JV, Bohlmann MC et al. (1993) Mitochondrial ribosomal RNA mutation associated with both antibiotic-induced and non-syndromic deafness. Nature Genetics 4: 289-94.

Pruzansky S, Lis EF (1958) Cephalometric roentgenography of infants: sedation, instrumentation and research. American Journal of Orthodontics 44: 159-65.

Pruzansky S (1973) Clinical investigation of the experiments of nature. ASHA Reports 8: 62-94.

Pruzansky S (1982) Craniofacial surgery: the experiment on nature's experiment: Review of three patients operated by Paul Tessier. European Journal of Orthodontics 4: 151-9.

Puffenberger EG, Kauffman ER, Bolk S et al. (1990) Identification of mutations in the *COL4A5* collagen gene in Alport syndrome. Science 248: 1224-7.

Puffenberger EG, Kauffman ER, Bolk S et al. (1994) Identity-by-descent and association mapping of a recessive gene for Hirschsprung disease on human chromosome 13q22. Human Molecular Genetics 3: 1217-25.

Puffenberger EG, Hosoda K, Washington SS et al. (1994) A missense mutation of the endothelin-B receptor gene in multigenic Hirschsprung's disease. Cell 79: 1257-66.

Ramsay HAW, Linthicum Jr FH (1994) Mixed hearing loss in otosclerosis: indication for long-term follow-up. American Journal of Otology 15: 536-8.

Raskind WH, Williams CA, Hudson LD, Bird TD (1991) Complete deletion of the proteolipid protein gene (PLP) in a family with X-linked Pelizaeus-Merzbacher disease. American Journal of Human Genetics 49:1355-60.

Read AP (1989) Medical Genetics: an illustrated outline. Philadelphia: Gower Medical Publishing. p 100.

Read AP, Foy C, Newton V, Harris R (1990). Assignment of Waardenburg Syndrome type 1 I 2q37. Journal of Medical Genetics 27: 652-3.

Read AP, van Heyningen V (1994) *PAX* genes in human developmental anomalies. Seminars in Developmental Biology 5: 323-32.

Reardon W (1992) Genetic deafness. Journal of Medical Genetics 29: 521-6.

Reardon W, Pembrey M (1990) The genetics of deafness. Archives of Disease in Childhood 65: 1196-7.

Reardon W, Middleton-Price HR, Sandkuijl L et al. (1991) A multipedigree linkage study of X-linked deafness: linkage to Xq13-q21 and evidence for genetic heterogeneity. Genomics 11: 885-94.

Reardon W, Middleton-Price HR, Malcolm S et al. (1992) Clinical and genetic heterogeneity in X-linked deafness. British Journal of Audiology 26: 109-14.

Reardon W, Roberts S, Phelps PD et al. (1992) Phenotypic evidence for a common pathogenesis in X-linked pedigrees and in Xq13-q21 deletion related deafness. American Journal of Medical Genetics 44: 513-7.

Reardon W, Ross RJM, Sweeney MG et al. (1992) Diabetes mellitus associated with a pathogenic point mutation in mitochondrial DNA. Lancet 340: 1376-9.

Reardon W, Bellman S, Phelps P, Pembrey M, Luxon LM (1993) Neuro-otological function in X-linked hearing loss: a multipedigree assessment and correlation with other clinical parameters. Acta Otolaryngologica 113: 706-14.

Reardon W, Winter RM, Rutland P, Pulleyn LJ, Jones BM, Malcolm S (1994) Mutations in the fibroblast growth factor receptor 2 gene cause Crouzon syndrome. Nature Genetics 8: 98-103.

Reardon W, Harding AE (1995) Mitochondrial genetics and deafness. Journal of Audiological Medicine 4: 40-51.

Reed WB, Stone VM, Boder E, Ziprkowski L (1967) Pigmentary disorders in association with congenital deafness. Archives of Dermatology 95: 176-86.

Reeves RH, Citron MP (1994) Mouse chromosome 16. Mammalian Genome 5: 229-37.

Reid FM, Vernham GA, Jacobs HT (1994) A novel mitochondrial point mutation in a maternal pedigree with sensorineural deafness. Human Mutation 3: 243-7.

Resnik JI, Kinney MB, Kawamoto HK (1990) The effects of rigid fixation on cranial growth. Annals of Plastic Surgery 25: 372-74.

Riedner ED, Levin LS, Holliday MJ (1980) Hearing patterns in dominant osteogenesis imperfecta. Archives of Otolaryngology 106: 737-40.

Rimoin DI, Edgerton MT (1967) Genetic and clinical heterogeneity in the oral-facial-digital syndromes. Journal of Pediatrics 71: 94-104.

Robertson NG, Khetarpal U, Gutierrez-Espeleta GA, Bieber FR, Morton CC (1994) Isolation of novel and known genes from a human fetal cochlear cDNA library using subtractive hybridisation and differential screening. Genomics 23: 42-50.

Rogers BO (1964) Berry-Treacher Collins syndrome: a review of 200 cases. British Journal of Plastic Surgery 17, 109-37.

Rommens, JM, Iannuzzi MC, Kerem B-S et al. (1989) Identification of the cystic fibrosis gene: chromosome walking and jumping. Science 245: 1059-65.

Rose CSP, King AAJ, Summers D et al. (1994) Localization of the genetic locus for Saethre-Chotzen syndrome to a 6 cM region of chromosome 7 using four cases with apparently balanced translocations at 7p21.2. Human Molecular Genetics 3: 1405-8.

Rose SP, Conneally PM, Nance WE (1977) Genetic analysis of childhood deafness. In Bess FH (Ed) Childhood Deafness. New York: Grune and Stratton. pp 19-36.

Rosenfeld PJ, Cowley GS, McGee TL, Sandberg MA, Berson EL, Dryja TP (1992) A null mutation in the rhodopsin gene causes rod photoreceptor dysfunction and autosomal recessive retinitis pigmentosa. Nature Genetics 1: 209-13.

Rosenthal N (1994) Molecular medicine – regulation of gene expression. New England Journal of Medicine 331: 231-3.

Rotig A, Cormier V, Chatelain P (1993) Deletion of mitochondrial DNA in a case of early-onset diabetes mellitus, optic atrophy, and deafness (Wolfram syndrome, MIM 222300). Journal of Clinical Investigation 91: 1095-8.

Rouleau GA, Seizinger BR, Wertelecki W et al. (1987) Genetic linkage of bilateral acoustic neurofibromatosis to a DNA marker on chromosome 22. Nature 329: 246-8.

Rouleau GA, Merel P, Lutchman M et al. (1993) Alteration in a new gene encoding a putative membrane-organizing protein causes neurofibromatosis type II. Nature 363: 515-21.

Rowland LP (1988) Dystrophin: a triumph of reverse genetics and the end of the beginning. New England Journal of Medicine 318: 1392-4.

Ruben RJ (1991) The history of the genetics of hearing impairment. In Ruben RJ, van der Water TR, Steel KP (Eds) Genetics of hearing impairment. Annals of New York Academy of Science, 630: 6-15.

Ruben RJ, Rozycki DL (1971) Clinical aspects of genetic deafness. Annals of Otology, Rhinology and Laryngology 80: 255-63.

Rubenstein JLR, Brice AEJ, Ciaranello RS, Denney D, Porteus MH, Usdin TB (1990) Subtractive hybridisation system using single-stranded phagemids with directional inserts. Nucleic Acids Research 18, 4833-42.

Rüedi L, Spoendlin H (1957) Die Histologie der otosklerotischen Stapesankylose im Hinblick auf die chirurgische Mobilisation des Steigb.gels. Bibliographia Oto-rhino-laryngologica Fasc. 4: 1.

Russell IJ, Sellick PM (1978) Intracellular studies of hair cells in the mammalian cochlea. Journal of Physiology (London) 284: 261-90.

Ruttledge MH, Narod SA, Dumanski JP et al. (1993) Presymptomatic diagnosis for neurofibromatosis II with chromosome 22 markers. Neurology 43: 1753-60.

Ryan AF, Batcher S, Brumm D, Lin L, O'Driscoll K, Harris JP (1993) Cloning genes from an inner ear cDNA library. Archives of Otolaryngology and Head and Neck Surgery 119: 1217-20.

Sambrook J, Fritsch EF, Maniatis T (1987) Molecular Cloning. A Laboratory Manual. 2nd edn. Cold Spring Harbor: Cold Spring Harbor Laboratories Press.

Samii M, Turel KE, Penkert G (1985) Management of seventh and eight nerve involvement by cerebellopontine angle tumours. Clinical Neurosurgery 32: 242-72.

Sandberg L, Terkildsen K (1965) Caloric tests in deaf children. Archives of Otolaryngology 81: 352-4.

Sank D (1963) In Family and Mental Health Problems in a Deaf Population (Eds Rainer JD, Altschuler KZ, Kallmann EJ). New York: Columbia University Press. pp 28-81.

Sankila EM, Pakarinen L, Kaariainen H et al. (1995) Assignment of an Usher syndrome type III (USH3) gene to chromosome 3q. Human Molecular Genetics 4: 93-8.

Sataloff RT, Schiebel BR, Spiegel JR (1987) Morquio's syndrome. American Journal of Otolaryngology 8: 443-9.

Schaap T, Gapany-Gapanavicius B (1978) The genetics of otosclerosis: distorted sex ratio. American Journal of Human Genetics 30: 59-64.

Schachern PA (1984) Mucopolysaccharidosis 1-H (Hurler's syndrome) and human temporal bone histopathology. Annals of Otorhinolaryngology 93: 65-69.

Scheer AA (1967) Correction of congenital middle ear deformities. Archives of Otolaryngology 85: 55-63.

Schinzel A (1994) The Human Cytogenetics Database. Oxford: Oxford University Press.

Schleurin W (1935) Uber die vererbung der Pigmentdegeneration der Netzhaut und ihre Verbreitung in Württemburg und Hohenzollern. Klinischer Monatsblat für Augenheilkunde 94: 761-92.

Schmidt E (1933) Erblichkeit und Gravidität bei der Otosklerose. Archive von Ohr, Nase und Kehlheilkunde 136: 188.

Schneider C, King RM, Philipson L (1988) Genes specifically expressed at growth arrest of mammalian cells. Cell 54: 787-93.

Schneider KW (1937) Untersuchungen einer mit hereditärer degenerativer Innenohrschwerhörigkeit stark belasteten Sippe. Zeitschrift fur Hals, Nase und Ohrenheilkunde 42: 314-20.

Schuknecht HF (1974) Pathology of the Ear. Cambridge: Harvard University Press.

Schuknecht HF, Kirchner JC (1974) Cochlear otosclerosis: fact or fantasy? Laryngoscope 84: 766-82.

Schweinfest CW, Henderson KW, Gu J-R et al. (1990) Subtraction hybridisation cDNA libraries from colon carcinoma and hepatic cancer. Genet Anal Techn Appl 7: 64-70.

Scott DA, Carmi R, Elbedour K, Duyk GM, Stone EM, Sheffield VC (1995) Nonsyndromic autosomal recessive deafness is linked to the DFNB1 locus in a large inbred Bedouin family from Israel. American Journal of Human Genetics 57: 965-8.

Scott HS, Ashton LJ, Eyre HJ et al. (1990) Chromosomal localization of the human alpha-L-iduronidase gene (IDUA) to 4p16.3. American Journal of Human Genetics 47: 802-7.

Seizinger BR, Martuzai RL, Gusella JF (1986) Loss of genes on chromosome 22 in tumorigenesis of human acoustic neuroma. Nature 322: 644-7.

Sellars S, Beighton P (1983) Childhood deafness in Southern Africa. Journal of Laryngology and Otology 97: 885-9.

Sensi A, Bettoli V Calzolari E (1994) Vohwinkel syndrome. American Journal of Medical Genetics 50: 201-3.

Shah KN, Dalal SJ, Sheth PN, Joshi NC, Ambani LM (1981) White forelock, pigmentary disorder of the irides and long segment Hirschsprung disease: possible variant of Waardenburg syndrome. Journal of Pediatrics 99: 432-5.

Shambaugh G (1930) Statistical studies of children in public schools for deaf. Archives of Otolaryngology 12: 190-245.

Shambaugh GE (1949) Fenestration operation for otosclerosis. Acta Otolaryngologica, Supplement 79.

Shambaugh GE (1952) Developmental anomalies of the sound conducting apparatus and their surgical correction. Annals of Otology, Rhinology and Laryngology 61: 873-87.

Shambaugh GE (1965) Clinical diagnosis of cochlear (labyrinthine) otosclerosis. Laryngoscope 75: 1558.

Shambaugh GE Jr, Scott A (1964) Sodium fluoride for arrest of otosclerosis. Archives of Otolaryngology 80: 263-70.

Shapiro J, Stome M, Crocker A (1985) Airway obstruction and sleep apnea in Hurler and Hunter syndrome. Annals of Otorhinolaryngology 94: 458-61.

Sheffield VC, Kraiem Z, Beck JC et al (1996) Pendred Syndrome maps to chromosome 7q, 21-34 and is caused by an intrinsic defect in thyroid iodine organification. Nature Genetics 12, 424-426.

Shiang R, Bell G, Divelhiss JE (1987) Mapping of ADH3, EGF and IL2 in a patient with Riegers-like phenotype and 4q23-q27 deletion. American Journal of Human Genetics 41: 185.

Shiang R, Thompson LM, Zhu Y-Z et al. (1994) Mutations in the transmembrane domain of FGFR3 cause the most common form of dwarfism, achondroplasia. Cell 78: 335-42.

Shiloh Y, Litvak G, Ziv Y et al. (1990) Genetic mapping of X-linked albinism-deafness syndrome (ADFN) to Xq26.3-q27.1. American Journal of Human Genetics 47: 20-7.

Shoffner JM, Lott MT, Lezza AMS, Seibel P, Ballinger SW, Wallace DC (1990) Myoclonic epilepsy and ragged-red fiber disease (MERRF) is associated with a mitochondrial DNA tRNA^{Lys} mutation. Cell 61: 931-7.

Shoffner JM, Brown M, Huoponen K et al. (1994) A mitochondrial DNA mutation associated with maternally inherited Parkinson disease and deafness. American Journal of Human Genetics 55: 1417 (abstract).

Siebenmann F (1912) Totaler Knocherner Verschluss beider Labyrinthfenster und Labyrinthitis serosa infolge progressiver Spongiosierung. Verhandlungen der Deutscher Otologischen Gesellschaft 21: 267.

Sill AM, Prenger VL, Stick MJ, Phillips SL, Boughman JA, Arnos KS (1992) A genetic study of hearing loss in an adult population. American Journal of Human Genetics 51: A159.

Sill AM, Stick MJ, Prenger VL, Phillips SL, Boughman JA, Arnos KS (1994) Genetic epidemiologic study of hearing loss in an adult population. American Journal of Medical Genetics 54: 149-53.

Sirimanna T, Meredith R, Reardon W, Meyer-Bisch C, Stephens D (1992) Detection of carriers of Usher syndrome type II. Paper presented at the 21st International Congress of Audiology, Morioka, Japan.

Sirimanna KS, France E, Stephens SDG (1995) Alport's syndrome: can the carriers be identified by audiometry? Clinical Otolaryngology 20: 158-63.

Sive HL, St John T (1988) A simple subtractive hybridisation technique employing photoactivatable biotin and phenol extraction. Nucleic Acids Research 16: 10937.

Smeets HJM, Melenhorst JJ, Lemmink HH et al. (1992) Mutations in the COL4A5 gene leading to different types of Alport syndrome. Kidney International 42: 83-8.

Smith AB (1939) Unilateral hereditary deafness. Lancet ii:1172-3.

Smith PG, Dyches TJ, Loomis RA (1984) Clinical aspects of branchio-oto-renal syndrome. Otolaryngology and Head and Neck Surgery 92: 468-75.

Smith RJH, Coppage KB, Ankerstjerne JK (1992) Localization of the gene for branchio-oto-renal syndrome to chromosome 8q. Genomics 14: 841-844.

Smith RJH, Lee EC, Kimberling WJ et al. (1992) Localization of two genes for Usher syndrome type I to chromosome 11. Genomics 14, 995-1002.

Smith RJH, Berlin CI, Hejtmancik JF et al. (1994) Clinical diagnosis of the Usher syndromes. Usher Syndrome Consortium. American Journal of Medical Genetics 50: 32-8.

Smith RJH, Fukushima K, Ramesh A et al. (1995) Identifying loci for recessive nonsyndromic hearing loss using consanguineous nuclear families. In Proceedings of 2nd International Conference on The Molecular Biology of Hearing and Deafness, Bethesda. p 21

Smith S (1991) Recurrence risks. In Ruben RJ, van der Water TR, Steel KP (Eds) Genetics of hearing impairment. Annals of New York Academy of Science 630: 203-11.

Smith SD (1995) Overview of genetic auditory syndromes. Journal of the American Academy of Audiology 6: 1-14.

Snik AFM, Teunissen E, Cremers CWRJ (1994) Speech recognition in patients after successful surgery for unilateral congenital ear anomalies. Laryngoscope 104: 1029-34.

Snik AFM, Hombergen GCJH, Mylanus EAM, Cremers CWRJ (1995) Airbone gap in patients with X-linked stapes gusher syndrome. American Journal of Otology 16: 241-6.

Solc CF, Derfler BH, Duyk GM, Corey DP (1995) Molecular cloning of myosins from the bullfrog saccular macula: a candidate for the hair cell adaptation motor. Auditory Neuroscience 1: 63-76.

Soong NW, Hinton DR, Cortopassi G, Arnheim N (1992) Mosaicism for a specific somatic mitochondrial DNA mutation in adult human brain. Nature Genetics 2: 318-23.

Southard JL, Dickie MM (1970) Jackson circler. Mouse Newsletter 42: 30.

Sparkes RS, Graham CB (1972) Camurati-Engelmann disease: genetics and clinical manifestations. Journal of Medical Genetics 9: 73-85.

Spoendlin, H. (1972) Innervation densities of the cochlea. Acta Otolaryngologica 73: 235-48.

Spoendlin H (1974) Congenital stapes ankylosis and fusion of carpal and tarsal bones as a dominant hereditary syndrome. Archives of Oto-Rhino-Laryngology 206: 173-9.

Spranger JW, Maroteaux P (1983) Genetic heterogeneity of spondyloepiphyseal dysplasia congenita? American Journal of Medical Genetics 14: 601-2.

Spranger J, Beighton P, Giedion A et al. (1992) International classification of osteochondrodysplasias. American Journal of Medical Genetics 44: 223-9.

Spritz RA, Holmes SA, Berg SZ, Nordlund JJ, Fukai K (1993) A recurrent deletion in the KIT (mast/stem cell growth factor receptor) proto-oncogene is a frequent cause of human piebaldism. Human Molecular Genetics 2: 1499-1500.

Stahle J, Stahle CH, Arenberg JK (1978) Incidence of Menière's disease. Archives of Otolaryngology 104: 99-102.

Stebbins WC, McGinn CS, Feitosa AG et al. (1981) Animal models in the study of ototoxic hearing loss. In Lerner SA, Matz GL, Hawkins JE jr (Eds) Aminoglycoside Ototoxicity, Boston: Little, Brown and Co. pp 5-25.

Steel KP (1991) Similarities between mice and humans with hereditary deafness. Annals of the New York Academy of Sciences 630: 68-79.

Steel KP (1995) Inherited hearing defects in mice. Annual Reviews of Genetics 29: 675-701.

Steel KP, Bock GR (1983) Hereditary inner-ear abnormalities in animals: relationships with human abnormalities. Archives of Otolaryngology 109: 22-9.

Steel KP, Harvey D (1992) Development of auditory function in mutant mice. In Romand R (Ed) Development of Auditory and Vestibular Systems Vol. 2. Amsterdam: Elsevier Press. pp 221-42.

Steel KP, Smith RJH (1992) Normal hearing in Splotch (Sp/+), the mouse homologue of Waardenburg syndrome type 1. Nature Genetics 2: 75-9.

Steel KP, Brown SDM (1994) Genes and deafness. Trends in Genetics 10: 428-35.

Steel KP, Barkway C, Bock GR (1987) Strial dysfunction in mice with cochleo-saccular abnormalities. Hearing Research 27: 11-26.

Steel KP, Davidson DR, Jackson IJ (1992) TRP-2/DT, a new early melanoblast marker, shows that steel growth factor (c-kit ligand) is a survival factor. Development 115: 1111-9.

Steel KP, Self T, Mahony M et al. (1995) Effects of myosin mutations on cochlear development and function. In Proceedings of 2nd International Conference on

The Molecular Biology of Hearing and Deafness, Bethesda. p 9.

Steele BC (1969) Congenital fixation of the stapes footplate. Acta Otolaryngologica supplement 245: 1-24.

Steinberg G (1938) Uber die Schwierigkeit der Diagnose und Beurteilung familiärer Schwerhörigkeit. Zeitschrift für Hals, Nase und Ohrenheilkunde 43: 501-24.

Steingrimsson E, Moore KJ, Lamoreux F et al. (1994) Molecular basis of mouse *microphthalmia* (*mi*) mutations helps explain their developmental and phenotypic consequences. Nature Genetics 8: 256-63.

Stephens SDG (1984) Hearing-aid selection: an integrated approach. British Journal of Audiology 18: 199-210

Stephens SDG (1985) Genetic hearing loss: a historical overview. Advances in Audiology 3: 3-17.

Stephens D, Meredith R, Sirimanna T, France L, Almqvist C, Haugen H (1995) The application of the Audioscan in the detection of carriers of genetic hearing loss. Audiology 34: 91-7.

Stern C (1950) The birth of genetics. Genetics 35, supplement.

Stevenson A, Cheeseman E (1956) Hereditary deaf mutism, with particular reference to Northern Ireland. Annals of Human Genetics 20: 177-207.

Stevenson RE, Hall JG, Goodman RM (1993) Human Malformations and Related Anomalies. Oxford Monographs on Medical Genetics no. 27. Oxford: Oxford University Press.

Strachan T, Read AP (1994) *PAX* genes. Current Opinions in Genetics and Development 4: 427-38.

Strachan T, Read AB, (1996) Human Molecular Genetics. Oxford: Bios Scientific

Strasnick B, Jacobson JT (1995) Teratogenic hearing loss. Journal of the American Academy of Audiology 6: 28-38.

Suga F, Hattler KW (1970) Physiological and histopathological correlates of hereditary deafness in animals. Laryngoscope 80: 81-104.

Sulik KK, Johnston MC, Smiley SJ, Speight HS, Jarvis BE (1987) Mandibulofacial dysostosis (Treacher Collins syndrome): a new proposal for its pathogenesis. American Journal of Medical Genetics 27: 359-72.

Suomalainen A, Kaukonen J, Timonen R et al. (1994) Nuclear gene causing multiple mtDNA deletions in autosomal dominant ophthalmoplegia maps to a distinct chromosomal region: involvement of both nuclear and mitochondrial DNA in a single disorder. American Journal of Human Genetics 55: 59 (abstract).

Suzuki H, Mashimo K (1972) Significance of the iodide perchlorate discharge test in patients with I^{131} treated and untreated hyperthyroidism. Journal of Clinical Endocrinology and Metabolism 34: 332-8.

Swaroop A, Xu J, Agarwal N, Weissman SM (1991) A simple and efficient cDNA library subtraction procedure: isolation of human retina-specific cDNA clones. Nucleic Acids Research 19: 1954.

Tabor JR (1961) Absence of the oval window. Archives of Otolaryngology 74, 515-21.

Tachibana M, Perez-Jurado LA, Nakavama A et al. (1994) Cloning of *MITF*, the human homolog of the mouse microphthalmia gene and assignment to chromosome 3p14.1-p12.3. Human Molecular Genetics 3: 553-7.

Takeda K, Sakurai A, De Groot LJ, Refetoff S (1992) Recessive inheritance of thyroid hormone resistance caused by complete deletion of the protein coding region of the thyroid hormone receptor β gene. Journal of Clinical Endocrinology and Metabolism 74: 49-55.

Talbot JM, Wilson DF (1994) Computed tomographic diagnosis of X-linked congenital mixed deafness fixation of the stapedial footplate and perilymphatic gusher.

American Journal of Otology 15: 177-82.

Tang A, Parnes LS (1994) X-linked progressive mixed hearing loss: computed tomography findings. Annals of Otology, Rhinology and Laryngology 103: 655-7.

Tassabehji M, Read AP, Newton VE et al. (1992) Waardenburg syndrome patients have mutations in the human homologue of the *Pax-3* paired box gene. Nature 355: 635-6.

Tassabehji M, Read AP, Newton VE et al. (1993) Mutations in the *PAX3* gene causing Waardenburg syndrome type I and type II. Nature Genetics 3: 26-30.

Tassabehji M, Newton VE, Read AP (1994) Waardenburg syndrome type II caused by mutations in the human microphthalmia (*MITF*) gene. Nature Genetics 8: 251-5.

Tassabehji M, Newton VE, Leverton K et al. (1994) *PAX3* gene structure and mutations: close analogies between Waardenburg syndrome and the *Splotch* mouse. Human Molecular Genetics 3: 1069-74.

Tassabehji M, Newton VE, Liu XZ et al. (1995) The Mutational spectrum in Waardenburg syndrome. Human Molecular Genetics 4: 2131-7.

Tavormina PL, Shiang R, Thompson LM et al. (1995) Thanatophoric dysplasia (types I and II) caused by distinct mutations in fibroblast growth factor receptor 3. Nature Genetics 9: 321-8.

Taylor IG, Hine W, Brasier V, Chiveralls K, Morris T (1975) A study of the causes of hearing loss in a population of deaf children with special reference to genetic factors. Journal of Laryngology and Otology 89: 899-914.

Tessier P, Guiot G, Rougerie, Delbert JP, Pastoriza J (1967) Osteotomies cranio-naso-orbito-facialies Hypertelorisme. Annales de Chirurgie Plastique 12: 103-12.

Tessier P (1967) Osteotomies totales de la face Syndrome de Crouzon, Syndrome d'Apert, oxycephalies, scaphocephalies, turricephalies. Annals de Chirurgie Plastique 12: 273-86.

Tessier P (1971) The definitive plastic surgical treatment of the severe facial deformities of craniofacial dysostosis. Plastic and Reconstructive Surgery 48: 419-42.

Tessier P (1971) Total Osteotomy of the middle third of the face for faciostenosis or sequelae of le Fort sequelae III. Plastic and Reconstructive Surgery 48: 533-41.

Tessier P (1972) Orbital hypertelorism I. Successive surgical attempts: Materials and Methods: causes and mechanism. Scandinavian Journal of Plastic and Reconstructive Surgery 6: 135- 55.

Tessier P (1973) Orbital hypertelorism II. Definitive treatment of orbital hypertelorism by craniofacial osteotomies. Scandinavian Journal of Plastic and Reconstructive Surgery 7: 39- 58.

Tessier P (1974) Experience in the treatment of orbital hypertelorism. Plastic and Reconstructive Surgery 53: 1-18.

Tessier P (1976) Orbital hypertelorism. In Symposium on Plastic Surgery in the Orbital Region. Saint Louis: Mosby. pp 255-67.

Tessier P (1985) Apert's syndrome: acrocephalo syndactyly type I. In Caronni E (Ed) Craniofacial Surgery. Boston: Little Brown. pp 280-303.

Tessier P (1986) Craniofacial surgery in syndromic craniosynostosis. In Cohen M (Ed) Craniosynostosis, Diagnosis, Evaluation and Management. New York: Raven Press. pp 321- 411.

Tessier P (1987) A foreword in the form of a warning. In Procedings of the First International Congress of the International Society of Craniomaxillofacial Surgery. Berlin: Springer.

Tessier P, Tulasne JF (1987) Treacher Collins Syndrome. In Proceedings of the First International Congress of the International Society of Craniomaxillofacial Surgery. Berlin: Springer. pp 369-89.

Tessier P, Tulasne JF (1989) Stability in correction of hypertelorbitism and Treacher Collins Syndrome. Clinics in Plastic Surgery 16: 195-204.

Teunissen E (1992) Major and minor congenital anomalies of the ear. Classification and surgical results. Thesis, University of Nijmegen.

Teunissen E, Cremers CWRJ (1993) Classification of middle ear anomalies: a report on 144 ears. Annals of Otology, Rhinology and Laryngology 102: 606-12.

Thieme ET (1957) A report of the occurrence of deaf-mutism and goiter in four of six siblings of a North American family. Annals of Surgery 146: 941-8.

Thompson A (1846) Notice of several cases of malformation of the external ear, together with experiments on the state of hearing in such persons. Monthly Journal of Medical Sciences 7: 420.

Thornton ARD, Phillips AJ (1992) Comparison of four vibrotactile aids. In Summers IR (Ed) Tactile Aids for the Hearing Impaired. London: Whurr. pp 231-51.

Thorpe P, Sellars SL, Beighton P (1974) X-linked deafness in a South African kindred. South African Medical Journal 48: 587-90.

Tinkle WJ (1933) Deafness as a eugenic problem. Journal of Heredity 24: 13-18.

Tishler PV (1979) Healthy female carriers for a gene for the Alport syndrome: importance for genetic counselling. Clinical Genetics 16: 291-4.

Tolan JF, Wilson HL (1958) Anomalies of the middle ear. Archives of Otolaryngology 68: 384-7.

Tranebjaerg L, Schwartz C, Eriksen H et al. (1995) A new X linked recessive deafness syndrome with blindness, dystonia, fractures, and mental deficiency is linked to Xq22. Journal of Medical Genetics 32: 257-63.

Tranebjaerg L, Moum T, Nilssen O et al. (1995) Genetic mapping of autosomal dominant deafness genes in 3 Norwegian families. In Proceedings of 2nd International Conference on The Molecular Biology of Hearing and Deafness, Bethesda. p 106.

Treacher Collins E (1900) Cases with symmetrical congenital notches in the outer part of each lid and defective development of the malar bones. Transactions of the Ophthalmological Society of the UK 20: 190-92.

Treacher Collins Syndrome Collaborative Group (1996) Positional cloning of a gene involved in the pathogenesis of Treacher Collins syndrome. Nature Genetics 12: 130-6.

Troffater JA, MacCollin MM, Rutter JL et al. (1993) A novel Moesin- , Ezrin-, Radixin-like gene is a candidate for the neurofibromatosis II tumor suppressor. Cell 72: 791-800.

Trotter WR (1960) The association of deafness with thyroid dysfunction. British Medical Bulletin 16: 92-8.

Tryggvason K, Zhou J, Hostikka SL, Shows TB (1993) Molecular genetics of Alport syndrome. Kidney International 43: 38-44.

Tyler RS (1993) Speech perception by children. In Tyler RS (Ed) Cochlear Implants: Audiological Foundations. California: Singular Publishing Group. pp 191-256.

Uchermann V (1869) De Dovstumme i Norge. Christiana: Cammermeyer.

Upfold LJ (1988) Children with hearing aids in the 1980s – aetiologies and severity of impairment. Ear and Hearing 9: 75-80.

Usher CH (1914) On the inheritance of retinitis pigmentosa with notes of cases. Royal London Ophthalmic Hospital Review 19: 130-6.

Valsalva AM (1704) De Aure Humana Tractatus. Utrecht.

van Aarem A, Cremers CWRJ, Pinckers AJLG, Huygen PLM, Hombergen GCJH, Kimberling WJ (1995) The Usher syndrome type IIa: clinical findings in obligate carriers. International Journal of Pediatric Otorhinolaryngology 31: 159-74.

van Buchem FS, Hadders HN, Hansen JF, Woldring MG (1962) Hyperostosis corti-calis generalisata: report of seven cases. American Journal of Medicine 33: 387-97.

van Camp G, van Thienen MN, Handig I et al. (1995a) Chromosome 13q deletion with Waardenburg syndrome: further evidence for a gene involved in neural crest function on 13q. Journal of Medical Genetics 32: 531-6.

van Camp G, Coucke P, Balemans W et al. (1995b) Localization of a gene for non-syndromic hearing loss (DFNA4) to chromosome 7p15. Human Molecular Genetics 4: 2159-64.

van Camp G, Coucke P, van Velzen D, Balemans W, Willems PJ (1995c) Linkage of progressive hearing loss of high tones to two loci. In Proceedings of 2nd International Conference on The Molecular Biology of Hearing and Deafness, Bethesda. p 67.

van Camp KJ, Margolis RH, Wilson RH, Creten WL, Shanks JE (1986) Principles of Tympanometry. Rockville, MD: ASHA Press.

van den Ouweland JMW, Lemkes HHPJ, Ruitenbeek W et al. (1992) Mutation in mito-chondrial tRNA$^{Leu(UUR)}$ gene in a large pedigree with maternally transmitted type II diabetes mellitus and deafness. Nature Genetics 1: 368-71.

Vanderbilt University Hereditary Deafness Study Group (1968) Dominantly inherit-ed low-frequency hearing loss. Archives of Otolaryngology 88: 242-50.

van der Meulen JC (1979) Medial faciotomy. British Journal of Plastic Surgery 32: 339-42.

van Gelder RN, von Zastrow ME, Yool A, Dement WC, Barchas JD, Eberwine JH (1990) Amplified RNA synthesized from limited quantities of heterogeneous cDNA. Proceedings of the National Academy of Sciences of the USA 87: 1663-7.

Vanniasegeram I, Tungland OP, Bellmann S (1993) A five year review of children with deafness in a multi-ethnic community. Journal of Audiological Medicine 2: 9-19.

van Rijn P, Cremers CWRJ (1988) Surgery for congenital deafness in Klippel-Feil syn-drome. Annals of Otology 97: 347-52.

van Rijn PM (1989) Causes of early childhood deafness. Thesis: University of Nijmegen.

van Rijn PM, Cremers CWRJ (1991) Causes of childhood deafness at a Dutch school for the hearing-impaired. Annals of Otology, Rhinology and Laryngology 100: 903-8.

van Widdershoven J, Moonens L, Assmann K, Cremers C (1983) Renal disorders in the branchio-oto-renal syndrome. Helvetica Paediatrica Acta 38: 513-22.

van Woude JP, Wijnands MC, Mourad-Baars PEC et al. (1986) A patient with dup(10p)del(8q) and Pendred syndrome. American Journal of Medical Genetics 24: 211-7.

Vartianen E, Karjalainen S, Nuutinen J, Suntioinen S, Pellinen P (1994) Effect of drinking water fluoridation on hearing of patients with otosclerosis in a low flu-oride area: a follow-up study. American Journal of Otology 15: 545-8.

Vassart G, Dumot JE, Refetoff S (1995) Thyroid disorders. In: Scriver CR, Beaudet A, Sly WS, Valle D (Eds) The inherited basis of metabolic disease. 7th edn. New York: McGraw-Hill, pp 2883-928.

Veske A, Oehlmann R, Younus F, Mohyuddin A, Müller-Myhsok B, Mehdi SQ, et al. (1996) Autosomal recessive non-syndromic deafness locus (DFNB8) maps on chromosome 21q22 in a large consanguineous kindred from Pakistan. Human Molecular Genetics 5: 165-8.

Vickery A (1981) The diagnosis of malignancy in dyshormonogenetic goitre. Clinics in Endocrinology and Metabolism 10: 317-35.

Villard L, Gecz J, Mattéi JF etal. (1996) XNP mutation in a large family with Juberg-

Marsilli syndrome Nature Genetics 12, 359-360.

Vincent C, Kalatzis V, Compain S et al. (1994) A proposed new contiguous gene syndrome on 8q consists of Branchio-Oto-Renal (BOR) syndrome, Duane syndrome, a dominant form of hydrocephalus and trapeze aplasia: implications for the mapping of the BOR gene. Human Molecular Genetics 3: 1859-66.

Virolainen E (1972) Vestibular disturbances in clinical otosclerosis. Acta Otolaryngologica Supplement: 306.

von Graefe A (1858) Vereinzelte Beobachtungen und Bemerkungen: Exceptionelles Verhalten des Gesichtfeldes bei Pigmentartung der Netzhaut. von Graefe's Archive der klinische und experimentelle Ophthalmologie 4: 250-3.

Waardenburg PJ (1951) A new syndrome combining developmental anomalies of the eyelids, eyebrows and nose root with pigmentary defects of the iris and head hair and with congenital deafness. American Journal of Human Genetics 3: 195-253.

Waelsch SG (1991) Genetics of Hearing Impairment. In Ruben RJ, van der Water TR, Steel KP (Eds) Genetics of hearing impairment. Annals of New York Academy of Science, 630: 3-5.

Wagenaar M, Ter Rahe B, van Aarem A et al. (1995) Clinical findings in obligate carriers of type I Usher's syndrome. American Journal of Medical Genetics (in press).

Wallace MR, Marchuk DA, Andersen LB et al. (1990) Type I neurofibromatosis gene: identification of a large transcript disrupted in three NF1 patients. Science 249: 181-6.

Wallis C, Ballo R, Wallis G, Beighton P, Goldblatt J (1988) X-linked mixed deafness with stapes fixation in a Mauritian kindred: linkage to Xq probe pDP34. Genomics 3: 299-301.

Wang CR, Loveland BE, Fischer-Lindahl K (1991) H-2M3 encodes the MHC class I molecule presenting the maternally transmitted antigen of the mouse. Cell 66: 335-45.

Wang Y, Treat K, Schroer RJ, O'Brien JE, Stevenson RE, Schwartz CE (1994) Localization of Branchio-oto-Renal (BOR) syndrome to a 3 Mb region of chromosome 8q. American Journal of Medical Genetics 51: 169-75.

Watson C, Gaunt L, Evans G, Harris R, Strachan T (1993) A germinal interstitial deletion maps the locus for type II neurofibromatosis to the interval between D22S6 and LIF (leukaemia inhibitory factor). Human Molecular Genetics 2: 701-4.

Weaver DD, Cohen MM, Smith DW (1974) The tricho-rhinophalangeal syndrome. Journal of Medical Genetics 11: 312-4.

Weber BA (1982) Comparison of auditory brain stem response latency norms for premature infants. Ear and Hearing 3: 257-62.

Weber BA (1994) Auditory brainstem response: Threshold estimation and auditory screening. in Katz (Ed) Handbook of Clinical Audiology.

Weber M (1935) Otosklerose und Umbau der Labyrinthkapsel. Leipzig: Poeschel and Trepte.

Weil D, Blanchard S, Kaplan J et al. (1995) Defective myosin VIIa gene responsible for Usher syndrome type IB. Nature 374: 60-61.

Weil D, Lévy G, Sahly I et al. (1996) Human myosin VIIa responsible for the Usher 1B syndrome: a predicted membrane-associated motor protein expressed in developing sensory epithelia. Proceedings of the National Academy of Sciences of the USA (in press).

Weinberg W (1925) Methoden und Technik der Statistik mit besonderer Berücksichtigung der Sozialbiologie. In Gottstein A, Schlossmann A, Teleky L, (Eds) Handbuch der Sozialbiologie. Berlin: Springer.

Wellesley D, Goldblatt J (1992) A new form of X-linked high frequency sensorineural deafness. Clinical Genetics 41: 79-81.

Wertelecki W, Rouleau GA, Superneau DW et al. (1988) Neurofibromatosis II: clinical and DNA linkage studies of a large kindred. New England Journal of Medicine 319: 278-83.

Whiteley CH (1992) Mucopolysaccharidoses. In Beighton P (Ed) McKusick's Heritable Disorders of Connective Tissue. 5th edn. St Louis: Mosby.

Wijmenga C, Sandkuijl LA, Moerer P et al. (1992) Genetic linkage map of facioscapulohumeral muscular dystrophy and five polymorphic loci on chromosome 4q35-qter. American Journal of Human Genetics 51: 411-5.

Wilcox ER (1992) Strategies for constructing a guinea pig organ of Corti cDNA library and its potential use. Otolaryngological Clinics of North America, 25: 1011-6.

Wilcox ER, Fex J (1992) Construction of a cDNA library from microdissected guinea pig organ of Corti. Hearing Research 62: 124-6.

Wilde WR (1853) Practical Observation on Aural Surgery and the Nature and the Treatment of Diseases of the Ear. Philadelphia: Blanchard and Lea.

Wildervanck L (1957) Audiometric examination of parents of children deaf from birth. Archives of Otolaryngology 65: 280-95.

Wilkie AOM, Slaney SF, Oldridge M et al. (1995) Apert syndrome results from localised mutations of FGFR2 and is allelic with Crouzon syndrome. Nature Genetics 9: 165-71.

Wilkinson WB, Poswillo DE (1991) Asymmetry in mandibulofacial dysostosis. Journal of Craniofacial Genetics and Developmental Biology 11: 41-7.

Williams ED (1979) The aetiology of thyroid tumours. Clinics in Endocrinology and Metabolism 8: 193-207.

Winata S, Arhya N, Moeljopawiro S et al. (1995) Congenital non-syndromal autosomal recessive deafness in Bengkala, an isolated Balinese village. Journal of Medical Genetics 32: 336-43.

Winship I, Gericke, Beighton P (1984) X-linked inheritance of ocular albinism with late onset sensorineural deafness. American Journal of Medical Genetics 19: 797-803.

Winter R, Baraitser M (1993) London Dysmorphology Database. Oxford: Oxford University Press.

Wishart JH (1820) Case of tumours in the skull, dura mater and brain. Edinburgh Medical and Surgical Journal 18: 393-7.

Worth HM, Wollin DG (1966) Hyperostosis corticalis generalisata congenita. Journal of Canadian Association of Radiologists 17: 67-74.

Yoo TJ (1984) Etiopathogenesis of otosclerosis: a hypothesis. Annals of Otology, Rhinology and Laryngology 93: 28-33.

Young PF, Eldridge RC, Nager GT, Deland FH, McNew J (1971) Hereditary bilateral acoustic neuroma (central neurofibromatosis). Birth Defects Original Article Series 7: 73-86.

Zang KD (1982) Cytological and cytogenetic studies on human meningioma. Cancer Genetics and Cytogenetics 6: 249-74.

Zechner G, Moser M (1987) Otosclerosis and mucopolysaccharidosis. Acta Otolaryngologica 103: 384-6.

Zeviani M (1992) Nucleus-driven mutations of human mitochondrial DNA. Journal of Inherited Metabolic Disease 15: 456-71.

Zhou J, Mochizuki T, Smeets H et al. (1993) Deletion of the paired $\alpha 5$(IV) and $\alpha 6$(IV) collagen genes in inherited smooth muscle tumors. Science 261: 1167-9.

Zlotogora J, Lerer I, Bar-David S, Ergaz Z, Abielovich D (1995) Homozygosity for

Waardenburg syndrome. American Journal of Human Genetics 56: 1173-8.

Zühlke D (1969) Der Steigbügelersatz bei Ohrfehlbildungen. Archive der Ohr-, Nasen- und Kehl-Heilkunde 194: 609-12.

Index